Consciousness
& healing

Integral Approaches to
Mind-Body Medicine

Consciousness & healing

Integral Approaches to Mind-Body Medicine

Marilyn Schlitz, PhD
Vice President for Research and Education
Institute of Noetic Sciences
Petaluma, California

Tina Amorok, MA, PsyD candidate
Research Associate
Institute of Noetic Sciences
Petaluma, California

With
Marc S. Micozzi, MD, PhD
Executive Director
Jefferson-Myrna Brind Center of Integrative Medicine
Thomas Jefferson University Hospital
Philadelphia, Pennsylvania;
Director
Policy Institute for Integrative Medicine
Bethesda, Maryland

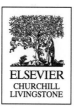

ELSEVIER
CHURCHILL
LIVINGSTONE

ELSEVIER
CHURCHILL
LIVINGSTONE

11830 Westline Industrial Drive
St. Louis, Missouri 63146

CONSCIOUSNESS AND HEALING: INTEGRAL   0-443-06800-3
APPROACHES TO MIND-BODY MEDICINE
Copyright © 2005, Elsevier Inc.

NOTICE

Complementary Medicine is an ever-changing field. Standard safety precautions must be followed, but as new research and clinical experience broaden our knowledge, changes in treatment and drug therapy may become necessary or appropriate. Readers are advised to check the most current product information provided by the manufacturer of each drug to be administered to verify the recommended dose, the method and duration of administration, and contraindications. It is the responsibility of the licensed prescriber, relying on experience and knowledge of the patient, to determine dosages and the best treatment for each individual patient. Neither the publisher nor the authors assume any liability for any injury and/or damage to persons or property arising from this publication.

The Publisher

International Standard Book Number 0-443-06800-3
Publishing Director: Linda Duncan
Editor: Kellie Fitzpatrick
Developmental Editor: Jennifer Watrous
Editorial Assistants: Kendra Bailey and Elizabeth Gadberry
Publishing Services Manager: Pat Joiner
Project Manager: David Stein
Senior Designer: Amy Buxton
Cover Art: Zoe Hersey©

Printed in the United States of America

Last digit is the print number: 9 8 7 6 5 4 3 2 1

CONTRIBUTORS

ALEXANDER W. ASTIN, PhD
Allan M. Cartter Professor Emeritus
  Education
University of California, Los Angeles
Los Angeles, California

JOHN A. ASTIN, PhD
Research Scientist, California Pacific
  Medical Center
San Francisco, California

DAVID H. BEGAY, PhD
Adjunct Professor, Department of
  Physics and Astronomy
Northern Arizona University
Flagstaff, Arizona;
Vice-President, Indigenous Education
  Institute Department
Salt Lake City, Utah

WILLIAM BENDA, MD
Associate Research Scientist, Institute
  for Children, Youth, and Families
Graduate Fellow, Program in
  Integrative Medicine
Department of Internal Medicine
University of Arizona
Tucson, Arizona

THOMAS BERRY, PhD
Author, *Dream of the Earth*
Emeritus Professor, History of
  Religions
Fordham University
Bronx, New York;
Past Director, Riverdale Center of
  Religious Research,
Riverdale, New York

WILLIAM BRAUD, PhD
Professor of Psychology, Institute of
  Transpersonal Psychology
Palo Alto, California

DEEPAK CHOPRA, MD
Author, *Book of Secrets*
Carlsbad, California

SARAH A. CONN, PhD
Instructor in Psychology, Department
  of Psychiatry
Harvard University
Cambridge, Massachusetts;
Professor, Boston Architectural Center
Boston, Massachusetts

ELLIOTT S. DACHER, MD
Aquinnah, Massachusetts

HARRIS DIENSTFREY
Sharon, Connecticut

LARRY DOSSEY, MD
Executive Editor, *Explore: The Journal
of Science and Healing*
Author of many books on
consciousness, spirituality, and
healing

HENRY E. DREHER, MA
Faculty Member, Cancer Guides TM
Training Program
Center for Mind-Body Medicine
Washington, DC;
Director, Cancer Guide Consultations
New York, New York

LOREN ESKENAZI, MD
Clinical Faculty, Stanford University
San Francisco, California

LAWRENCE E. GEORGE, MD
Director, Department of Integral
Medicine
Integral University
Associate Faculty, Department of
Family Medicine
University of Colorado
Denver, Colorado;
American Academy of Family Practice
Leawood, Kansas

JAMES S. GORDON, MD
Clinical Professor of Psychiatry,
Department of Psychiatry
Georgetown University School of
Medicine
Founder and Director, The Center for
Mind-Body Medicine
Washington, DC

STANISLAV GROF, MD
Visiting Faculty, Philosophy,
Cosmology, and Consciousness
California Institute of Integral Studies
(CIIS)
San Francisco, California;
Visiting Faculty, Pacifica Graduate
Santa Barbara, California

ANNA HALPRIN, PhD (hon.)
Co-Founder, Former Director (with
Daria Halprin), Tamalpa Institute
for Body Base Expressive Art
Therapy
Founder, Dancers' Workshop of San
Francisco
Tamalpa Institute
Kentfield, California

WILLIS HARMAN, PhD (Deceased)
Former President of the Institute of
Noetic Sciences
Former Professor of Engineering-
Economic Systems, Stanford
University
San Francisco, California;
Former Researcher, SRI International
Menlo Park, California
Author, *Global Mind Change and
Creative Work*, among other books

CARYLE HIRSHBERG
Consultant, Program in Integrative
Medicine
College of Medicine
University of Arizona
Tucson, Arizona;
Consultant, Institute of Noetic
Sciences
Petaluma, California

GAIL BERNICE HOLLAND
Author and Journalist
Former Associate Editor of *IONS
  Review*

TOM JANISSE, MD, MBA
Assistant Regional Medical Director
Editor-In-Chief and Publisher, *The
  Permanente Journal*
Northwest Permanente
Portland, Oregon

DON HANLON JOHNSON, PhD
Professor, School of Professional
  Psychology
California Institute of Integral Studies
  (CIIS)
San Francisco, California

JON KABAT-ZINN, PhD
Professor of Medicine Emeritus
Founding Executive Director of the
  Center for Mindfulness in
  Medicine, Health Care, and Society
Founder and Former Director, Stress
  Reduction Clinic
University of Massachusetts Medical
  School
Worcester, Massachusetts;
Scientist, Writer, and Meditation
  Teacher
Senior Advisor to the Consortium of
  Academic Health Centers on
  Integrative Medicine
Board Member of the Mind and Life
  Institute

ROBERT M. KENNY, MBA, PhD
Associate Professor, Master of Arts
  Program
Transformative Leadership
California Institute of Integral Studies
  (CIIS)
San Francisco, California;
Founder and Principal, Leaderful
  Teams Organizational Consulting
Seattle, Washington;
Co-Founder and Principal, Bluff
  House Leadership Retreats
Seattle, Washington

SUMEDHA KHANNA, MD
Executive Director, Healing Well
  Associates
Gualala, California

STANLEY KRIPPNER, PhD
Professor of Psychology, Saybrook
  Graduate School and Research
  Center
San Francisco, California

MICHAEL LERNER, PhD
President, Commonweal
Bolinas, California

CONTRIBUTORS

DAVID MICHAEL LEVIN, PhD
Professor, Department of Philosophy
Northwestern University
Evanston, Illinois
Author, *Gestures Befitting the Measure:*
Physiognomies of Ethical Life (2005);
The Philosopher's Gaze (1999)
Editor, *Sites of Vision* (1999), *Language*
Beyond Postmodernism (1997)

JEFF LEVIN, PhD, MPH
Scientist and Author
Valley Falls, Kansas

RONDI LIGHTMARK, MA
Rhinecliff, New York

FREDERIC LUSKIN, PhD
Senior Fellow, Stanford University
Center on Conflict and
Negotiation
Associate Professor, Institute of
Transpersonal Psychology
Palo Alto, California

BETSY MacGREGOR, MD
Beth Israel Medical Center
New York, New York

NANCY C. MARYBOY, PhD
Adjunct Professor, Department of
Physics and Astronomy
Northern Arizona University
Flagstaff, Arizona;
President, Indigenous Education
Institute
Bluff, Utah

ELIZABETH LLOYD MAYER,
PhD
Clinical Professor, Psychology
Department
University of California at Berkeley
Berkeley, California;
Clinical Professor, Psychiatry
Department
University of California Medical
Center
San Francisco, California;
Senior Research Scholar,
International Consciousness
Research Laboratories
Princeton University
Princeton, New Jersey;
Training and Supervising
Psychoanalyst, San Francisco
Psychoanalytic Institute
San Francisco, California

RICHARD B. MILES
President, Health Frontiers
San Rafael, California

MARY MOHS, LVN, MA
Director, Awakening: A Center for
Exploring Living and Dying
Brentwood, California

REV. WAYNE MULLER
M. Div. Harvard
Founder and President, Bread for the
Journey International
Mill Valley, California

JAMES O'DEA, MIA
President, Institute of Noetic Sciences
Petaluma, California

DEAN ORNISH, MD
President and Director, Preventive
  Medicine Research Institute
Sausalito, California;
Clinical Professor of Medicine,
  University of California, San
  Francisco
San Francisco, California

JOSEPH CHILTON PEARCE, MA
Faber, Virginia

CANDACE B. PERT, PhD
Research Professor, Department of
  Physiology and Biophysics
Georgetown University
Washington, DC

YIFANG QIAN, MD, PhD
Research Consultant, Research
  Institute
California Pacific Medical Center
San Francisco, California

MAUREEN REDL, MFT
Founder and Director,
  Voices of Healing
Private Practice in Transpersonal
  Psychotherapy
Mill Valley, California

RACHEL NAOMI REMEN, MD
Clinical Professor, Family and
  Community Medicine
University of California, San
  Francisco School of Medicine
Founder and Director, Institute for
  the Study of Health and Illness
Commonweal
Bolinas, California

MICHAEL R. RUFF, PhD
Research Associate Professor,
  Department of Physiology and
  Biophysics
Georgetown University
Washington, DC

MICHAEL SAMUELS, MD
Instructor, Institute of Holistic
  Studies
San Francisco State University
San Francisco, California;
Board, Center for Arts and Healing
  Research and Education
University of Florida
Gainesville, Florida;
Director, Art as a Healing Force
Bolinas, California

ALLEN C. SHERMAN, PhD
Director of Behavioral Medicine
Associate Professor, Otolaryngology
University of Arkansas for Medical
  Sciences
Little Rock, Arkansas

BAHMAN A.K. SHIRAZI, PhD
Director of Graduate Studies,
California Institute of Integral
Studies (CIIS)
San Francisco, California;
Adjunct Faculty, School of Liberal
Arts
John F. Kennedy University
Pleasant Hill, California

STEPHANIE SIMONTON-
ATCHLEY, PhD
Associate Professor, Arkansas Cancer
Research Center
University of Arkansas for Medical
Sciences
Little Rock, Arkansas

SOGYAL RINPOCHE
Recognized as an incarnation of
Lerab Lingpa Tertön Sogyal who
was teacher to the Thirteenth Dalai
Lama
Student of Jamyang Khyentse Chökyi
Lodrö, the most outstanding
Tibetan Buddhist Master of the
Twentieth Century
Studied Comparative Religion at
Cambridge University
Renowned Teacher of Tibetan
Buddhism for nearly 30 years
Author of the highly-acclaimed and
ground-breaking book, *The Tibetan
Book of Living and Dying*

BROTHER DAVID STEINDL-
RAST, OSB, PhD
www.Gratefulness.org
Ithaca, New York

WILLIAM B. STEWART, MD
Medical Director, Institute for Health
and Healing
California Pacific Medical Center
San Francisco, California;
Marin Community Health
Marin, California;
Mills-Peninsula Health Services
San Mateo, California

BRIAN SWIMME, PhD
Mathematical Cosmology Professor
Philosophy, Cosmology, and
Consciousness
California Institute of Integral Studies
(CIIS)
San Francisco, California

RON VALLE, PhD
Director, Awakening: A Center for
Exploring Living and Dying
Brentwood, California

FRANCES VAUGHAN, PhD
Psychologist and Author
Independent Practice
Mill Valley, California

ROGER WALSH, MD, PhD
Professor of Psychiatry, Philosophy,
and Anthropology
Adjunct Professor of Religious
Studies
University of California Medical
School
Irvine, California

CONTRIBUTORS

JEAN WATSON, PhD, RN, HNC, FAAN
Distinguished Professor of Nursing
Murchinson-Scovill Endowed Chair in Caring Science
University of Colorado Health Sciences Center School of Nursing
Denver, Colorado

KAREN WYATT, MD, ABHM
Associate Director, Department of Integral Medicine
Integral University
Denver, Colorado;
Diplomate, American Board of Holistic Medicine
Makawao, Hawaii

MICHAEL J. YEDIDIA, PhD
Professor, Robert F. Wagner Graduate School of Public Service
New York University
New York, New York

GARRET YOUNT, PhD
Scientist, Research Institute
California Pacific Medical Center
San Francisco, California

HONGLIN ZHANG, MD
Professor, Office of Qigong Research
China Academy of Traditional Chinese Medicine
Beijing, P.R. China

We dedicate this book in loving memory to the pioneering works of Winston (Wink) Franklin, Willis Harman, Nola Lewis, Brendan O'Regan, Helene Smith, and Elizabeth Targ, whose lives were dedicated to the exploration of this great mystery we call healing.

"We are explorers and the most compelling frontier of our time is human consciousness. Our quest is the integration of science and spirituality, a vision that reminds us of our connectedness to the inner self, to each other, and to the Earth."

—Edgar Mitchell,
Founder of The Institute of Noetic Sciences

The Integral Vision of Healing

It always struck me as interesting that a major tenet in the Hippocratic Oath, an oath that in various forms has been taken by many physicians around the world for almost 2,000 years, is simply, "First, do no harm."

The positive injunctions are few; but that negative injunction jumps right out at you. Why would it even be necessary to ask a future physician to promise something like that? Hippocrates understood that, of all the power a physician has, much of it is enormously positive and beneficial. One item needs most to be checked: the almost unprecedented capacity to harm a person, legally. In several versions of the Hippocratic Oath, it is clear that there are two ways to do harm: errors of commission and errors of omission. A physician can harm a patient with what he knows; but even more so, with what he doesn't.

The aim of integral medicine can be stated simply as the desire to lessen the harm done by both of those types of errors. Therefore, medicine may more effectively set the stage for the extraordinary miracle of healing that, 2000 years later, none of us yet fully understands.

Stated more positively, the aim of integral medicine is to utilize as complete and as comprehensive an approach as possible in treating any illness—while remaining constrained by the pragmatic realities of time, insurance limitations, and office management. The integral medicine that is rapidly developing today has moved significantly beyond early attempts in this area, variously known as "holistic," "allopathic," "alternative," and "complementary." Although some of the components of those pioneering efforts are retained, integral medicine is being launched from a platform much wider in its reach, more grounded in empirical research, and more effectively related to comprehensive models of human psychology and consciousness. But it is helpful to remember that an integral medicine differs in significant ways from both conventional and complementary medicine, while attempting to include the enduring and effective elements of each.

What does such an integral medicine look like? And how can it effectively be applied given the economic and pragmatic constraints of today's world? The following essays are attempts to address such questions. Before outlining some of their ground-breaking conclusions, let's set the stage by considering some of the traditional problems and dilemmas faced by most medical and health-care professionals.

THE DILEMMAS FACING MEDICINE

Everybody knows the first dilemma, because for years it was drummed into medical students: "Don't get emotionally involved with your patients." At the time, it was certainly not a cruel and uncaring injunction to treat people like objects; it was a genuine and sincere attempt to bring a dispassionate and scientific approach to healing illness. Becoming emotionally involved with a patient not only clouded the physician's judgment, it constantly drained the physician and accordingly seemed to harm the patient.

And yet, beginning in earnest a decade or two ago, there was an explosion of hard empirical research showing that positively enlisting various emotional factors—on the part of the heath-care practitioner as well as the patient—has a profoundly affirmative effect on the treatment, in many cases not only reducing recovery time but medical costs as well. Nor was this a case of "needy" patients doing better if somebody held their hands. Controlled studies consistently show that, if certain emotional and affective elements are engaged in the healing process, positive effects tend to be seen across all types of patients. Put bluntly, not becoming emotionally involved in some ways could not only increase medical costs but significantly harm the patient. What's a poor doctor to do?

Medical schools across the country began viewing this research warily. The whole thing had too much of a "New-Age" ring to it for most conventional medical practitioners. Trying to introduce these "subjective" factors was the opposite of what modern medicine ought to be doing. Nonetheless, virtually all medical schools were forced to confront this issue when research showed that patients were bypassing conventional medicine and spending some two billion dollars annually on types of health-care that did not ignore these subjective factors. Over two thirds of medical schools now have courses in complementary medicine. Part of integral medicine is an attempt to find a framework that can allow both of those approaches—conventional and complementary—to exist in a form that embarrasses neither.

A second common dilemma faced by medical practitioners is the very difficult problem that has become popularly known as "Cartesian dualism," or the mind-body problem. For all its high-minded philosophical accoutrements, this dualism may be simply seen as this: right now you most likely feel that you have some sort of consciousness and free will, and yet physical science proceeds as if reality is a closed materialistic system. Even if philosophically you are a materialist, you have to constantly translate every experience you have into materialistic terms, because that is simply not how your experience arrives. Physicalism, in other words, violates the grain of how the world naturally presents itself (not to mention the fact that the majority of philosophers in the area simply do not believe that consciousness can be reduced to eliminative materialism). And yet a conventional physician is more or less forced to treat a patient as if the patient were essentially a biophysical or material system—medications, surgery, radiation—one physical intervention after another. Their patients, when it comes to science-based medicine, are physical machines, and yet in their own awareness they do not feel that they are a physical machine—and neither do their patients. The "Cartesian" problem in the conventional practice of medicine is that they treat a patient as if he or she were a physical machine, when they all know otherwise.

A third common dilemma faced by conventional medicine is that of compliance. It is now estimated that in many cases a majority of treatment failures are due to lack of patient compliance with the prescribed medical intervention (from taking pills to following a recommended diet). Patient compliance has always fallen into the rather nebulous area of "subjective psychology"—exactly the area ruled out by the biophysical model of medicine. Once again, the very core practices of biophysical medicine are rendered ineffective precisely by those factors deemed not central to the model.

A fourth dilemma faced by health-care practitioners is rarely spoken about, but it is a topic always lurking in the background: just where do we locate illness? And where do we locate the causes of any illness? It is simply impossible to draw a boundary around any disease entity, let alone its causes. Arteriosclerotic heart disease has many contributing factors, including diet, with primary culprits including trans-fatty acids, now thought to directly contribute to thousands of deaths annually but nonetheless widespread ingredients in virtually every packaged food product in this country. Or take the number of hormone-like synthetic chemicals, now numbering in the tens of thousands, around 10% of which are known carcinogens. Can any person be healthy if the biosphere is sick? From this uncomfortable perspective, it appears that a physician, when treating any patient, is being asked to fix one small link in a thoroughly diseased chain of events.

Psychiatrists face this painful dilemma all the time. A teenager comes to the office for treatment of anxiety neurosis; it soon becomes obvious that it is not so much the teenager who is sick as his family, with an abusive father and alcoholic mother. Where is the illness "located"? Not to mention the fact that this teenager has to pass through metal detectors every day in school in order to make sure that he is not carrying an Uzi machine gun. And so what's the poor psychiatrist to do? Medicate the kid, of course.

This dilemma is simply that, just as in some mysterious way everything is connected to everything else, so all illness is somehow deeply embedded in networks, systems, and chains of pathology, with any individual patient being something like a canary in the proverbial mine shaft, picking up the systemic illness a bit earlier than others and having the good sense to drop dead first.

Whether or not any particular health-care practitioner explicitly thinks of illness as being part of larger (and possibly diseased) systems in the world, there is usually the gnawing sense that one's efforts at health-care are not much different from being a surgeon in a MASH unit during a war: the medic patches them up and sends them right back out on the battlefield to catch the next bullet. The intrinsic insanity of the situation—this impossible *Catch-22* job—seems to be felt to some degree by all sensitive health-care professionals.

Related to that difficult issue of how to define or even locate "illness" is the converse and equally impossible dilemma: what do we mean by "health"? Once it is understood that a human being is not simply an assemblage of physical parts, but contains emotional, mental, and spiritual dimensions that cannot be reduced without remainder to material processes, then what exactly does "health" mean in such a multidimensional being? How many levels of being—physical, emotional, mental, spiritual—should a doctor treat? Can I be healthy if I am spiritually malnourished? "Well, as a physician, that is not, and cannot be, my primary concern." But that is the same agonizing dilemma. By saying that those areas are not the concern of physicians, we are by default pledging allegiance to the old materialist version of medicine, thus forcing ourselves to treat a person according to a model that both the doctor and the patients know is incomplete. And there is the painful dilemma: as a health-care professional, you might indeed have to specialize in one particular area and ignore and compartmentalize all others; but as a human being, you simply cannot do so. The more effective one is as a conventional physician or health professional of any kind, the more he or she may struggle as a human being.

INTEGRAL THEORY AND PRACTICE

Integral medicine is designed, in part, to help with those dilemmas, not only as they affect the patient or client, but as they affect the physician and health-care practitioner. Integral medicine is also, of course, a way to more effectively and efficiently help patients. But it is, first and foremost, a way to help the health-care professional handle all of those pressing problems and painful dilemmas.

This is one of the defining ways that sets integral medicine apart from both conventional medicine and alternative medicine. It is sometimes said that conventional medicine treats the illness and alternative medicine treats the person. That's fine, and I personally believe both of those tenets are very important. But integral medicine goes one step further: it treats the illness, the person, and the physician.

Here it is useful to make a distinction between what might be called "an integral approach" and an "integrally informed approach." As we will see, both of these play an important role in integral medicine, although the former applies more to the patient, and the latter to the health-care professional. While an integral approach can more effectively help the patient, an integrally informed approach can more effectively help the healer.

All of the dilemmas mentioned above are variations on a common theme: the nature of a human being and his or her relation to a larger scheme of things. It might seem at this point that we are taking an unnecessary detour through philosophy, psychology, metaphysics, or some other alarmingly irrelevant field. The whole point about any truly integral approach is that it touches bases with as many important areas of research as possible before returning very quickly to the specific issues and applications of a given practice, in this case, medicine. Fortunately, the results of this particular detour can be summarized fairly simply and succinctly, with its direct relevance to medicine quickly established.

An integral approach means, in a sense, the "view from 50,000 feet." It is a panoramic look at the modes of inquiry (or the tools of knowledge acquisition) that human beings use, and have used, for decades and sometimes centuries. An integral approach is based on one central idea: no human mind can be 100% wrong. Or, we might say, nobody is smart enough to be wrong all the time. And that means, when it comes to deciding which approaches, methodologies, epistemologies, or ways of knowing are "correct," the answer can only be, "All of them." That is, all of the numerous practices or paradigms of human inquiry—including physics, chemistry, hermeneutics, collaborative inquiry, meditation, neuroscience, vision quest, phenomenology, structuralism, subtle energy research, systems theory, shamanic voyaging, chaos theory, and developmental psychology. All of those modes of inquiry have an important piece of the overall puzzle of a total existence that includes, among other things, health and illness, doctors and patients, and sickness and healing.

So an integral approach does not start by asking, for example, "Which of those methodologies are right and which are wrong?," but instead asks, "What kind of a universe is it that allows all of those practices to arise in the first place?" Since no mind can produce 100% error, this inescapably means that all of those approaches have at least some partial truths to offer an integral conference. The really interesting question is, what type of framework can we devise that finds a place for the important if partial truths of all of those methodologies?

If we found such an integral framework, we would hope to have an impact on the practice of medicine. The difficult dilemmas faced by medical practitioners who, in effect, are presently forced to be less than integral in their medical practice—while nevertheless feeling the strain and inner turmoil of wishing to be as whole and as integral as they can as human beings? And wishing to bring that *integrity* to an *integrally informed* practice of medicine? Is it really necessary that the more I become a doctor, the less I become a human? Or is there some way to practice medicine that surrenders not one ounce of the rigorously scientific, empirical, and clinical dimensions that will always be a cornerstone of any modern scientific system of health care, but also makes room, in a coherent fashion, for all of those other dimensions of being-in-the-world, dimensions that, if ignored or repressed, not only subtract from one's humanity but from being a truly effective physician?

To show what is involved, here is an example of how an integral approach has been used in psychology; the example is directly relevant because it is in the dimensions of psychology and consciousness that an integral approach has much to offer conventional medicine.

There are at least a dozen major schools of psychology, East and West, ancient and modern. There are the more "external" and "objective" approaches to consciousness, such as neuroscience, cognitive science, chaos and complexity theory, behaviorism, and neuropharmacology. There are the more "interior" or "subjective" approaches, such as depth psychology, meditation, guided imagery, and phenomenology. There are the "social" approaches that emphasize the relational nature of consciousness, including family therapy, systems theory, and social psychology. And there are the avant-garde approaches, including subtle energy research, metanormal and paranormal capacities, and transpersonal states and stages of consciousness.

When I first began studying psychology and consciousness, it was still common practice to pick one (or at most two) of those schools, decide that those were basically the correct approaches, and then spend the rest of one's professional life vigorously attacking the other ten schools. But as integral perspectives began to have an effect on the field, the central question in psychology and consciousness studies changed from, "Which of those 12 schools is the best or most accurate approach?," to "Why is it that all 12 of those schools exist in the first place?"

Nobody is smart enough to be wrong all the time. The implication was clear: if we are ever to have anything resembling a comprehensive, inclusive, integral view of psychology and consciousness, there is one and only one thing that we know for sure: it will include all 12 of those schools. Hundreds of thousands of decent men and women around the world are *already* practicing neuroscience, or psychiatric pharmacology, or meditation, or subtle energy research, or transpersonal psychology, or contemplation, or chaos and complexity theories. For the most part, they are responsible, sincere, and concerned men and women of integrity, and they honestly believe that the practice of their chosen field is making a positive and helpful contribution to humanity. I believe them. And I hope you do, too. It is not a matter of whether they can do that, or should do that, or are mistaken to be doing that. It is simply the case that they are already doing that, and are doing so in knowledge communities that have passed their knowledge forward for decades or even centuries, all of them contributing in invaluable ways to the sum total of understanding of what it means to be a human in the world.

So the really interesting question in psychology and consciousness studies soon becomes, "What theoretical framework can account for the important, if partial, truths of all 12 of those schools?" And then, "Once we have some sort of integral and nonexclusionary theory, how can that *integral theory* be put into *integral practice?*"

In psychology and consciousness studies, here is one result of such an integral approach. If you put all 12 of those important schools of psychology on the table; if you assume that they all have an important piece of the overall puzzle; if you then ask, "What must be the nature of the human psyche in order that all of those approaches are focusing on some important aspect of it?," one of the conclusions that you reach is that the human psyche must contain various dimensions or domains in order for the above methodologies to exist in the first place.

The type of integral psychology that I am most familiar with condenses all of those "necessities" down into five of the most important dimensions or components of the psyche, which are called quadrants, levels, lines, states, and types. A few of the following chapters present a general outline of this version of integral psychology, so here I can be mercifully brief—but the point, in any event, is that if we have a more integral psychology, we might very well be getting closer to what it means to be an integral psychologist.

"Quadrants" is merely shorthand for first-, second-, and third-person perspectives. All major human languages have first-, second-, and third-person pronouns (*first person*: I, we; *second person*: you, all of you; *third person*: him, her, them, they, it, its). The simplest and least derogatory explanation for that is: those pronouns represent real and enduring dimensions of experience and reality, dimensions that language itself has therefore adapted to and included during evolution. The first-person dimensions of being-in-the-world include, among other things, the interior "I," self-identity, art and aesthetic expression, meditation, depth psychology, guided imagery, introspection, contemplative prayer, normal and altered states of consciousness, and interior phenomenology. The second-person dimensions of being-in-the-world involve, among other things, the ways that a "you" and an "I" can come together and form a "we" (which is how "you" and "we" are sometimes treated together as second person), and thus second-person dimensions include culture, hermeneutics, mutual understanding, morality (or how we treat each other with regard), inter-subjectivity in all its dimensions, and communication itself. The third-person dimensions of being-in-the-world include the more "objective" approaches to reality, which do not use "I-language" or "we-language" but rather "it-language"—namely, the more scientific approaches that focus on those third-person dimensions of being-in-the-world—approaches that include physics, chemistry, neuroscience, pharmacology, and so on. These "it" approaches are sometimes subdivided into individual and systems approaches, giving us the sciences that focus on an individual or its subcomponents (the more "atomistic" versions of science, including physics, molecular biology, etc.) and those that focus on the collective (such as the numerous forms of systems theory, ecology, and complexity theory). These two approaches are often summarized as "it" (singular) and "its" (plural, collective, systems).

So the quadrants (I, we, it, and its) are just a simple way to keep track of the four major dimensions of being-in-the-world that are not only embedded in all major languages—and are therefore already present and fully operating in both you and your patients—but dimensions of reality that have been intensely investigated by literally hundreds of major paradigms, practices, methodologies, and modes of inquiry. These dimensions of being-in-the-world are most simply summarized as self (I), culture (we), and nature (it). Or art, morals, and science. Or the beautiful, the good, and the true. Or simply I, we, and it. And the interesting point is that, as far as we can tell, none of those dimensions can be reduced without remainder to the others (which is why, as a scientist, one might try to focus exclusively on the "it" dimension of reality, but as a human being, he or she cannot do so without rupturing the fabric of experience).

Of course, for centuries reductionists representing every quadrant have tried to reduce the other three quadrants to subtle variations on their own, only to be met with one salient failure after another. The materialist is an "I" who spends his time trying to prove that "I's" don't exist; a subjective idealist is an "I" who looks at "its" and tries to prove that they don't exist; a postmodern constructivist tries to prove that both "I's" and "its" are nothing but social constructions of a "we." Overall, one gets the sense of four limbs of a body each arguing that the others don't exist, a situation probably best summarized by Lovejoy as, "There is no human stupidity that has not found its champion." But in any event, such a reductionistic endeavor is simply not interesting to an integrally informed practitioner, because nobody is smart enough to be wrong all the time.

If you look at these four quadrants, embedded in all natural languages, it soon becomes apparent that there is a simple symmetry involved. "I," "we," "it," and "its" represent the interior and the exterior of the individual and the collective (Figure 1). The Left-Hand or interior dimensions (of I and we, or the first- and second-person dimensions of being-in-the-world) are "invisible," in that they can't be seen with the senses (e.g., mathematics, logic, mutual understanding, love, compassion, introspection, meditation, guided imagery, normal and altered states of consciousness). The Right-Hand or exterior dimensions (of it and its) can be seen with the senses, in that they are the objective or third-person dimensions of being-in-the-world, including atoms, molecules, cells, organisms, ecosystems, and so on. If the Left and Right Hand quadrants

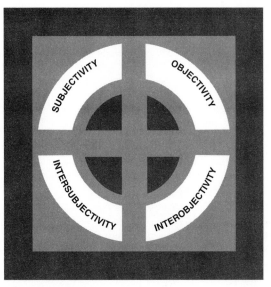

Figure 1 Wilber's four quadrants.

represent interior and exterior realities, the upper and lower quadrants represent the individual (I, it) and the collective (we, its).

Now the implication of that simple scheme is that all four of those dimensions inextricably go together, if for no other reason than that you cannot have an inside without an outside, nor a singular without a plural (which is probably why reductionism has had such a consistent history of failure). This scheme becomes quite intriguing because it can be directly related to the practice of medicine. If you simply use the quadrants alone, and lay them out on a table (Figure 2), it becomes obvious that conventional medicine has focused almost exclusively on one of the quadrants—namely, on the Upper-Right quadrant, or the third-person singular dimension of being-in-the-world. In other words, conventional medicine has focused almost entirely on the individual organism and the objective physical dimensions of that organism (including its anatomy, physiology, and organ systems, and the effects of physical interventions from drugs to surgery)—all of the "it" dimensions of a person, which are definitely real and definitely a crucial part of health. This dimension represents only one fourth of the overall story presenting itself in the physician's office.

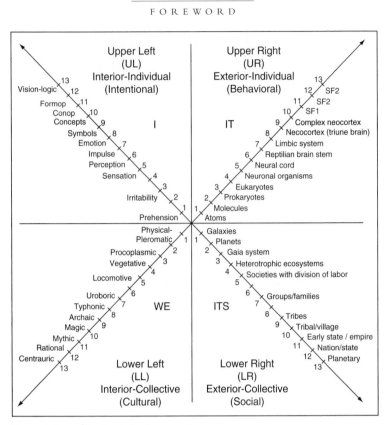

Figure 2 Some details of the four quadrants.

Physicians and their patients have these four dimensions always available and always functioning in any event. However, in their practice of medicine, they are only "allowed" to use or treat one fourth of the actual condition, and some sort of rupture has occurred somewhere. Both practitioners and their patients can *feel* it, can feel this fracture in the Kosmos called "going to the doctor."

It is perhaps obvious that many alternative and complementary approaches to medicine are, in their own ways, attempting to include the other three quadrants neglected by conventional medicine. For example, many alternative approaches attempt to include the important dimensions of the Upper Left (or "I"), including meditation, guided imagery, relaxation techniques, visualization, contemplative prayer, and so on. Other approaches attempt to include the importance of social systems (or the Lower Right), and thus see health issues in a larger context of ecological systems and environmental toxins, social systems and their ills, and the complex networks that involve all living creatures. Other complementary approaches draw attention to the finer dimensions of the Upper Right, such as the subtle energies that seem to surround and permeate the gross physical organism. Still other complementary approaches add the importance of the Lower-Left quadrant or "we"—the importance of culture, of a supportive network of intersubjective understanding (including communication between the doctor, patient, family, and friends), along with support groups or group therapy.

Although it is true, for example, that women with breast cancer who join support groups often have a 30% longer survival rate than those who don't, interpersonal culture is a good in itself. It is a very real and very important quadrant or dimension of being-in-the-world. One engages that dimension not simply because it makes the physical organism sustain itself longer, but because it exercises a profound, wonderful, deep dimension of being and consciousness. The fact that people get healthier when they do so is simply to say that comprehensive is better.

Examples abound. An integral framework suggests that every state of consciousness in the individual "I" has a corresponding brain state in the physical organism (or the individual "it"). Physicians can treat a brain state with pharmacology or neurosurgery; they treat mind states and consciousness with depth psychology and meditation. It is not necessary that as a neurosurgeon, or a family practitioner, they somehow use depth psychology and meditation in their practice (although they certainly can if they wish).

However, it is the case that an integrally informed medical practitioner is aware of the actual dimensions of being and consciousness that are present in his or her patients. Thus can the practitioner tell when patients might need Prozac or when they might need meditation—or both. As it is now, most illnesses in other quadrants are treated with tools that effectively address only the physical organism. Diseases of the soul are treated with antibiotics, because the patients demand something.

While most holistic or alternative frameworks acknowledge the importance of those four quadrants or dimensions (intentional, behavioral, social, and cultural), an integral framework continues to expand its heuristic scope by also acknowledging levels, lines, states, and types. This framework is not merely eclectic, which is present in most alternative or holistic approaches (and which simply asserts that everything is connected to everything else), but integral (or a coherent system that specifically indicates how everything is connected to everything else). Here I will give only a few quick examples to illustrate what is involved, and then return to what an "integrally informed" medical practice might entail.

Among specialists in the interior dimensions of the individual (the "I" or the Upper-Left quadrant), we find a general consensus that there are *stages* of consciousness, *states* of consciousness, and *types* of consciousness. Because events in any one quadrant reverberate through all of the quadrants (with health or illness in one tending to induce health or illness in the others), an integral framework gives us a way to begin to correlate the effects of different aspects of consciousness on organic health and illness. The impact of altered *states of consciousness* on health and healing has been documented from shamanic times to today's psychoneuroimmunology. There are several empirical studies on those approaches presented in this volume. Just as important is the existence of *stages of consciousness*. The documented stages or waves of consciousness appear to span a spectrum from sensory to mental to spiritual; from pre-personal to personal to transpersonal; from subconscious to self-conscious to superconscious. When the ancients talked about a spectrum of consciousness ranging from matter to body to mind to soul to spirit, it seems that they were giving voice to one version of this great spectrum of potentials—physical, emotional, mental, and spiritual—potentials that, like the quadrants, effectively resist reductionism.*

---

*Yes, I know, the attempt to reduce spirit to matter is another folly that has not lacked its champions. But try as one might, one simply cannot reduce spirit to combinations and permutations of "frisky dirt." And why this dirt would get right up and start writing poetry has never really been made clear by materialists of any flavor. It's not just that such reductionism violates the grain of the given, it is that it invariably fails on its own terms, importing in an implicit fashion the very things that it attempts to explain away. William James called reductionism "genius backed by prejudice"—it takes genius to be able to make that philosophical game even seem to make sense, and it takes prejudice to want to do it in any event. A more integrally informed practitioner simply sets aside any reductionistic prejudice and, in throwing the theoretical net as wide as possible so as to miss the fewest open secrets, acknowledges what human beings have known pretty much from day one: we all have physical, emotional, mental, and spiritual dimensions of being and awareness.

Moreover, it appears that each of those dimensions, levels, or waves can exist in healthy or diseased forms. There are not only more ways to be healthy than conventional medicine recognizes, there are more ways to be sick, too.

Of course these ways are always intertwined, but there does indeed seem to be physical health, emotional health, mental health, and spiritual health, expressing the levels, stages, or waves of this extraordinary spectrum. Likewise, there seems to be physical illness, emotional illness, mental illness, and spiritual illness. As we will see, this great spectrum of health and sickness becomes of keen interest to an integral practitioner.

Through this spectrum of consciousness with its stages or waves run numerous different streams. That is, there appear to be at least two dozen relatively independent developmental lines or streams that progress through the developmental levels or waves of consciousness. These developmental lines include the cognitive line (studied by, e.g., Robert Kegan, Patricia Arlin), the interpersonal line (e.g., William Selman, Cheryl Armon), that of values (Clare Graves), self-identity (Jane Loevinger), stages of faith (James Fowler), morals (Lawrence Kohlberg, Carol Gilligan), needs (Abraham Maslow), among others. These developmental lines or streams are sometimes called "intelligences" in a manner made well-known by Howard Gardner (e.g., emotional intelligence, musical intelligence, kinesthetic intelligence, cognitive intelligence). The important phenomenon known as "waves and streams" (or "levels and lines") simply means that a person can be at a fairly high level of development in some lines (such as cognitive), at a medium level of development in other lines (such as interpersonal), and at a fairly low level in yet others (such as moral). This also makes intuitive sense in that we all know individuals who are, say, highly intelligent but not very ethical, or people who are highly advanced in some skills and not as developed in others (an extreme example being the "idiot savant"). An integral psychology makes room for all of those factors.

And all of those factors come urgently and unavoidably into play, not just in heath and healing, but in the entire arena of what it means to practice medicine, not one mechanic to one machine, not one plumber to one broken faucet, but one human being to another. What if in our little black medical bag we had—not 20 pills, two scalpels, and an orthopedic hammer—but also all quadrants, all waves, all streams, all states, and all types? What if our medical bag included a more comprehensive and integral map of the human being who has come for help, such that you can engage in a truly integral diagnosis covering all the known bases of what might be ailing?

"Ah, but unfortunately all of those factors are not my concern. As physicians, we must focus on organic health and illness." However, these are our concerns, because in this culture, when anybody gets really sick, everybody tells them the same thing: "You better see a doctor." If you are *really* sick, in virtually *any* area, you do not go to a rabbi, a priest, or a massage therapist. You go to a doctor.

Again what's a poor doctor to do? Most general practitioners tell us that in well over half of their cases, there is nothing physically wrong with the patient. What that really means is that there is nothing wrong in the Upper-Right quadrant, because there is clearly something wrong in one of the other quadrants (or the other levels or lines or states). Again, it is not necessary that a family practitioner be able to treat all of the illnesses in all of the quadrants or levels or states. Specialization will always be necessary to some degree. But if we aspire to be integrally informed medical practitioners, we will at least be familiar with the diseases and treatments in the other quadrants and dimensions. An "integral medical practice" is a practice that makes room for the entire panoply of effective treatments across all quadrants and dimensions of human health and illness. There do indeed appear to be physical, emotional, mental, and spiritual waves of being and awareness, each of them possessing an "I" and a "we" and an "it" dimension. Through those waves of existence appear to run cognitive streams and self-identity streams and value streams and artistic streams, all rushing and roiling across that extraordinary spectrum from subconscious to self-conscious to superconscious. And it now appears more than likely that every single one of those variables is at work in every single case of health and illness, sickness and recovery, healer and healed.

The crucial ingredient in any integral medical practice is not the integral medical bag itself—with all the conventional pills, and the orthodox surgery, and the subtle energy medicine, and the acupuncture needles—but the holder of that bag. Integrally informed health-care practitioners, the doctors and nurses and therapists, have opened themselves to an entire spectrum of consciousness—matter to body to mind to soul to spirit—and who have thereby acknowledged what seems to be happening in any event. Body and mind and spirit are operating in self and culture and nature, and thus health and healing, sickness and wholeness, are all bound up in a multidimensional tapestry that cannot be cut into without loss.

An integrally informed medical practice changes the practitioners first; they can then decide which of the treatments—conventional, alternative, complementary, and/or holistic—they wish to utilize, individually and collectively when practicing medicine with integrity. It may include adding new treatments, conventional and alternative; or more conscientiously referring patients to other-quadrant practitioners when an integral diagnosis so indicates; or becoming part of a medical group or center that specializes in integral treatments (by having staff specialists in the various quadrants, states, and levels of health and illness). The only item that is constant in all of these scenarios is the transformed practitioner. It is the physician or other health professional who is healed and wholed first, not merely by learning new and complementary techniques, but by inhabiting a new consciousness that makes room for new techniques; and how that integrity then expresses itself in an integrally informed medical practice might vary considerably.

The advantage of integrally informed medical practice over both conventional and holistic approaches may now be a little more clear. The problem with many alternative, complementary, or holistic practices is that, for all their noble intent and sincere efforts, they often end up simply creating a bigger "grab bag" of treatments without an integrally informed diagnosis or treatment plan. Too often this results in the sense that if I prescribe both doxycycline and Chinese herbs, I am being holistic. Or every radiation treatment gets 15 minutes of guided imagery. The problem with that approach, in my opinion, is that it too often focuses merely on increasing the number and types of treatments in the little black bag, and hence falls into what amounts to the same objectifying tool-kit approach, but now with more types of pills and hammers. That often opens the otherwise sincere holistic practitioner to forms of treatment that are ineffective or even regressive, simply because everything must be included. To say that none of these alternatives are 100% wrong is not to say that they are 100%

right. Integral approaches can be very rigorous in standards of evidence and efficacy, a rigor that some holistic approaches let go of too quickly in an attempt to be "all inclusive." A genuinely comprehensive medical practice does not have to include leeches, eye of newt, or dragon dung, no matter what Eastern name is attached to them.

The net result of this tension between conventional and alternative approaches is that physicians and nurses today are very unhappy with the present state of conventional medicine and yet they often distrust the holistic alternatives. They know conventional medicine is limiting them personally and in the healing they can offer the sick. Yet they may suspect that too much of alternative and holistic approaches have abandoned evidence and rigor in a show of what amounts to a medical version of politically correct thinking: "nobody wants to marginalize leeches."

An integrally informed medical practice does not neglect the types of effective treatments that can or should be included in a comprehensive medical treatment. But all of that, truly, comes after the transformation in the practitioners themselves. The one thing that will have changed in adopting an integral approach is their own awareness, their own consciousness, their own map of human possibilities—this map that has dramatically expanded from organic interventions to caring for a human being in all of his or her extraordinary richness across an entire spectrum that runs from dust to deity, from dirt to divinity, even from here and now. An integrally informed medical practitioner is one who has let the most amount of the Kosmos into his or her mind, finds thereby the most potentials for health and healing and compassionate care, and brings that Big Mind to his or her practice in a way that inculcates both more confidence and more humility, all at once.

HUMBLE BEGINNINGS

Integral medicine is in its infancy. As such, the medical and health-care practitioners who are helping to forge an integral practice are on a voyage of incredible discovery, arguably one of the most important that the millennia-old profession of medicine has ever made. In the following chapters you will see some of these important pioneering efforts. Taken together, they cover aspects of virtually all of the quadrants, levels, lines, states, and types. There are exciting chapters on leading-edge science in the objective or "it" dimensions, including recent research on neuropeptides and other organic communication systems; spontaneous healing and mechanisms of self-repair; the bodily components of healing and their future evolution; empirical evidence on the existence and effects of subtle energies and their role in health and energy medicine. (Please note the strong emphasis that is given to empirical evidence and scientific grounding in these areas. Eye of newt, for example, goes into the little black bag, if and only if there is reproducible scientific evidence that it works.) I personally believe that subtle energy medicine is on the verge of scientific breakthroughs that alone could revolutionize the objective dimensions of medical care.

There are also chapters on the vast territory of the "I" dimension with all its waves, streams, and states—including the role of mental factors in organic health and illness; the many ways that the mind and body can neither be reduced to each other nor separated from each other; the nature of conscious healing; ways to transform illness by involving both higher states and stages of consciousness; and ways that the health-care professional can transform his or her own consciousness as well, particularly through service and transformational engagement—the entire spectrum of "opening your heart: anatomically, emotionally, spiritually."

There are likewise important chapters on the "we" dimension of health and illness, including cross-cultural perspectives on sickness and healing; participatory medicine; relational medicine; the many ways that each "I" and "it" are nestled in layers of "we"—that is, both subjects and objects arise in cultural backgrounds of intersubjectivity that play an enormously influential role in health and sickness (dimensions made all the more important by the degree of neglect usually accorded them, in conventional and alternative approaches alike). As theoreticians from Heidegger to Habermas have demonstrated, these cultural "we's" cannot be reduced to the terms of systems theory (or social "its"), nor can they be captured by "I" or "it" approaches, but must be addressed in their own terms, with their own techniques, in their own ways—ways that any integrally informed practitioner would want to be familiar with. In the last analysis, the doctor-patient relationship is not one "I" operating on a slab of "it," but an extraordinary "we" for which the term "sacred" is very likely the only accurate adjective. It is from that sacred "we" that all healing arises as a miracle of love and grace that perhaps thankfully none of us will ever understand. (If we did, perhaps we would mess it up rather badly.) Medicine, when it works, will always be riding a wave of miracle and mystery, of which nothing is more mysterious and miraculous than a "we."

There are significant chapters on the important role played by social systems, the self-organizing systems of dynamic "its," the networks of ecological connectivity that leave no individual untouched. This includes chapters on ecological health, the ecozoic era, the web of life and what it means for us all—the many ways that we are linked not just intersubjectively in cultures of "we" but interobjectively in systems of dynamic processes. Notice that these interlocking systems (such as the web of life) are always described in third-person plural terms (because they are indeed systems of dynamic and interrelated its). The whole point is that every "it" and "its" has "I" and "we" correlates, and all of those dimensions need to be taken into account in any integral approach to medicine. Although intentional "I's" and cultural "we's" cannot be reduced to, or explained by, social systems of ecological processes, they cannot exist without them, either. The web of life covers only one quadrant, but a quadrant all too often neglected in a focus on individual health.

All of those important dimensions of integral medicine are addressed in the following chapters. Because various integral approaches are all in their infancy, it goes without saying that not all theorists in this volume will agree with each other. Certainly not everybody would agree with the version or the terminology that I have been using in this introduction, nor should they. Have you ever seen those maps that the early European explorers made of the Americas—where Cuba is the size of Siberia and Florida extends all the way to Brazil? And on the indigenous side of the Atlantic as well—have you ever seen the similar maps the Aztecs made of the new territories they were exploring? That view is almost certainly what our present maps of an integral medicine look like. But that is simply all the more reason to push forward in this extraordinary exploration.

The following chapters are the maps of intrepid explorers pushing into a new territory that can only dimly be seen forming on the horizon of our integral conversations. This is why it is especially important that all of these approaches be put on the table and held with a gesture of respect, with one integral guideline kept gently in mind: nobody is smart enough to be wrong all the time. In this extraordinary endeavor, everybody has a piece of the integral puzzle, and thus what we are looking for is a framework that can coherently include the most number of approaches without pathologizing the alternatives.

This book, then, is not the last word in integral medicine, but merely a humble beginning. It is the opening of a dialogue too long ignored, the calling forth of extraordinary potentials too long denied, the acknowledging of a healing love too long left unspoken. Integral medicine is an acknowledgment of the Kosmos in all of its radiant richness; and thus—in some mysterious way that every true physician knows in the depths of the compassionate heart—an integrally informed practitioner is one through whom the Kosmos heals. One in whom the entire spectrum of consciousness is allowed to speak and shout its truths; one who puts self aside in the healing gesture and lets the entire universe come rushing through—matter to body to mind to soul to spirit—in self and culture and nature. The panoramic vista opened to the integrally informed practitioner restructures his or her own being and consciousness, turning the practitioner into something of a beautiful, tender, hollow bamboo reed. The reed is hollow to resonate with the sound of the entire Kosmos washing upon the shores of the soul, wild and radiant in all its dimensions, overflowing in a healing gesture that leaves no sentient being untouched, a gesture that every now and then glances at that Oath hanging on the wall, knowing that, in this integral regard, no sacred promises have been broken in this office.

Ken Wilber

The Integral Impulse: An Emerging Model for Health and Healing

Centuries ago, adventurers exploring the frontiers of our planet discovered, again and again, that they lived in a wider world than previously assumed. During this period, the art of mapmaking made tremendous strides. Fictitious lines of latitude and longitude became as important to navigators as the force of currents and the direction of winds. Perceptions of the world changed as new tools were discovered and new ideas unfolded.

More recently, the quest to understand the universe and our place in it follows a similar pushing of boundaries with its own inventive mapmaking. New maps are being made to reflect new discoveries: The universe now appears, if not infinite, at least infinitely complex. Astonishing scientific advances have been made in our mastery of the outer world—we have seen astronauts walk on the moon, collected data about the physical structure of Jupiter, invented a computer chess champion named Deep Blue, and cloned a sheep named Dolly. Such advances are displays of humankind's generative ability to transform physical reality.

Yet this primary focus of modern science on the objective, material world has come at a cost—frequently obscuring what is meaningful and valuable in human experience. Since the rise of modern science, Western culture has assumed a separation between consciousness and matter, between mind and body, between humans and nature, between spirituality and science. These dualisms, deeply troublesome for science and philosophy, were also incorporated into the historical development of Western medicine.

AN INTEGRAL VISION

While science has contributed to our understanding and treatment of disease, it has also served to limit the development of a model in which personal relationships, emotions, meaning, and belief systems are viewed as fundamental points of connection between body, mind, spirit, society, and nature. For increasing numbers of health-care consumers and professionals alike, the biomedical model fails to offer a system for understanding the fullness of lived experience—minimizing or negating completely the possibility for human transcendence in the face of illness and disease.

A significant barrier to the integration of inner and outer approaches to reality is the seeming incongruity between, on the one hand, the ontology and epistemology of physical science and, on the other hand, those of the spiritual traditions. As they are commonly conceived, religion and science are indeed incompatible. But if properly understood and properly enlarged, these two realms may be incorporated within a framework that is at once true to their distinctions and yet comprehensive of both. It is such an inclusiveness that is called for in this book.

The emergence of such an integral perspective in medicine can be traced to the work of Indian mystic and political leader, Sri Aurobindo (1951). It is based on an intuitive understanding of life and ultimate reality as undivided wholeness. The greatest aspiration of Indian Yoga is to realize the ultimate ground of existence (Brahman) in which Nature and Spirit are unified. Integral thinking is based on unity-in-diversity. Franklin Merrell-Wolf (1994) captured the essence of this integral impulse in his conviction that "science, in the sense of knowing fully, cannot be restricted to objective material, but must, as well, be open to other possibilities of awareness."

Recognition that the scientific quest is incomplete without data from many domains of inquiry, and without various kinds of knowing, has grown since the teachings of Aurobindo. Through the writings of such scholars as Haridas Chaudhari (1977), Indra Sen (1986), Michael Murphy (1992), and Ken Wilber (1995), integral philosophy today represents a dynamic integration of the scientific, phenomenological, and dialectical methods of the West and the self-analytical, psycho-integrative, non–dual value disciplines of the East. Integralism speaks to its very own evolution occurring on individual and collective levels.

British philosopher C.D. Broad (1953) set a high standard for non-exclusive science when he insisted that the quest for genuine knowledge involves two closely connected intellectual activities: synopsis and synthesis.

"Synopsis is the deliberate viewing together of aspects of human experience which, for one reason or another, are generally kept apart. . . . The object of synopsis is to try to find out how these various aspects are interrelated. Synthesis is the attempt to apply a coherent set of concepts and principles which cover satisfactorily all the regions of fact which have been viewed synoptically."

Broad's framework goes beyond merely making it possible to view together disparate realms of experience. It becomes clear that our capacity to comprehend new possibilities for human advance indeed depends on a willingness to deliberately view together our physiological, emotional, cognitive, social, ecological, and spiritual processes—and more, a willingness to formulate comprehensive theories sufficiently robust to ask crucial questions about the relationship between consciousness and the physical world.

A CALL FOR INTEGRAL MEDICINE

The first attempts to bring an integral approach to medicine were advanced more than 20 years ago in a book entitled *Mind, Body & Health: Toward an Integral Medicine*, by James Gordon, Dennis Jaffe, and David Bresler (1984). Speaking to the many challenges of Western medicine, they noted that integral medicine practitioners were rediscovering the healing potentiality of the doctor-patient relationship. Being concerned with the whole person rather than the disease, the authors called on health professionals to consider the possibility of a universal life force as manifested mentally, physically, and spiritually, which is benevolent and at the ground of human development and healing.

Today, we see that the state of medicine continues to shake at its very foundations. Recognizing that health-care is in a time of crisis—crisis of care, confidence, and cost—we are being called on to make our system more humane, effective, and empowering of the patient. A reevaluation and revisioning of the theoretical underpinnings of modern medicine is called for, as we seek to create a new map. And although there is no universal consensus on just what this new map looks like, we suggest in the pages that follow that it includes the mapmaker, as both a product and a participant in that which he or she seeks to know and represent.

This integral perspective calls for deep change within the practitioners and the patients as together we embark on a transformation in worldview. Ken Wilber writes in his introduction to this book: "The crucial ingredient in any integral medical practice is not the integral medical bag itself—with all the conventional pills, and the orthodox surgery, and the subtle energy medicine, and the acupuncture needles—but the holder of that bag. Integrally informed health-care practitioners, the doctors and nurses and therapists, have opened themselves to an entire spectrum of consciousness—matter to body to mind to soul to spirit—and who have thereby acknowledged what seems to be happening in any event. Body and mind and spirit are operating in self, culture, and nature, and thus health and healing, sickness and wholeness, are all bound up in a multidimensional tapestry that cannot be cut into without loss." This view of an "engaged epistemology" can be seen clearly in the formulation of an integral healing model, uniting the many dimensions of human consciousness.

KEY TENETS OF INTEGRAL MEDICINE
As we prepared this collection of essays, we identified the following as key tenets of the integral impulse currently emerging within modern healthcare.

1. Integral medicine does not just refer to the science of diagnosing, treating, or preventing disease and damage of the body or mind, but to a medicine that *heals*. It is a dynamic, holistic, life-long process that exists in widening and deepening relationships with self, culture, and nature. Integral medicine is about transformation, growth, and the restoration of wholeness. Health is seen not as the absence of disease, but as a process by which individuals maintain their ability to develop meaning systems that allow them to function, heal, and grow in the face of changes in themselves, their relationships, and the world.
2. Consciousness is a process that involves our awareness of ourselves and the world, including our thoughts, feelings, sensations, identity, and worldviews. In essence, consciousness involves the fundamental characteristics of human nature and experience and therefore shapes our

understanding of disease, illness, health, and well-being. Body, mind, and spirit interact in shaping the individual, developmental, and evolutionary potentials of human beings.

3. An integral perspective requires a deep examination of our core assumptions about reality and our place in it. Standard science holds that objective truth is arrived at through discovery of causal laws of the natural world that exists independently for all time, and for all human beings. When it comes to the human condition, an integral perspective suggests that so-called objectivity may need to be fundamentally transformed and that, in fact, no science and no medicine is possible independent of consciousness.

4. An integral methodology includes both objective, subjective, and intersubjective approaches to understanding human experience. A conjoining of divergent methods and approaches is needed to map the role of consciousness in health and healing—science has a place just as self-reflection and inner knowing have parts to play. This viewpoint necessarily dismisses dogmatic reduction of reality to only that which can be seen and measured. Indeed, the integral perspective emphasizes that a focus on the material basis of reality may not be the only or even the best way to look at issues inherent in healing.

5. Integral medicine involves a deep appreciation for the multiple cultural perspectives and approaches that contribute to the fullness of healing as a complex, dynamic, and multifaceted phenomenon. Therefore, it is crucial to honor and appropriately integrate the world's wisdom and healing traditions and their diverse and often contradictory epistemologies.

6. Harnessing our desire for health and healing as well as their will to live is as significant to an integral medicine as the role of scientific information and technology.

7. The key to an integral approach is not the contents of the medical bag, but the holder of the bag—one who has opened herself to the multidimensional nature of healing, including body, mind, soul, spirit, culture, and nature. This includes opening to the experience of suffering as it provides a catalyst for transformation; this is true for patients, health professionals, society and the institutions that serve us, and ultimately— our relationship to our sacred ground of being. An expanded view of

the person is called for in which the biological, phenomenological, cultural, and transpersonal come together in meaningful synergy.

8. The well-being of the planet's ecosystems is required for the well-being of the human. Despite medical science and technology, humans cannot be well in a sick society or on a sick planet. Integral medicine is concerned with transforming human consciousness to create life enhancing ways of being in the world. This calls for deep social and ecological healing.

9. Life is the greatest teacher. Our ability to see the way to a new approach requires deep humility in the face of wonder and mystery. Gratefulness, love, and compassion are essential tools to an inclusive and full-hearted healing system.

CONTRIBUTIONS FROM THE NOETIC SCIENCES

This book is the result of more than three decades of research on consciousness and healing at the Institute of Noetic Sciences (IONS). Noetic is derived from the Greek word *nous,* which may be translated as mind or direct ways of knowing. The Institute of Noetic Sciences, founded in 1973 by the Apollo 14 astronaut, Edgar Mitchell, seeks to further the explorations of conventional science through rigorous inquiry into aspects of reality—mind, consciousness, spirit—that include, yet potentially transcend, physical phenomena. A guiding premise of the research and educational programs is that the interface of inner experience and the outer world may provide the greatest opportunity for breakthroughs in our understanding of health and healing.

In the mid-1970s, the Institute of Noetic Sciences initiated a modest internal program of research on the inner mechanisms of the healing response. At that time, the notion that consciousness-related factors—including cognitive processes and emotional states—could play any role in bodily health and the healing of disease was both novel and unacceptable in mainstream biomedical thinking. Medicine focused largely on the physical aspects of disease.

Much has changed in these three decades. Mind-body medicine has come of age and we have increasing recognition, grounded in serious and disciplined research, that we all possess an innate healing system. The efficacy of this system rests on the premise that mind, brain, and spirit act in concert when healing occurs. As a "metasystem," it responds to symbolic processes as well as physical stimuli, perhaps acting in coordination with previously known systems (such as the immune or endocrine systems), but not limited to them.

Stimulated by the promise of this new perspective, and by new developments in the field of consciousness studies, the Institute of Noetic Sciences today continues to nurture the development of mind-body medicine—conducting and sponsoring research that expands our understanding of the effects of consciousness on our bodies, minds, and spirits. As we seek to harness the healing system, we are exploring the potential role of factors such as faith, prayer, intention, subtle energies, and biofields. With new data in hand, we are revising the map of our human capacities and offering a new vision of what we are capable of becoming.

FEATURES OF OUR INTEGRAL PERSPECTIVE

This book is organized into five major sections, with contributions in each by pioneers in the emerging field of consciousness and healing. In Section One we begin by considering the implications of an integral perspective for health and healing. We recognize that integral medicine promotes an approach embedded in the scientific dimension that epitomizes the best in modern health-care, while equally recognizing that human beings possess emotional, spiritual, and relational dimensions that are essential in the diagnosis and treatment of disease and the cultivation of wellness. Inherent in our quest for an integral approach is the recognition that a full system shift is needed to bring about the changes that are called for at this time. Such a transformation requires each of us to look within, reflecting on our own purpose and meaning. From this position, we are better able to take the actions needed to change our worldviews.

Section Two seeks to explore the nature of the healing system. We overview recent developments in mind-body medicine. These include new perspectives on the body, a revisioning of illness as a transformative process, and an appreciation of the various stages of the life process that are fundamental aspects of the integral healing journey. While these emerging subfields are not well-known within modern medicine, the potential results have far-reaching implications, suggesting that consciousness may be a far more extended causal agent than even the proponents of mind-body medicine have previously considered.

Section Three reaches out to embrace other dimensions of the healing system. Religion and spirituality have become important, though underresearched, domains of the noetic sciences. Epidemiological data reveal that better health is correlated with religious participation. Clinical benefits, including lowered levels of stress, substance abuse, suicide, depression, and hypertension, have been reported as correlates to religious and spiritual participation. Various factors have been identified to help account for healthpromoting effects of spirituality, including social support, lifestyle, altruism, and a connection to the transpersonal. There is increasing interest in the influence of prayer on healing, not only prayer for someone offered at the bedside, but also intercessory prayer at a distance. Again, we begin to find markers for the expanding role of consciousness in healing.

Section Four focuses on the multiple ways of knowing that are involved in an integral approach to health and healing. Healing practices, and the medical systems that deliver them, are based on cultural assumptions about the nature of the human body, the sources of illness, and appropriate medical responses to the challenges of disease. These may vary, depending on the way we model reality. With the increasing popularity of alternative medical practices in the United States, biomedicine is being forced to view health and healing within broader cultural contexts. Here we have another opportunity to examine our assumptions about health and healing and the role of our respective worldviews in shaping our healing experiences.

In Section Five we turn our attention to the various challenges currently facing Western medicine. Economic factors, an increasing burden of chronic illness, and higher levels of physician and patient dissatisfaction provide further indicators that our health-care system is in the process of significant change. Envisioning a new story entails a long view and a large vision. This emerging perspective includes transformation at the personal, social, and ecological levels of our experience. What is called for is a shift in consciousness: one that leads to a more expanded, humanistic, and lifeaffirming map to guide ourselves and future generations.

Ultimately, we see this book as a call to action for health professionals and patients alike. Medicine is in trouble. Each of us carries the responsibility to help craft a new, more fitting map. As Roger Walsh writes so beautifully in his essay in Section Three: "Our world is in grave trouble, we all know this. Our world is in grave, grave trouble. But our world also rests in good hands, because, actually, it rests in yours." Simply by taking the time to consider an integral perspective, we are helping to hospice an old paradigm that is ceasing to work. In so doing, we must be gentle with ourselves, with each other, and with a system of medicine that is struggling with its very existence. Change can be hard. But it is also revitalizing and ultimately transformative.

Just as one paradigm dies, so another will be born. For this, we may enthusiastically offer ourselves up as midwives. As we engage in this endeavor to bring a new life into the world, we are not alone. Together we can change the future. As noted by Michael Murphy and George Leonard in their book, *The Life We Are Given*, "Through transformative practices. . . we can share the most fundamental tendencies of the world's unfoldment—to expand, create, and give rise to more conscious forms of life. Like evolution itself, we can bring forth new possibilities for growth, new worlds for further exploration." And so, finally, we offer this book as a gesture of friendship and support for your own integral healing journey.

Marilyn Schlitz

References

Aurobindo S: *The Life Divine*, New York, 1951, Sri Aurobindo Library.
Broad CD: *Religion, Philosophy and Psychical Research*, 1953, Harcourt Brace, p 8.
Chaudhuri H: *The Evolution of Integral Consciousness*, Wheaton, Ill, 1977, Quest Books.
Gordon J, Jaffe D, Bresler D: *Mind, Body & Health: Toward an Integral Medicine*, New York, 1984, Human Sciences Press.
Leonard G, Murphy M: *The Life We Are Given*, New York, 1995, Tarcher/Putnam Books.
Merrell-Wolf F: *Experience and Philosophy: A Personal Record of Transformation and a Discussion of Transcendental Consciousness*, Albany, NY, 1994, SUNY Press, pp 305-306.
Mitchell E: *The Way of the Explorer*, New York, 1996, GP Putnam's Sons.
Murphy M: *The Future of the Body: Explorations Into the Further Evolution of Human Nature*, Los Angeles, 1992, Tarcher.
Sen I: *Integral Psychology: The Psychological System of Sri Aurobindo*, Pondicherry, India, 1986, Sri Aurobindo Ashram Trust.
Wilber K: *Sex, Ecology, Spirituality. The Spirit of Evolution*, Boston, MA, 1995, Shambhala Publications.

ACKNOWLEDGMENTS

This book is the product of over 30 years of groundbreaking work by frontier scientists and leaders in the field of health-care—each offering direction for a new model of health and healing. We are in their debt. In particular we are grateful to:

Each of the authors of this anthology who contributed their love, labor, and wisdom in their extraordinary chapters in the book and on the companion DVD. The doctors who shared their wisdom and experience through their rich interviews on the DVD. Everyone who contributed essays that in the end we were unable to include; we had to make some tough choices. Christian deQuincey and Barbara McNeill, who edit the IONS quarterly magazine from which some of the essays were drawn. The artists who contributed their images to lend beauty and grace to our work. Steve and David Gordon at Sequoia Records, whose music adds to the color and texture of our DVD. And to our colleagues, friends, and mentors who have encouraged us in many ways. These include: David Bresler, Daniel Brooke, Renata Brownbridge, Ken Corr, Dan Drasin, Bob Duggan, Kelly Durkin, Charlene Farrell, Stephen Francis, Winston Franklin, James Gordon, Richard Grossinger, Willis Harman, Michael Heumann, Ivan Illich, Dennis Jaffe, Lou Judson, Nola Lewis, Ted Mallon, Jenny Mathews, Caroline McEver, Edgar Mitchell, James O'Dea, Brendan O'Regan, Dean Radin, Helene Smith, Elisabeth Targ, Keith Thompson, and Cassandra Vieten.

We are grateful to our editorial team at Churchill Livingstone: Kellie Fitzpatrick, Jennifer Watrous, and Kendra Bailey, who have always been encouraging, helpful, and a pleasure to collaborate with on this book.

And finally, we'd like to wholeheartedly acknowledge the financial stewardship we received in the early stages of this research: The Carl & Roberta Deutsch Foundation, The Lucy Gonda Foundation, The Mallon Family Foundation, and one other anonymous angel who helped guide this book to fruition.

ABOUT THE INSTITUTE OF NOETIC SCIENCES

For 30 years **The Institute of Noetic Sciences** has been at the forefront of research and education into consciousness, health and healing, creativity, and the expansion of our human potentials. The word Noetic comes from the ancient Greek word *nous*. It refers to "inner knowing." This involves direct and immediate access to knowledge beyond what is available to our normal senses and powers of reason. Hatched in the mind of astronaut Edgar Mitchell after a visionary experience in space, Noetic Sciences has expanded the frontiers of science, as well as helped to empower major shifts in our philosophies and social structures. Today, Noetic Sciences is an international non-profit organization with 28,000 members and 300 community groups worldwide, all working together to foster a global shift in consciousness. Our educational programs explore frontier research and forge links between divergent ideas and disciplines, as well as illuminate familiar territory with fresh understanding. Our research programs are based on the premise that understanding the relationship between inner experience and the outer world holds great transformational potential. In the field of medicine, IONS' research team uses the tools of laboratory science, field studies, applied and clinical research, publications, conferences, and transformational learning media to help catalyze the emergence of a more sustainable, integrated, and life-enhancing model of medicine. For more information, to become a member, or to make a contribution to Noetic Sciences, please call us toll free at (877) 769-4667 or visit www.noetic.org.

CONTENTS

CONTENTS

CONTENTS

Part Three

CONTENTS

Part Four

Part Five

ENVISIONING A NEW STORY FOR
HEALTH AND HEALING, 435
Marilyn Schlitz
Tina Amorok
Marc S. Micozzi

SECTION ONE
Transformations of Medicine

C O N T E N T S

CONTENTS

SECTION FOUR
Social Healing

DVD CONTENTS

50-Minute Documentary of Interviews with the
Following Integral Medicine Health Professionals: Mitchell
Krucoff, Larry Dossey, Marie Mulligan, John Astin,
Tom Janisse, Paul Choi, and Stanley Krippner

Nine Additional Essays:

1

The Dark Side of Consciousness and the
Therapeutic Relationship
LARRY DOSSEY

2

Returning the Soul to Medical Education
GAIL BERNICE HOLLAND

3

Creating Healing Teams, Organizations and Societies
ROBERT M. KENNY

4

Eight Motifs of Dying: An Investigation Into Dying and the
Inner Life
BETSY MacGREGOR
MICHAEL J. YEDIDIA

Text versions of these bonus DVD essays
are posted at http://www.noetic.org.

Integral Health and Healing Resources

Book and DVD Essay References

Consciousness
& *healing*

Integral Approaches to
Mind-Body Medicine

Part One

DEFINING
INTEGRAL
MEDICINE

MARILYN SCHLITZ

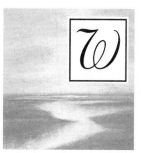

hat will health care become in the twenty-first century? Contemporary biomedicine and the systems that govern its delivery are in a period of unprecedented change. But change toward what? Among many health professionals, researchers, and patients, there is a growing conviction that we urgently need a new system that is grounded in healing, a more sophisticated model than the current one that often forcibly fits standard allopathic medicine and alternative therapies under one roof, with integration largely left to the patients rather than the practitioners.

This anthology reflects a new and evolving model—*integral medicine*. This approach is grounded in integral philosophy. The central tenet of integral philosophy is that of a comprehensive view of reality. Integral medicine promotes an approach embedded in the scientific dimension that epitomizes the best in modern health care, while equally recognizing that human beings possess emotional, spiritual, and relational dimensions that are essential in the diagnosis and treatment of disease and the cultivation of wellness.

DEFINING INTEGRAL MEDICINE

We seek to define this new field in this section and throughout this book. We hear first from internal medicine practitioner Elliott Dacher, who positions integral medicine within the broader arena of the post-modern worldview. Here we see that transformation of self and society is at the core of the integral model. Dacher identifies an expansion in consciousness as the foundation of a postmodern integral medicine. As the key component, consciousness shifts our healing efforts and results from a change that expands the range and scope of what is possible, to a change that actually transforms the entire landscape. As Dacher notes, this viewpoint embraces "all previous perspectives and approaches to health and healing while simultaneously transcending them in the creation of a fundamentally new vision." Through the full development of consciousness we will rediscover the inner aspects of healing—wholeness, peace, love, joy, and wisdom, and once embraced, Dacher writes that we can weave the inner with the outer aspects of healing practice, and create a new medicine.

An important function of this book is the building of a bridge from our currently evolving paradigm, integrative medicine, to yet another, integral medicine. William Benda, a specialist in family medicine, notes that the union of conventional and alternative medical theory and practice surfaced in the late twentieth century as the field of integrative medicine. Integral medicine represents the next step in health care, as it seems to incorporate all dimensions of healing, from physical to spiritual, and ecological to cosmological. Benda writes, "As such, it is more a template for the evolution of medical philosophy than a therapeutic approach. This evolution is not only necessary but inevitable and fundamental to solving the conundrum that is our current healthcare system."

Drawing on the rich psychosocial literature, health psychologists John and Alexander Astin note that there is something lacking in a model of health that neglects the role of inner experience. This is true of both the patient and the healer. According to the father-and-son team, we have also failed to fully recognize the value of collective experiences as they shape our health and well-being. The authors suggest that the fragmentation in medicine is due to the lack of a conceptual framework that draws together the scope of biopsychosociocultural variables. Drawing on philosopher Ken Wilber's writings, they argue that an integral approach will help to clarify otherwise vague concepts such as "holistic" and "integrative."

The new integral model of medicine that is emerging acknowledges human potentials for healing and self-awareness that link it with the larger story of our time. As such, this approach takes "mind-body medicine" to the next level, one that integrates spiritual dimensions fully into our understanding of how the body works in health and illness. Integral medicine reconciles the long-standing split between noetic (interior) aspects of experience and the physical and objective aspects that characterize science-based medicine. In so doing, it places medicine at the leading edge of a transformation emerging in multiple dimensions of human experience, an ontological shift illustrated through the specific research information, clinical experience, and personal understandings that are offered here.

Towards a Post-Modern Integral Medicine

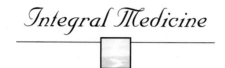

ELLIOTT S. DACHER

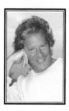

THERE IS GREAT FERVOR IN the health field. New ideas, innovative programs, and hope are everywhere, and today's rapid changes seem to have a momentum of their own. States are providing licensure to new categories of health practitioners; medical schools are offering programs on holistic healing; the National Center for Complementary and Alternative Medicine at the National Institutes of Health (NIH) is funding research on complementary therapies; insurance carriers are beginning to offer reimbursement for these therapies; and the Internet is overflowing with information and informal dialogues.

Confronted with the complexities of lifestyle- and stress-related degenerative diseases; addictive disorders, anxiety, depression, and their physical counterparts; dissatisfaction with the overuse of pharmacological and interventionist therapies; and a rising antipathy with professional arrogance and authority along with a growing demand for high-level health, conventional medicine has finally reached its limitations. There is now a broad-based consensus that change is both necessary and desirable. But the current pace of change has allowed both practitioners and the general public little opportunity for reflection and evaluation. As a result, there has been a lack of significant discourse in regard to the extent and the direction of change. Motivated by very real concerns yet conditioned by old patterns of thought, fired up with enthusiasm and hope yet compelled by complex professional and financial interests, and carried along by a seemingly unstoppable momentum, we simply assume that our current initiatives are taking us in a beneficial and innovative direction. As a result, we have failed to ask the critical questions whose answers can either reassure us about our current efforts or cause us to reconsider them. Consider these two simple but basic questions:

- What will be the distinguishing elements that will characterize an expanded and revitalized approach to health and healing—a postmodern integral medicine?
- Do our current initiatives reflect and support the full development of these essential elements?

PAST AND FUTURE GATHERED TOGETHER

The first question, one that deals with the essential characteristics of a newly emerging worldview, must be considered in the context of our unique historical moment. Today we find ourselves living in an extraordinary in-between time, a sort of gap in time that has been created by the decline of our previously unquestioned optimism and faith in the 500-year tenure of modernism and the emergence of a new postmodern integral viewpoint. As practitioners and individuals in search of a more meaningful approach to health and healing, we rarely concern ourselves with these larger cultural movements, issues we usually leave to historians, social scientists, and philosophers. Yet at times of great transformation we cannot afford to do so. Only to the extent that we can accurately understand the historical forces that are driving and shaping our times can we effectively embrace and align ourselves with these forces rather than unknowingly undermine them with potentially misguided efforts.

Westerners' cultural history can largely be traced to Hellenistic Greece. This meeting of the ancient mythological world and the emerging world of rational inquiry gave rise to an extraordinary culture that for a brief period of time sustained a precarious yet highly creative balance between sensory-based and intuitive knowledge—the outer and inner ways of knowing. The outer way investigates the world and attains its knowledge through the sensory-based intellectual analysis of what is considered an "objective" pre-given world. In contrast, the inner way uses the first-person investigative tools of reflection and meditation to uncover an experiential knowledge of the "lived world," the subjective experience. One of the most important achievements of Hellenistic Greece was the rise of Aesclepian medicine, an amalgam of the rudimentary elements of a scientific medicine interwoven with knowledge of the inner healing capacities—a prototype for the reunion of the matured inner and outer aspects of healing that is the essential movement that is unfolding in our time.

Several centuries later this union of rational and intuitive knowledge was sundered apart with the rise of the monotheistic Christian mythos. Faith, scripture, and external authority replaced rational inquiry and inner exploration as the primary route to knowledge, healing, and health. But the rise of a monochromatic perspective in either personal psychology or cultural history always empowers its suppressed counter-balancing force that invariably re-emerges from the shadow, forcing the decline of the previously dominant perspective. It is in this manner that the dominance of the Christian era and its emphasis on external authority eventually declined, giving way to the Copernican revolution and the modern era with its rational analytic exploration of the outer world, an extraordinary epoch which was to last for 500 years and is only now beginning its decline as a dominant perspective.

Initiated by Copernicus and completed by Kepler, Galileo, and Descartes, this paradigm shift engaged the western world in a compensatory yet equally monotheistic worldview, one that was sensory-based and "objective." It assumed that humans are parachuted into a pre-given world whose intricacies could be accurately known through our natural senses and our extended senses—our sophisticated technology. This powerfully pragmatic worldview has been highly successful in elucidating the mechanistic aspects of nature, but it has left us with a disenchanted and devitalized world, one that is devoid of meaning and purpose.

We have denied and devalued all inner ways of knowing, leaving ourselves with no way to grasp or understand the groundless and mechanical world we have so brilliantly envisioned with our science. The result is the epidemic anxiety of our age—a lostness, an emptiness, an alienation from ourselves and our world that is reflected in our mind, body, spirit, and social institutions. It has become increasingly apparent than an understanding of life acquired solely through a sensory-based outer knowledge cannot in itself provide us with a progressive and endless improvement in the quality of our health and our lives. For this we need something else. We need to expand our consciousness and regain a rich inner life. This leap in consciousness will provide us with the knowledge and capacities that are required for a larger healing and health. To understand this is to comprehend that the changes we must now envision are fundamental rather than cosmetic and as much historically compelled as chosen. We either grow larger in our consciousness or our science and medicine will remain much the same, irrespective of our sincere efforts to change it through the addition of more therapies and remedies.

I would like to set forth the four elements that will characterize and distinguish a post-modern integral medicine, both serving to align us with the historical imperatives of our time and guiding us in our efforts to move beyond the limits of our current medical model.

1. AN EXPANDED CONSCIOUSNESS

An expansion in consciousness is the foundation of a post-modern integral medicine. It is the key component that shifts our efforts and results from horizontal change that merely expands the range and scope of what is to vertical change that transforms the entire landscape, embracing all previous perspectives and approaches to health and healing while simultaneously transcending them in the creation of a fundamentally new vision. Through the exploration and full development of consciousness we will at first rediscover the profound and denied inner aspects of healing—wholeness, peace, love, joy, and wisdom—and then seamlessly interweave the two traditional aspects of healing—outer and inner—into a new medicine.

2. HOLISM

The modern worldview assumes that outer reality is pre-given, objectified, impersonal, measurable, quantifiable, and ultimately knowable through our sensory perceptions. The post-modern view does not make this assumption. Objective and subjective, outer and inner, are seen as inseparable and seamless experiences, with each shaping the other in an ongoing circularity of movement. This interconnectedness of outer and inner is a middle way that denies the extremes of a purely sensory-based objective world and its antithesis, a radical subjectivism. Holism asserts the ultimate oneness of experience, viewing the objective and subjective as two aspects of the same reality. To reach this understanding and to know it directly heals our alienation from self, others, and the illusion of a pre-given world.

3. INTENTIONALITY

The modern worldview postulates that all phenomena are caused by unchanging universal laws that exist independently of human consciousness. In essence, causality is seen as physically based and upward in its direction. The post-modern perspective validates and legitimizes the causal nature of consciousness that is individually willed and downward in direction. In validating both downward and upward causation we affirm and expand our understanding of the mind-body unity and simultaneously affirm and expand our capacity for self-regulation. Here causality, "upward and downward," is seen as a seamless interconnectedness of experience that lays the foundation for an integral medicine that reflects the complex and dynamic flow of forces, biological and intentional, that define the human experience and open the possibility of a larger life and health.

4. A LARGER SELF

The modern worldview has assigned great importance to individualism, an ideal that has too often been degraded into a self-indulgent, egoistic, and aggressive quest for power and material gain. The post-modern worldview revitalizes and deepens the meaning of individualism by asserting the significance of the individual's search for authenticity through self-knowledge and a deepening consciousness while simultaneously affirming the larger goal of self-development: the transcendence of the self-grasping sense of "I" and the discovery of a deeper and more authentic ground of being that knows and lives our interconnectedness with all of life. It is this deeper, more expansive, and impersonal self that is the only agent that can fully comprehend and integrate the inner and outer forces of healing into a seamless embodied whole. The formula for a post-modern integral medicine is as follows: larger consciousness, larger self, larger medicine.

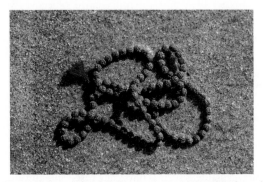

A, "Rudraksha on Beach." (Courtesy David "Dudi" Shmueli.)

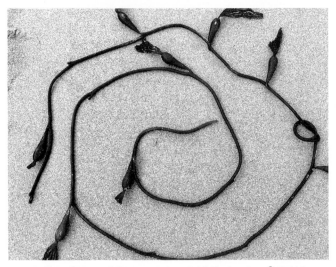

B, "Spiral Dance." (Courtesy Convivial Design, Inc. © 2004.)

A SHIFT IN WORLDVIEW OR MORE OF THE SAME

With these new perspectives in mind, let's consider our second question: Are our current efforts expressing and supporting these perspectives, these four viewpoints that characterize fundamental change? Consider the following recent attempts to expand our ideas about health and healing.

- John Travis, M.D., opened the first wellness center in the late 1970s in Mill Valley, California. Influenced by Halbert Dunn's book *High Level Wellness*, Travis' concept of wellness sought to expand our ideas about health beyond the customary focus on preventing and curing disease to include a concern for the promotion of well-being. Health and healing were seen as a personal affair, a psychosocial process of education and lifestyle change.

- The idea of holism, first described by Jan Smuts in his 1920s book *Holism and Evolution*, was revived in the 1980s by individuals and practitioners seeking a broader vision of health and healing. As a concept, holism expressed the view that life at all levels is organized as a unity. Although reductionism had been successful in explaining the mechanistic workings of nature, it was increasingly seen as a limited and partial approach to knowledge, an approach that distracted us from a more comprehensive and ecological view of the human condition that offered a more meaningful, vital, and enchanted view of nature.

- In the 1980s alternative and complementary practices and mind-body strategies for self-regulation began to emerge as a further expression of the rapid changes in our ideas about health care. Naturopaths, chiropractors, acupuncturists, and others sought and achieved state licensure and began the initial steps towards full integration into the mainstream of institutionalized health care, a process aimed at achieving conventional acceptability and consensual validation. The Office of Alternative Medicine (later the National Center for Complementary and Alternative Medicine) was established at the NIH to examine the efficacy and appropriateness of these diverse approaches to health and healing.

Each of these initiatives were honest attempts by sincere individuals and institutions to bring change to an entrenched health care system, one that no longer seemed effective in dealing with present-day problems and sensibilities and was at odds with the emerging post-modern viewpoint. Let's examine the results of each of these efforts.

The idea of wellness was rapidly integrated into our culture. But as it entered the mainstream of our cultural life, and particularly when it was integrated into existing health care institutions, wellness was reduced to four physically based issues: nutrition, smoking cessation, fitness, and stress management. Its fundamental emphasis on personal development and its psychosocial framework and values were largely jettisoned. And with its assimilation into the larger culture it was reshaped until it more resembled traditional preventive approaches, packaged as generic commodities carrying the "wellness" label, than the dramatic shift in perspective envisioned by Travis.

The idea of holism suffered a similar fate. As a philosophy, holism evolved as a counterforce to atomistic and reductionistic perspectives. Sixty years after Smuts defined this concept, his vision was reduced to packaged commodities that could be bought and sold with labels such as "holistic medicine," "holistic dentistry," and so on. And further, it became a marketable credential that was self-applied by a diverse group of practitioners who confused humanism and an expanded repertoire of remedies and practices with holism. And even in the case of those practices that evolved from a more comprehensive framework, the "holistic" components rapidly receded in importance or were completely discarded as they were secularized and reduced to disease-oriented treatments. As we are discovering, this is the cost of integrating into and accommodating to the institutional structures of mainstream health care whose perspectives are solidly embedded in the traditions of the modern worldview. It is the price of cultural acceptability and third-party reimbursement.

Alternative and complementary approaches to health and healing, however valuable in diversifying our treatment options, have similarly failed to significantly alter our existing worldview. Conventional and alternative practitioners too often use their specific expertise to prescribe techniques, practices, drugs, or supplements for the purpose of repairing or fixing an abnormality. The professional defines the approach solely within the context of his or her professional domain, and the prescribed treatment is external rather than internal. The individual is a more or less passive recipient of the therapeutic process, gaining little in the way of personal insight or additional self-healing capacities. Because all of us are conditioned to turn to authoritarian structures and external remedies at times of adversity, we often demand and easily accommodate to the treatment model, conventional or alternative. There are always individual practitioners whose practices reflect a substantial shift in perspective (both conventional and alternative healers can access holistic principles within their traditions), but this remains an individual prerogative in distinction to a cultural shift.

The answer to our second question is now apparent. With few exceptions these and similar efforts have ultimately failed in their implementation to explicitly and consistently express the perspectives that characterize a post-modern integral medicine, perspectives that alone can take us in the direction of fundamental change. So why has this happened? The answer is clear. Old perspectives and parochial interests are powerful and enduring. They silently and effectively reshape our efforts to more or less conform to existing conventions, incorporating and reshaping them until they accommodate to the assumptions of the existing worldview. Without a defining leap in consciousness all we do is expand the range and scope of what is, deluding ourselves in thinking we are creating fundamental change.

Because each of these initiatives explored new approaches and perspectives, they have been useful endeavors. But so far they have failed at fundamental change. As a result, these initiatives have largely fallen within the hegemony of the existing values, perspectives, and practices, falling far short of taking us in the direction of a post-modern integral medicine. Wellness became prevention, holism became an empty word, alternative approaches became alternative treatments, and mind-body strategies became relaxation techniques. The powerful influence of the existing worldview subtly but surely changes us before we can change it, and our efforts fall short of embodying the perspectives of the emerging post-modern viewpoint. Overcoming ourselves and our deeply conditioned and often unconscious assumptions is a difficult task.

A POST-MODERN INTEGRAL MEDICINE

So how do we assure fundamental change? How do we align ourselves with the future? First, we must clearly articulate the perspectives that we choose to assert, then carefully design and embed them into innovative programs, and finally measure the success of these programs by their demonstrated capacity to foster these perspectives. To accomplish this goal these perspectives must gain priority over our conditioned thoughts and actions and our parochial professional interests. The changes that will result from such an effort will not be an accumulation of new ideas and practices that are subtly but assuredly reshaped to resemble the past, but rather a fundamental revision of our approach to health and healing.

The central components of a post-modern integral medicine—an expanded consciousness, holism, intentionality, and a larger self—arise dependent upon the first factor, a leap in consciousness that takes us beyond the limitations of the rational analytic mind. This is at first a personal quest. So it is the individual (in contrast to professionals and institutions) that becomes the agent of change that will take us towards a post-modern integral medicine. Directly engaged in the historical process of actively integrating and living a new worldview, we ourselves are transformed by our quest for a larger consciousness, life, and health.

It follows from this that initiatives that result in an expansion and extension of professionalism and their monopoly over knowledge, conventional or alternative, expropriate power and possibility from the individual and run counter to the values of a post-modern medicine. Practitioners and their therapies will remain an important component of a person-centered and consciousness-centered post-modern integral medicine, but not a dominant one. They will be a valuable resource to individuals who are actively engaged in composing their lives, defining their personal visions of health, and using life's adversities as a doorway to a larger consciousness and expanded inner healing capacities.

Because we are still living in the gap between worldviews, we can only catch glimpses of what the full flowering of what this new medicine will look like. Yet there is much to gain from these glimpses. Let's consider two programs: the Dean Ornish Lifestyle Intervention Program and the Planetree Hospital Unit and Consumer Education Program. In examining each of these programs we can measure them against the perspectives that will characterize a post-modern medicine.

In 1977 Dr. Dean Ornish began to explore an alternative, non-pharmacological approach to atherosclerotic heart disease. The central elements of his program included a low-fat diet, meditation, yoga, exercise, and psychological counseling and support. When I visited this program I had an opportunity to join an evening meeting and to speak in some detail with several of the participants. What most impressed me was the extent to which these individuals had become empowered in the pursuit of their own healing. They had developed a repertoire of new skills, resources, and capacities; gained insight into their lives and relationships; cultivated a more expansive understanding of health and disease; learned to make conscious and self-directed choices; and accomplished each of these goals within the context of a supportive community. As a result of these experiences, the participants extended the scope of their personal autonomy, expanded consciousness and self-knowledge, and created new options. Each of these valued outcomes was built into the ongoing program. By transforming their approach to health and healing, they had simultaneously transformed themselves.

The goal of Ornish's program, as I view it, is to support the personal growth and development of the participants so they can assert their primary role in the healing process, recovering from illness and promoting vital and healthy lives. Ultimately the professional fades into the background, and the individual and his or her experience become the central factor in health and healing. This is not a treatment program in the way we have previously conceptualized treatment. My sense is that it begins to express the elements of a new medicine.

Let's look at another example, the Planetree model. In 1977 Angelica Thieriot, an Argentinian, was hospitalized during a visit to San Francisco. Although impressed by the technology, she was appalled by her hospital care. As a result of this experience, she approached the chief of medicine at the Pacific Presbyterian Medical Center in San Francisco with the idea of creating a model program, a program that would respond to the needs of the individual by supporting personal autonomy.

In 1981 the first Planetree Health Resource Center opened. This consumer library was designed to assist individuals in acquiring up-to-date medical information that would enable them to be active and informed participants in the healing process. The center maintained a library, subject files on conventional and alternative health care, access to the National Library of Medicine's search service, selected bibliographies, and listings of national and local organizations and support groups.

In 1985 the first Planetree hospital unit was established. In each of the patient's rooms the colors, lighting, carpeting, and other details were specifically designed so that the healing needs of individuals could be met. The patients had full access to their medical records and were encouraged to add their observations, feelings, and responses to their files. The new unit provided kitchen facilities, flexible visiting hours, and a health educator. Alternative practitioners were permitted within the hospital setting, and patients had the option of wearing their own clothes, robes, and pajamas. In what is for most individuals a highly vulnerable circumstance, the Planetree program focused on enhancing personal autonomy, expanding the individual's knowledge and capacities, and allowing for a pluralistic approach to the healing process.

When I visited the Planetree hospital unit and consumer library, the difference was clear. I did not feel I was visiting a treatment facility but rather a healing center, one that was focused on the individual. Patients could leave the hospital more informed, aware, resourceful, empowered, and autonomous, a unique experience in health and healing. This project is another example of how post-modern perspectives, when designed into the core of a program, can begin to support the emergence of a fundamentally new kind of medicine.

Yet each of these programs is only a first step in the right direction. In their early phase they are more a movement away from the limitations of an exclusively reductionistic and professional-centered treatment program than a full embodiment of the perspectives of an integral medicine. The complete unfolding of an integral medicine requires much more. It requires the full development of the inner aspects of healing, which results from a leap in consciousness that is brought about through reflection, study, meditation, and other related practices.

This personal transformation is then extended into the three other realms of the human experience—our physical body, our personal relationships, and our social values and institutions. As we have already discussed, the interconnectedness of mind and body ensures that a leap in consciousness will result in a corresponding shift in our physiology towards a more a natural state that significantly alters the modern epidemic of stress related dis-ease and distress. And as we transform ourselves, we will simultaneously transform and heal our relationships through the infusion of empathic listening, kindness, patience, and a more selfless love that are the qualities that emerge from an expanded consciousness. Finally, we will discover that collective social change comes about not by pressure exerted by the smaller self but rather by the infusion into our culture of the values exemplified by the transformation of our own life. So we can see that a fully developed post-modern integral medicine, driven by a personal leap in consciousness, extends into and heals all aspects of the interconnected human experience.

It is difficult to be a midwife to a new vision. Each of us was born, socialized, and educated to live within and to honor the existing viewpoint, a set of perspectives whose basic assumptions are unstated and silent yet at the same time relentlessly compelling. The science and particularly the medicine associated with this viewpoint have taught us to seek the remedies for our problems outside of ourselves, to distrust our inherent healing capacities, and to look towards the professional as the singular authority on issues of health and healing. An understanding of our historical moment would suggest that a post-modern integral medicine will be defined and directed by the individual. Its focus will be the development of consciousness and the inner healing dimensions as a prelude to the seamless integration of the outer and inner aspects of healing.

Thomas Kuhn, in his seminal book *The Structure of Scientific Revolutions*, said: "The transition from a paradigm in crisis to a new one . . . is far from a cumulative process, one achieved by an articulation or extension of the old paradigm. Rather it is a reconstruction of the field from new fundamentals, a reconstruction that changes some of the field's most elementary theoretical generalizations . . . . When the transition is complete, the profession will have changed its view of the field, its methods, and its goals."[1] It is time that we step back and begin to speak about fundamentals, about the perspectives that define our lives and our work. Such a conversation will surely assist us in creating and successfully implementing the fundamental changes that are now awaiting us. The result will be an uncommon life and health that will emerge from a post-modern integral medicine. Its foundation will be an expansion in consciousness. Its focus will be human flourishing rather than human survival.

References for this essay are located on the DVD accompanying this book.

An Integral Approach to Medicine *

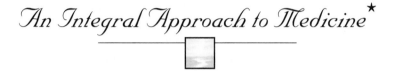

JOHN A. ASTIN
ALEXANDER W. ASTIN

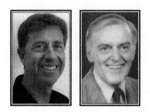

IN THIS ARTICLE WE SUGGEST that despite decades of compelling research in such fields as behavioral medicine and mind-body medicine, a more integral, less fragmented approach is still needed. We argue that one of the obstacles to realizing a more holistic-oriented medicine (i.e., biopsychosociocultural) has been the lack of a comprehensive conceptual framework. We therefore propose the application in medicine of modern-day philosopher Ken Wilber's four-quadrant model, which interfaces the dimensions of interior and exterior with those of the individual and collective. The article suggests that Wilber's framework offers a simple yet elegant heuristic tool for conceptualizing health and illness, investigating the efficacy of different treatment modalities, exploring the multifactorial

*Adapted from Astin JA, Astin AW: An Integral Approach to Medicine, *Altern Ther Health Med* 8(2):70-75, 2002.

nature of disease, and informing both research methodology and medical education. We further argue that this model has relevance for both the complementary and alternative as well as conventional medical fields, offering researchers, clinicians, and educators a way to clarify and operationalize otherwise vague concepts such as "holistic" and "integrative."

In 2000, Richard Sloan and colleagues[1] published a commentary in the *New England Journal of Medicine* in which they argued that physicians should not discuss issues of religion and spirituality with patients because they lack the requisite training to do so and because these issues are intensely private and personal and should not be the domain or province of physicians. These authors were concerned that discussions about patients' spiritual lives (and even worse, prescribing religious activities for patients) raise ethical issues of potential coercion and may ultimately serve to trivialize religion. They argued that just as physicians should not advise patients to marry simply because studies have found that marriage is associated with better health, physicians should not ask patients about their religious lives or prescribe religious activities regardless of the level of empirical evidence[2] suggesting that religious involvement is associated with improved health. They hold that, like marital status, the spiritual life of a patient is private territory into which physicians should not venture.

Although we are sympathetic with a number of the issues raised by Sloan and colleagues, we believe that their concerns point to an even larger meta-issue or question. If, as these authors suggest, certain domains of the human experience should not be the focus of physicians' clinical interest and inquiry, precisely which areas should be and how are such determinations to be made? For example, one could argue that because the emotional experiences of patients are private matters, they should not be the concern of physicians whose sole job it is to care for the physical well-being of patients. However, research[3-5] has demonstrated that in many instances psychosocial factors are of profound relevance to physical health. Therefore, as pointed out more than 20 years ago by Engel[6] in his seminal paper, there are significant limitations to a medical model that explains and treats physical health problems solely or even primarily in terms of biological or genetic factors while neglecting the role of psychological, social, and environmental factors in determining health outcomes.

Our own observations suggest that despite decades of research in fields as diverse as health psychology, behavioral medicine, and medical sociology, medicine by and large has not wholly embraced the biopsychosocial model.[7-13] We believe that concerns such as those voiced by Sloan et al reflect the continued dominance of a paradigm in medicine and science that too often fails to consider adequately or to integrate the complex dimensions of human lives.

We have reflected on ways that research and practice in our respective fields of medicine and education could become more integrative; that is, less fractured, more whole. We have found the work of a modern-day philosopher, Ken Wilber, to be extraordinarily useful. In the remainder of this article, we introduce the reader to Wilber's integral theory and discuss its practical and theoretical relevance for the field of medicine.

WILBER'S INTEGRAL THEORY

We cannot do justice either to the whole of Wilber's work or to his critics[12] in this short article. Our purpose here is to describe the foundations of his four-quadrant theoretical model, then to explore how this conceptual framework might be relevant to medicine in terms of moving the field in a more integral direction.

In a series of books compiled in an eight-volume collection,[13] Wilber has proposed a model that attempts to integrate the research findings and conceptual insights of researchers, social critics, scholars, and philosophers across an array of intellectual disciplines. Based on his extensive analysis[14-16] of these different areas of human knowledge and inquiry, Wilber suggests that all phenomena can be organized into four general domains that are formed by interfacing the two dichotomies of individual versus collective and interior versus exterior. The four quadrants (Figure 1) that comprise his integral model are as follows:

- Upper left: the interiors of individuals (thoughts, feelings, values)
- Upper right: the exteriors of individuals (atoms, molecules, behaviors)
- Lower left: the interior of the collective (shared cultural beliefs, intersubjective understanding)
- Lower right: the exterior of the collective (ecosystems, tribes, nation-states)

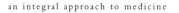

Upper Left Interior-Individual • Feelings • Meanings • Concepts • Beliefs	Upper Right Exterior-Individual • Organs • Tissues • Cells • Behavior
Lower Left Interior-Collective • Shared meanings • Cultural beliefs • Shared worldviews • Value subcultures	Lower Right Exterior-Collective • Social structures • Families, tribes • Ecosystems • Communities

Figure 1 Wilber's four-quadrant integral model.

These four dimensions rely on different modes of inquiry and require different descriptive language. The individual interior is described in the first-person singular (e.g., "I feel sad"). The collective interior is described in the first-person plural (e.g., "we understand one another"). Both the individual and collective exterior are described in the third person (e.g., "it weighs 2 pounds" or "that country has a population of 2 million").

APPLICATIONS OF WILBER'S MODEL TO MEDICINE

Wilber's four-quadrant model can serve as a simple yet elegant framework or heuristic device for addressing issues in health care. If adopted, the model may increase the chances that practitioners, educators, and researchers will consider the range of potentially relevant interior and exterior etiological factors as well as clinical outcomes.

According to Wilber, phenomena manifest to some extent in all four quadrants; in addition, the quadrants can and often are causally related, such that changes in one produce changes in the others. Therefore, just as neoplastic growth or the administration of a medication can produce changes in interior states such as moods, so can changes in interior states produce exterior changes in behavior or neurotransmitter functions. Thus, as research suggests,[17,18] the upper-left, individual–interior domain includes mental-emotional states, such as hostility or depressive mood, that also may have direct effects on disease states (Figure 3).

Upper Left Interior-Individual • Meditation, guided imagery • Expressive/supportive group therapy • Coping skills training for pain	**Upper Right** • Exterior-Individual • Radiation, chemotherapy • Dietary changes • Use of herbal medicines
Lower Left Interior-Collective • Consideration of the potential effect of cultural beliefs (e.g., causes of disease, different treatment approaches, perceived efficacy)	**Lower Right** Exterior-Collective • Financial resources available • Third-party coverage for treatments • Creation of social structures that provide emotional support

Figure 2 Four-quadrant model applied to cancer: treatment variables.

Upper Left Interior-Individual • Mood states • Beliefs, attitudes	**Upper Right** Exterior-Individual • Genetic abnormalities • Immune disregulation • Health behaviors
Lower Left Interior-Collective • Cultural beliefs regarding the value of preventive health care practices, such as dietary habits	**Lower Right** Exterior-Collective • Environmental toxins • Lack of economic resources for preventive screening and early detection

Figure 3 Four-quadrant model applied to cancer: multifactorial causes of disease.

As illustrated in Figures 2 and 3, the disease of cancer also has both interior and exterior collective aspects. In Wilber's lower-left quadrant, one finds various cultural conceptions and shared beliefs about cancer, such as "It's incurable; she will die" or "How did she cause her cancer?" or "She didn't eat the right foods" or "It runs in the family," and so on. Cultural beliefs also may causally influence cancer and other disease states as well as treatment outcomes. For example, in our society, the shared cultural belief that doctors can cure may, in and of itself, directly influence physiological function and disease states such as cancer. Similarly, the ubiquitous placebo effect demonstrates the power of cultural beliefs (as in "the medicine will cure") to influence physical processes. In other societies, shared cultural beliefs—for example, voodoo or "the evil eye"—may play some role in influencing disease states and recovery within those particular cultures. In Wilber's lower-right quadrant, the disease of cancer has very tangible and observable causes and manifestations, from the presence of environmental toxins[19] to its effects on families' social and economic functioning. The types of treatments for the disease that are afforded research funding also are influenced by powerful social-structural (lower-right quadrant) forces such as lobby groups, which wield significant power and influence in governmental funding decisions, and economic forces such as pharmaceutical companies, which may be motivated primarily by profit concerns.

Applying Wilber's Model: Specific Examples

Here we consider how Wilber's model might be used to deepen our understanding of an array of issues relevant to medicine by examining two phenomena: the placebo effect and doctor-patient communication.

THE PLACEBO EFFECT. The four quadrants can provide an elegant framework for understanding the complexity of and possible explanatory mechanisms for the placebo effect. For example, in a hypothetical clinical trial, subjects are administered a drug such as fluoxetine (Prozac) or an inactive substance, a placebo. The administration and taking of the pill or placebo are upper-right quadrant, exterior phenomena, as are the biochemical changes that may result, either direct pharmacological effects or effects mediated by the patient's belief or expectation. However, the subjective experience of one's own mental states (hopelessness, low motivation, sadness) and any changes or fluctuations that arise in these are upper-left quadrant, interior phenomena.

To briefly illustrate how this framework can be applied, we will examine cancer across each of the quadrants. Figure 2 addresses treatment considerations, and Figure 3 deals with causes of disease.

At the individual level, cancer has interior and exterior dimensions. In the upper-right quadrant of Figure 3, one can observe changes in immune parameters, the abnormal replication of cells, the disruption of organ function, and so on. Causes within this quadrant may involve genetic or biochemical defects that lead to a breakdown in immune function. These exteriors have what Wilber calls "simple location," meaning they can be observed empirically through the senses or extensions, such as microscopes or ultrasound devices.

However, the disease also has interior dimensions that historically have been underemphasized in medicine.

In Wilber's upper-left quadrant (see Figure 3), a diagnosis of cancer is experienced subjectively with such states as pain, fear, anxiety, dread, depression, despair, terror, uncertainty, and hope. And whereas these internal reactions may register in some way externally by changes in blood chemistry in the brain or alterations in behavior, they cannot be reduced to mere exteriors. In other words, individuals do not experience despair and terror as changes in neurotransmitters, but as powerful internal, subjective, upper-left quadrant states. When patients or friends with cancer speak of their despair, terror, or hope, we understand what they mean intersubjectively, through the medium of language. Although the words and tears may be viewed as movements of air across the ear canal (i.e., they may be described in "it" language), their meaning is understood at an entirely different level—one that also must be described in "I" or "we" language, precisely because such internal states do not have simple location. To illustrate, one cannot weigh the meaning of a person's words with the same empirical tools with which one measures the weight of his or her body.

Taking an active medication or placebo, however, also occurs within social (lower-right) and cultural (lower-left) contexts, which are potentially important sources of the individual (upper-left) beliefs that ultimately may produce placebo effects; that is, different cultural contexts may well determine which activities (e.g., taking a pill, having a shaman offer prayers) ultimately produce expectations of healing.

In addition, these lower quadrants may play other important roles in contributing to the placebo response. For example, an individual may develop certain expectations (upper-left quadrant) about the likely effects of the drug through conversations with others who have used it. Once the person has begun taking the medication (or participating in a drug trial in which he receives a placebo), he may talk with friends and family about his activities, why he is participating in a clinical trial, and how he feels it affects him. Such conversations, which involve communication and interpretation of shared meanings (lower-left quadrant), may in their own right serve a healing function.

While discussing the taking of a medication or placebo, the person ends up speaking about his interior mental-emotional state—depression, for example. He then receives verbal and nonverbal input, reinforcement, and guidance from others that alters mood, provides insight, and changes consciousness. In other words, the upper-right quadrant activity of taking a pill also occurs in the context of the other three quadrants in a series of complex, reciprocal interactions, all of which may ultimately lead to a biochemical (upper-right quadrant) or emotional (lower-left quadrant) therapeutic response, irrespective of whether the person is taking an active or inactive substance.

THE DOCTOR-PATIENT RELATIONSHIP. A careful examination of the dynamics of the doctor-patient relationship, with its potential difficulties and challenges, is critical to improving current clinical practice and educating future practitioners more effectively. In the upper-right quadrant, one might observe the number of minutes consumed by the clinical encounter, the amount of time physicians spend examining or talking and instructing versus listening to patients, and so on. In the upper-left quadrant, one finds the patient's subjective perceptions of the encounter, such as satisfaction or frustration; internal feelings, such as worry or anxiety about symptoms; and personal beliefs about the doctor, perhaps as an absolute authority figure. In this quadrant one also finds the practitioner's internal feelings about, perceptions of, and beliefs about the encounter (e.g., feelings of interest or boredom, irritation, empathy, preoccupation with personal problems), all of which significantly can affect the manner in which the physician behaves and communicates in the relationship and the way in which the patient responds (upper-right quadrant).

In the lower-left quadrant, both the patient and physician are also embedded in various cultural contexts that are likely to influence their relationship. For example, depending on the patient's cultural background, she may tend to either believe or question the power and authority of the doctor and, as already noted, these beliefs would very likely influence behaviors such as compliance, as well as the extent to which the patient relates more or less assertively and proactively with her doctor. Physicians are also influenced by cultural factors, including the social culture of biomedicine and medical training, that significantly can affect the manner in which they relate to patients. In the lower-right quadrant, one sees the potential effect of the setting (hospital, private office, home); various social structures, such as managed care; and economic demands and incentives that influence both the time spent with patients (upper-right quadrant) and the internal (upper-left quadrant) experiences of physicians (e.g., anger, powerlessness, frustration) that further affect the quality of their relationships with patients.

In short, when one considers the myriad aspects of the doctor-patient relationship suggested by the four-quadrant model, it becomes clear that each aspect has the potential to affect the quality of information elicited by the clinical encounter and, hence, the validity of the diagnosis, the treatment, and ultimately the course of the illness.

In these two examples, we have suggested that Wilber's four-quadrant model can further our understanding of different phenomena in medicine, because it provides a comprehensive framework for applying an integrative, interdisciplinary, multimethods approach. Applying this model thus encourages clinicians, researchers, and educators to pose a number of key questions:

- Are we looking at all four quadrants?
- How thoroughly have we incorporated the full range of potentially important variables within each quadrant?
- Are we considering the reciprocal influence of factors across quadrants?

Although it may not always be practical or feasible to examine all of the quadrants thoroughly in any given clinical situation or research endeavor, using Wilber's model encourages researchers, clinicians, and educators alike to be aware, at least, of those quadrants that are not being directly investigated (e.g., lower-left cultural factors, upper-left interior psychological states). To give but one example, whereas Sloan et al[1,20] may be partly correct that physicians should not attempt to tackle issues (such as spiritual or religious concerns) for which they are inadequately trained, Wilber's model suggests that practitioners at least should be cognizant of domains they may not be addressing and the possible implications to their patients of not doing so.

THE FOUR QUADRANTS AND THEIR RELEVANCE TO CAM

Wilber's four-quadrant model may not be exceptionally relevant to the emerging field of complementary and alternative medicine (CAM), because these ideas already are well understood and applied by many if not most CAM researchers and practitioners. Research suggests that a principal reason CAM therapies appeal to many patients is that they are perceived as intrinsically more holistic, addressing not just Wilber's upper-right quadrant (body), but also the psychosocial and spiritual dimensions represented by the other three quadrants.[21] However, these arguments notwithstanding, we believe there are a number of reasons the four quadrants may be as relevant for the CAM field as they are for conventional biomedicine.

1. Although many CAM therapies are, by nature, more likely to address nonphysical factors in human health and illness, this is not always the case. In fact, both the practice and study of CAM could easily become overly focused on the upper-right quadrant in the Wilber schema. Whereas we may find that St. John's wort, for example, has several distinct advantages over present-day pharmacological approaches to depression, this herb can be used by patients and practitioners alike as nonholistically as any drug, if they fail to consider adequately the role of psychological, spiritual, cultural, and social factors in the etiology and treatment of depression. Similarly, other prominent CAM therapies such as acupuncture and chiropractic can be exclusively studied and applied clinically in an upper-right quadrant, mechanistic, or reductionistic manner.

2. Whereas CAM therapies ultimately could be reduced to mere bodily or mechanical processes as denned by Wilber's upper-right quadrant, we also have witnessed the opposite problem of reducing

all health-related phenomena to the interior, upper-left quadrant; that is, because "consciousness creates reality," it has absolute power to influence physiology and health. Wilber's model demands that we instead consider and appreciate each of the four quadrants rather than reducing or defining any phenomenon exclusively in terms of its interior or exterior dimensions.

3. As Michael Lerner[22] has observed, despite significant contributions in recognizing the crucial importance of the upper-left quadrant, the CAM and mind-body communities have in many respects failed to consider adequately the crucial role that environmental and social factors, such as chemical toxins or poverty, also play in the genesis of many health-related problems. In fact, it could be argued that social, political, and environmental influences (lower-right quadrant) on human health similarly have been underappreciated by many conventional medical researchers and practitioners.

4. Recently, the term *integrative* has begun to replace earlier terms such as *complementary* and *alternative* when discussing the CAM field. However, what is frequently not clear is precisely what is meant by *integrative*. In other words, what is actually being integrated in integrative medicine? An implied if not explicit suggestion is that we are integrating complementary, alternative, and conventional medical approaches. However, as Weil[23] and others have pointed out, this is quite a narrow and limiting interpretation of integrative medicine.

Using the four-quadrant model as our heuristic tool, it could be argued that the most integrative health care would include those approaches, conventional or alternative, that most effectively integrate the widest and most complete array of factors that can influence human health and well-being. At the most basic level, Wilber's model suggests that what has become fragmented and therefore requires our integration—not just in medicine but in all fields (e.g., education, business, politics, law, art)—are the subjective and objective worlds, the interior and exterior dimensions of life and human experience. In many ways the quadrant model offers a simple yet elegant way to make more explicit the meaning of the term integrative, because it suggests the four broad domains—interior-psychospiritual, cultural, physical, and social-environmental—that must be addressed if any conventional or CAM therapeutic endeavor is to be considered truly integrative.

SUMMARY

In this chapter we have suggested that a more integral, less fragmented approach is still needed in medicine. We believe that one of the obstacles to embracing a more holistic (i.e., biopsychosociocultural) viewpoint has been the lack of a comprehensive conceptual framework. To fill this need we have proposed the application of modern-day philosopher Ken Wilber's four-quadrant model, which interfaces interior and exterior dimensions with the individual and collective levels. This model provides a powerful heuristic tool for conceptualizing health and illness, investigating the efficacy of different treatment modalities, exploring the multifactorial nature of disease, and informing research methodology and medical education. In short, we believe that Wilber's fourfold scheme offers researchers, clinicians, and educators a way to clarify otherwise vague concepts such as "holistic" and "integrative."

In many ways, an understanding of and grounding in Wilber's upper-right quadrant (e.g., biochemistry, physiology, genetics) was the hallmark of modern, biomedical science and practice for much of the twentieth century. And whereas this quadrant is of obvious and enormous importance and relevance in health, it is, so to speak, only one fourth of the story. As Wilber's integral theoretical work suggests, all medical conditions (as all phenomena in life) have causes and manifestations that can be seen across each of the four quadrants. To leave out or ignore any one of these dimensions or levels is to have a medicine that may, in the end, be incomplete.

ACKNOWLEDGMENT

Research for this article was supported by National Institutes of Health grant 5-P50-AT0084-03.

References for this essay are located on the DVD accompanying this book.

From Integrative to Integral Medicine: A Leap of Faith

WILLIAM BENDA

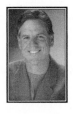

WHAT WILL MEDICINE become in the twenty-first century? This was the question put to each author contributing to this anthology, and in the following chapters you will encounter a collective vision of how mind, body, spirit, birth, death, relationships, cultures, politics, and ecologies influence our health and will hopefully influence health care in America.

In this chapter, I address the question of how one might build a bridge from our currently evolving paradigm, integrative medicine, to yet another, integral medicine, which is the focus of this anthology. Integrative medicine surfaced in the late twentieth century as a union of conventional and alternative medical theory and practice, just as conventional and alternative medicine arose from the fields of pharmacology, homeopathy, surgery, naturopathy, and countless other established disciplines.[1] Integral medicine proposes to be the next step in health care, one that incorporates all dimensions of healing, from physical to spiritual, and ecological to cosmological. As such, it is more a template for the evolution of medical philosophy than a therapeutic approach. This evolution is not only necessary but inevitable and fundamental to solving the conundrum that is our current health care system.

THE STATE OF THE NON-UNION—A HISTORICAL PERSPECTIVE

Although the argument of a holistic versus a reductionistic approach to health care appears to be a recent philosophical dispute, it has indeed a long and colorful history. We know that the Hygieans (holists) and the Aesculapians (reductionists) of ancient Greece passionately debated this issue centuries ago, and consensus has not been reached even over the intervening centuries. Nineteenth-century America in fact claimed no established medical orthodoxy—various and sundry practitioners applied their trade without the need for licensure or bureaucratic oversight.

By the end of the nineteenth and the beginning of the twentieth centuries, new technologies began to deliver the kind of scientific evidence that would give those adhering to reductionistic beliefs clinical, political, and economic authority; the initial code of the American Medical Association (AMA) excluded all "irregular" practitioners from membership. Continued advances in diagnostics and therapeutics, along with new vaccines and antibiotics to defeat infectious disease, drove additional nails into the coffins of nonallopathic professions, and those choosing not to become part of the system were subsequently forced underground. The now orthodox views of allopathic medicine directed health care policy through much of the twentieth century.[2]

Orthodoxy, whether religious, political, or medical, inevitably inspires revolution. Resistance to the allopathic mandate appeared by the end of World War II, taking firm root during the 1960s decade of dissent. Critics charged that medical institutionalism had placed its own welfare above that of the society it served by ignoring the obligation of self-regulation. The status quo response from the AMA on down was at first defensive, but to no avail. Unregulated fee for service, reimbursement through managed care, and costly defensive medicine had created a perfect storm in health care, and the old structures began to crumble.[3] A second and perhaps final blow arrived when public demand for "alternative" therapies accelerated erosion of orthodox medicine's primary political constituency, the patient. The national debate focusing on repair of the system became moot; the need for a complete re-evaluation of priorities and redesign of delivery became apparent.

Enter integrative medicine, and conventional and alternative practitioners began to negotiate a truce under this new flag. After extensive, passionate, and imaginative negotiations, integrative medicine proposed to define itself according to the following principles.

Integrative medicine:

1. Employs therapies drawn from all modalities, conventional or alternative, providing patients with individualized treatment plans optimized for their specific clinical situations
2. Recognizes and relies upon the innate healing capacity of the human body as primary to recovery of health
3. Emphasizes the importance of the relationship between practitioner and patient
4. Shares rather than dictates medical decisions; patients are informed of all possible options and given autonomy over their own health care choices.

There were, of course, shortfalls in the implementation of this new paradigm. The appearance of a multitude of therapeutic choices lacked coherence of delivery; informed consent did not imply informed choice. Centuries-old modalities did not lend themselves to scientific study, nor did many of their practitioners wish such validation, with its implied loss of self-regulation. There was no standardization of training in integrative medicine; indeed there were less than a handful of medical institutions willing to take the political heat of such an endeavor. Finally, and perhaps most importantly, the deepest philosophical tenets of the new field, such as attention to spirituality and physician self-inquiry, soon fell by the wayside or were never instituted in the first place.

Such growing pains soon caught the nation's attention. Although many welcomed this movement towards a more holistic approach, conflicts arose between ideologues on both sides. Voters and their money entered the fray, and politicians took note; the president created the White House Committee on Complementary and Alternative Medicine, Congress passed the Dietary Supplement Health and Education Act, and the National Institutes of Health established the National Center for Complementary and Alternative Medicine, bringing research funding for unconventional therapies under conventional medicine's sphere of influence.

Academia became partisan. Traditional medical journals published reports of adverse effects from botanical medicines while rejecting studies demonstrating positive clinical outcomes. Alternative medical journals cried foul, pointing to the pharmaceutical industry's influence on editorial decision-making. Twenty-two allopathic medical schools formed the Consortium of Academic Health Centers for Integrative Medicine, revamping medical school curricula to include unconventional therapeutic approaches. Chiropractic, acupuncture, and naturopathic training institutions sought increased legislative clout and state licensure. Meanwhile, traditional physicians feared losing patients to alternative practitioners. Alternative practitioners feared being co-opted by the orthodox system. Although the integration of alternative and conventional medicine was a step in the right direction, it has not yet given us the necessary redesign of our systems of health and healing, and this has proved disappointing to those who pioneered the movement.

Yet, creating a bridge from integrative to a more elegant and inspired health care paradigm does not require tearing down the present model and beginning anew. Fortunately, every possible combination of conventional and alternative and legislative and reimbursement tactics imaginable is currently being addressed by the proponents of integrative medicine, and one must be grateful for their dedicated and sustained efforts. Perhaps essential pieces of the bridge between the two medicines can be found in the following anthology of deep-rooted ideas and new constructs. Perhaps all this new field of endeavor needs to flourish is a catalyst, an energy source: the experience of noetic relationship—inner, subjective relationship—with one's self, with one another, and with one's environment.

ENTER INTEGRAL MEDICINE

I believe that all new paradigms follow a course of initiation, growth, plateau, and decline, followed by the next initiatory phase. Because the underlying impulse is evolutionary, such repetitive cycles do not close back upon themselves, but move upwards as a spiral—an endless reincarnation in the direction of theoretical perfection. The paradigm shift from integrative to integral medicine requires such an evolution, from the simplistic model of "body, mind, and spirit" into the more inclusive social, political, economic, metaphysical, ecological, and cosmological dimensions of health care. At the same time, the secret dimensions of self and other require equal status with the physical and objective foundations of science.

THROUGH THE LOOKING GLASS

Inner work is by definition intensely personal and, for the true healer, requires commitment across a lifetime. The ultimate goal is love and acceptance of the self, which leads to the ability to love and accept others. "Love thy neighbor as thyself" becomes not a simplistic platitude, but a prescription in the highest sense. Perhaps one might instead say, "Love thyself first in order to be able to love thy neighbor," for without an intact self there can be no true healing of another. When the intent to heal another comes from our place of inner knowing, we instinctively and automatically know what to do.

Bridging the gap from integrative to integral medicine through a commitment to personal work would only span half the chasm. While the mystic may focus primarily on inner work, the healer cannot ignore the social responsibilities inherent in his or her profession. We are both healers and professionals, and our failures are often more in the latter area than the former.[4]

As a physician, I must contend with complicated and obtrusive political, legal, and market forces—that is the price to pay for living within a social structure. However, even the greatest of healers is ineffective without the trust of the patient, and trust, in turn, is a direct reflection of the integrity of the healer. In order to contend with all of the forces that bear on me in today's world, I seek ethical simplicity in my practice, and I do so through adherence to three principles: primacy of patient welfare, assurance of patient autonomy, and attention to social equality.[5] It matters not should my desire for financial gain, position, or power lie one nanometer below what is best for those under my care—if the patient's welfare is the first priority when difficult decisions confront me, I will maintain the patient's trust. If I realize and accept that the patient is the ultimate master of his or her body, mind, and soul and am willing to relinquish control, the outcome is a sense of empowerment worthy of the word. Finally, if I apply the dictum of equality and social justice, regardless of color, gender, or social status, I fulfill the oath I took when I crossed the line from practitioner to healer.

There is great cause for optimism at this particular moment in our medical and social evolution. After years of eroded confidence, the public is once again seeking a trusting relationship, once again asking their health care professionals to take charge of the delivery of service and creation of policy.[6] The professional also desires to regain the authority and power that was foolishly abdicated to those with different priorities and opposing principles. For the first time in decades, the public and the healing professions are in agreement; should such synergy continue to grow and develop, no corporate or legislative institution will withstand its mandate. Patient and professional alike are returning, literally and figuratively, to a time when the physician sits at the bedside to hold the patient's hand, and the patient looks back with trust and faith.

BACK TO THE FUTURE

I have been asked to postulate a bridge spanning the paradigms of integrative and integral medicine and admit to a sense of futility inherent in such a humbling task. How can one possibly define what has not yet come to be? Yet the groundwork has already been laid for us, as each previous paradigm struggles to become the foundation for the next. Integrative medicine, still in its infancy, is being asked to mature more rapidly than any archetype before it; perhaps this is simply a reflection of these times of incredible change and evolution.

And yet build we must. I see great promise and longevity in the foundational tenets of all healing modalities, be they conventional or alternative or integrative. Integral medicine needs simply to resurrect what have been fundamental directives of all who have chosen to care for their fellow human—the search for inner truth and devotion to social justice. Physician heal thyself. And then love thy neighbor.

It has become clear that we healing professionals will never create a new paradigm alone. Integral medicine cannot exist without its integrative forebears, just as integrative medicine cannot exist without both conventional and alternative therapies to draw from, which, in turn, supply the context for each other's very existence. We are all part of a health care hologram—shine a light through one of us, and you will see an image of the whole.

In the end it really doesn't matter what name we give to this new paradigm. What matters is that the simple intent to discover the true meaning of healing requires application of both inner integrity and outer social consciousness, therefore contributing to the evolution of humankind as a whole. This is the mandate of integral medicine. Fortunately, we have as our guides women and men whose efforts to create a new world are offered in this unique collection of writings.

References for this essay are located on the DVD accompanying this book.

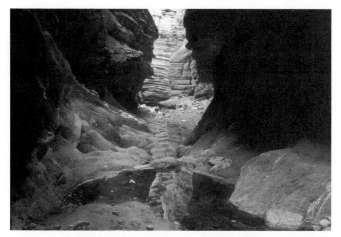

"Grand Canyon." (Courtesy Michael Eller.)

Part Two

MAPPING THE HEALING SYSTEM

MARILYN SCHLITZ
TINA AMOROK

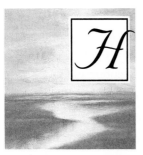 _ow do we heal?_ What inner processes direct self-repair, recovery, and the return to health when we are challenged by accident or illness? How do these processes interrelate with features of the outer world, such as cultural setting, social support, lifestyle choices, health care alternatives, and religious participation? Such questions hold deep personal meaning as well as profound scientific interest. No one is exempt from having a stake in their answers; from cut fingers to major medical catastrophes, we all experience the need for healing at one time or another in our lives.

Less than a decade ago, the notion that consciousness-related factors—including our thoughts and emotions—could play any role in bodily health and the healing of disease was both novel and unacceptable to mainstream medical thinking. Medicine focused largely on the physical aspects of healing and the growing armamentarium of techniques for treating conditions that were previously untreatable. Yet, curiously little was known about the overall process of healing, including mental and spiritual realms—in addition to its biological basis.

A deep split existed between those who studied healing and those who practiced mainstream medicine. This could be attributed to two factors. First, those who studied "healing" generally accorded primacy to the mind, whereas mainstream medicine virtually ignored any role the mind or spirit might play in affecting the course of an illness. In addition, the claims in alternative medicine tended to be somewhat overblown and were usually unaccompanied by the "gold standard" of scientific evidence: results from randomized, controlled, double-blind trials.

Today a convergence is occurring. There is a growing appreciation for the importance of mind-body-spirit as an integral whole. Unlike the nervous system, immune system, or endocrine systems, the healing system may act as a "meta-system" between the realms of mind and matter, responsive to symbolic processes as well as physical stimuli, perhaps acting in coordination with previously known systems (such as the immune or endocrine systems). While the "healing system" represents a hypothetical construct, several lines of evidence provide clues to its existence or to an understanding of its operation.

MIND-BODY MEDICINE

We consider some of these clues in this section. Harris Dienstfrey demonstrates how the mind is absent in most mind-body research following the scientific edifice of biomedicine, when in fact there is overwhelming evidence in placebo studies alone of the "mind's capacity to do in the body (some bodies) what any newly invented drug can do."

Researchers Candace B. Pert, Ph.D, Henry E. Dreher, MD, and Michael R. Ruff, Ph.D trace the emergence of neuropeptide research and the conceiving of the psychosomatic network and the biology of emotions. They review the current findings in psychoneuroimmunology and its allied fields, discussing its implications and future directions. In so doing, they raise critical questions. Can psychosocial factors influence fundamental oncogenic processes? What animates the neuropeptides in their flow patterns through the body? The authors argue that emotional expression in the healing system "may be the best available marker for a psychospiritual vitalization of the life force, however one defines such a phenomenon."

In a similar vein, the rapidly growing area of psychosocial or mind-body interventions on immune function and disease outcome in the cancer experience is overviewed by Stephanie Simonton-Atchley, Ph.D, and Allen Sherman, Ph.D. The authors discuss psychosocial risk factors and, conversely, who is most likely to benefit from mind-body interventions. In so doing, they explore psychological interventions to enhance immune function and enhance disease outcome. Simonton and Sherman stress the importance of continued research to confirm what behavioral, immune, and neuroendocrine mechanisms are involved.

NEW PERSPECTIVES ON THE BODY

In this next section, we will consider that how we view the body is an important aspect of how we formulate the healing system. As philosopher David Michael Levin points out, the body is more than an evolutionary biological entity; it is also part of a social and cultural context in which it is embedded. Therefore, we cannot separate the body of nature from the body of culture in medicine. Levin emphasizes that the interpretations and images of the human body have changed historically within the context of the history of medicine. Levin stresses the need for a more integral conceptualization and practice of medicine and for patients themselves to be freed from negativistic conceptualizations of the body—empowering themselves to imbue the body with their own meaningful experiences and awareness, as well as to honor the body's profound intelligence and transformative nature.

Philosopher Don Hanlon Johnson, a central figure in the somatics movement, emphasizes the importance and difficulty of trusting somatic subjective experiences in a culture and dominant paradigm that have infected us with distorted images, experiences, and concepts of the body. Johnson articulates why the disciplines within the field of somatics provide a more reliable basis for dealing with subjective experience, as he gives us a brief history of the somatics movement. Crucial at this point in integral medicine as well as to the field of somatics, Johnson states, is the need to develop adequate empirical methods to study the various modalities within their appropriate context.

Loren Eskenazi, a plastic surgeon in private practice, identifies the transformative nature of surgery—not only physically but also psychologically and spiritually. Eskenazi discusses the symbolic meaning of body manipulation in contemporary western culture and the longing and conditioning of those who engage in it. Her own training as a physician encouraged a mind-body split that finally gave way to a deeper understanding of the meaning of healing.

Following this, Anna Halprin, a dancer and pioneer in the expressive arts, and Michael Samuels, a physician, illuminate how mind-body science provides a bridge between the fields of expres-

sive arts and western medicine and supports the integration of both
our intuitive and rational knowledge about healing. They discuss
how an image or dance movement held in our consciousness and
responded to can alter our physiology in a second.

REVISIONING ILLNESS

A new model of medicine calls on us to examine our deepest
assumptions about healing. How do we define illness, and therefore
what is being healed? What meaning does illness hold for people,
and do these ascribed meanings influence health and illness?
Physician Larry Dossey addresses these issues in his essay "What
Does Illness Mean?" He considers the role of meaning in science
and the propensity to render nature and life itself meaningless. In
contrast, Dossey suggests that the popularity of alternative therapies
and therapists is largely due to the fact that they help people find
meaning in their lives when they need it most. Dossey writes, "No
matter how technologically effective modern medicine may be, if
it does not honor the place of meaning in illness it may lose the
allegiance of those it serves."

Caryle Hirshberg brings us up to date on the state of evidence
for spontaneous remissions from life-threatening diseases; she
demonstrates that through stories of healing, "the value of faith,
hope, and love can only be evaluated in relationship to the whole
person—body, mind, and spirit" and that they are "of immeasurable value to people faced with life-threatening disease."

Richard Miles, a pioneer in reforming medicine, explores how
our personal and collective beliefs about health and disease are
shaped by our worldviews. He chronicles this worldview as it has
changed in the last 100 years, describing the Supernatural Model,

Warrior Model, Self-Regulating Systems Model, and the now-emerging Integral Model, in which consciousness and intentionality are central organizing principles.

HONORING THE SPECTRUM OF LIFE

As we broaden our understanding of the healing system, we have included the stages of life development in our integral approach. Educator Joseph Chilton Pearce postulates that emotional deprivation and social anxiety in child-bearing and child-rearing result in compromises in neural structure and function in the unborn child. He argues that this affects personal and social relationships as well as intellectual ability, predisposing children toward anxiety and/or violence. Pearce's essay envisions a return to more emotionally nurturing practices and environments of childbirth and child-rearing.

Psychologists Ron Valle and Mary Mohs discuss how healing and wisdom emerge when we allow ourselves to consciously grieve and be open to the changes inherent in aging, as well as the array of feelings that are present throughout the aging process. Aging with awareness, they argue, involves inner work so to cultivate a "soul consciousness."

In a classic essay by cardiologist and visionary Deepak Chopra, we consider aging in the context of the superstition of materialism, in which we think of the body as something akin to a machine with consciousness as only a by-product. Based on his readings of spiritual texts and quantum physics, Chopra proposes that "we are discovering that our body is actually the objective experience of consciousness, just as our mind is the subjective experience of consciousness. But they're both inseparably one." He asserts that inherent in the experience of the timeless mind and the ageless body lies a doorway to healing.

Karen Wyatt discusses the end of life in her beautiful essay on her work as a hospice physician and the transformative nature of this practice. Understanding life to be a spiritual journey, one that is as temporal as it is precious, she critiques modern medicine's contribution to our societal denial of death and hence the possibility for transformation through embracing the nearness of death and bringing this awareness into every aspect of our lives. In the author's own words, "To truly participate in integral medicine we must open our own hearts to suffering and loss, to death in all its forms, to the perfection of this spiritual existence we have been asked to live out in physical bodies."

And finally, medical anthropologist Marilyn Schlitz examines the data concerning the possible survival of bodily death from the perspective of the world's religious and spiritual traditions, as well as from the vantage point of empirical science. Schlitz suggests that the scientific investigation of mediums, reincarnation, out-of-body experiences, and near-death experiences combine, creating a new image that sees death as a continuum rather than an end. Schlitz writes, "By reframing death, we may engage in levels of transpersonal growth that provide us with connections to the subtle, causal, and ultimate realms of reality."

$\mathcal{M}ind$ and $\mathcal{M}indlessness$ in $\mathcal{M}ind$-$\mathcal{B}ody$ $\mathcal{R}esearch$*

HARRIS DIENSTFREY

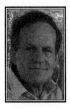

WHAT CAN THE MIND DO to treat or moderate illness and to sustain health? Anyone unfamiliar with mind-body research might assume that the field's primary interest was to explore this question. Such a presumption is clearly wrong. Most mind-body research stays a good body's length away from the mind. The research is framed and interpreted as if the mind—let's characterize it as a major decision-making process in the body—did not exist.

Consider the usual format of a mind-body study. A group of subjects are placed in (subjected to) a social situation. The situations commonly are instances of social support or stress. Sometimes the subjects are healthy, sometimes they are ill. Sometimes they have recovered from a disease and

*Adapted from Dienstfrey H: Mind and Mindlessness in Mind-Body Research, *ADV* 15: 229-233, 1999.

are at risk that the disease will reoccur. Sometimes they are injected with a virus or another illness-inducing source. Sometimes their immune systems are deliberately comprised. Whatever the particulars, the subjects matched with a comparable control group lack the particular feature the researchers want to study (no social support versus the social support of the experimental group, no compromised immune system versus the compromised immune system of the experimental group, and so on). The researchers then wait to see if there are measurable differences between the experimental and control groups in one or another health outcome.

Now, let us be clear about the import of such research—the predominant research in mind-body studies: It has achieved results that are revolutionary from the perspective of biomedicine. First of all, the research shows conclusively that nonbiological factors can have statistically significant, clinically important effects on physical health. Look at the findings on social support. Researchers of social support have repeatedly shown that social support (variously defined) is correlated with a lower risk for many health problems, including heart disease; that it diminishes the increased risks for various health problems that are otherwise associated with stress (variously defined); and that it is correlated with a lower risk for the reoccurrence of various health problems, including heart disease. These studies provide unambiguous evidence that a purely biological approach to health is deficient and that the presence or absence of a "psychosocial" factor (as it is currently called) like social support can have biological consequences robust enough to increase or diminish the likelihood of disease. This is not news that fits within the physiological reality of biomedicine.

Second of all, the predominant type of mind-body research has begun to show that biological ills, possibly even serious biological ills, can be positively affected by entirely nonbiological treatments like support groups and by techniques to manage stress and anger and to induce relaxation. For a medicine that has built its treatment approach on drugs, this is a discomforting piece of information.

Such work is continuing, and it seems clear to me that sooner or later the results will reconfigure medicine as we know it.

Note, though, to return to my starting point, that neither the mind nor anything like it is present in this work (with the regularly unnoticed exception of the learning involved in the capacity to develop the techniques that reduce stress, control anger, induce relaxation).

The absence of the mind is more gapingly clear in the analysis commonly offered to explain the results of such research. I call this analysis the pathways approach. To explain the effects of social support or stress or virtually any mind-body phenomenon, researchers posit a physiological pathway that somehow is activated by the event to which the subjects are subjected and that then, ultimately, leads to the particular health outcome that the researchers have been able to associate with the situation and condition under study. The details go like this: When this or that hormone or neurotransmitter is activated, it leads in turn to this or that physiological event, leading in turn to another event, and so on until the bridge is made to the health outcome measured in the subjects. No mind here clearly, or anything like it.

So absent is the mind that if you look carefully at such research, you can see a striking similarity with the germ theory research that established the biomedical approach to disease. While the initiating element in germ theory research is a physiological element and is a "psychosocial" factor in the predominant type of mind-body research, the format otherwise is the same: An organism is subjected to a good or bad thing (drug or germ in germ theory research, social support or stress in mind-body research), and the body responds, as it were, on its own. The body, in both cases, does what it does. The mind is not a factor. Additionally, just as germ theory posits that every disease has its individual causative element, so in the pathways approach it would seem that every health-affecting social situation— every so-called psychosocial factor—likely has its own physiological pathway. Each pathway, in any event, begins with a particular physiological activation and runs its course to a particular health outcome.

Do mind-body researchers know they are adopting a research form promoted by germ theory research? I doubt it. But I would say that, for various reasons, researchers feel comfortable with the body posited by germ theory research. It is the body that most of us have been conditioned to believe is The Body. This body for decades has been mindless. Why start fooling with a mind now if you can get along without it, as did the medical researchers who created the scientific edifice of biomedicine? The body with a mind? It is hard to imagine even what kind of body that would be.

So, with its body that feels "right" and in the absence of any model of a body with a mind, the format of germ theory research has become by default the basis for the predominant form of mind-body research.

What does it matter, one could ask? After all, I have already said that the findings of this predominant form of mind-body research is contributing to the probable reconfiguration of medicine. Why do we need to worry about the mind?

To begin with, consider the pathways that researchers posit to explain the findings of mind-body research. What starts this pathway? In germ theory, one can understand how a physical entity like a germ or a drug can initiate a physical process in the body. But how does a social situation, a psychosocial factor, initiate a physiological process in the body?

At the very least there has to be an intervening step, an acknowledgement that the social situation or psychosocial factor exists and that this existence has some meaning for the organism. There is no stress if there is no awareness in the organism, both that the stress exists and that the stress is unhappy news. For the people who, as the saying goes, thrive on stress, stress is happy news. It is a challenge. For other people, the same stress is like the impact of a 10-foot wave. It knocks them flat, leaves them gasping for air. The difference lies in an awareness within the organism. This awareness determines where stress does or does not exist and whether it is or is not a problem. I call this awareness the mind, or a property of the mind. You can call it what you like, but all of the findings of the mind-body research that have associated particular health outcomes with particular social situations exist only because an awareness within the organism recognizes and gives meaning to a situation. Awareness links body to mind and creates—the act ultimately is a choice, even if the choice is conditioned or "unconscious"— the assorted health outcomes associated with social support, stress, whatever. Without awareness, nothing can happen in mind-body research.

In part, I am making a methodological point. At the same time, I am talking about something more important, the mind and its powers. The fact is, the mind and its awarenesses and its powers make things happen in the body. We need to explore the mind not simply to understand the findings that already have been revealed by the current mainstream of mind-body research. We need to explore the mind and its powers because they are a constituent element of physical health. I know this, minimally,

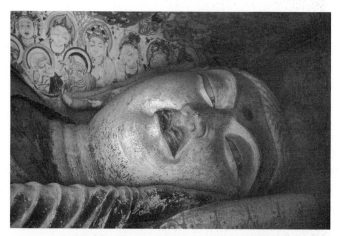

A, "Buddha Sleeping." (Courtesy Michael Eller.)

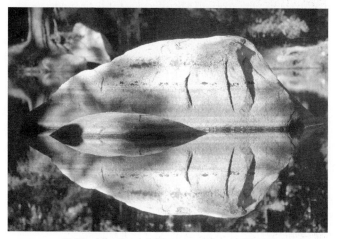

B, "Buddha Rock." (Courtesy Michael Eller.)

because the potentially revolutionary medical findings of mind-body research make no sense without the mind. More persuasively, I know it because there are two largely unattended sets of data that say so.

What are these two sources of data? As an introduction to the first set of data, I am happy to point out that whatever the main currents of mind-body research, there is at the periphery a steady trickle of studies that more or less directly explore the mind's effects on health. Three instances: In

1986, Henry Bennett,[1] studying a group of 94 surgical patients who were scheduled for spinal surgery, found that the patients who received preoperative information on how to move their blood from the site of their surgery lost 500 cubic centimeters of blood, while the patients who did not receive this information lost almost twice as much blood, 900 cubic centimeters, a statistically significant difference. In 1994, Lewis H. Mehl,[2] in a study of 100 pregnant women with fetuses in the breech position (face up rather than face down), found that when he encouraged the women under hypnotherapy to trust in their bodies and in nature and then explored with them any thoughts they had as to why their babies were in the breech position, 81 percent of the fetuses spontaneously converted, while in a matching control group of women who did not receive hypnotherapy, only 48 percent of the breech babies spontaneously converted, again a significant difference.* In 1998, Jon Kabat-Zinn and colleagues[3] found that a small group of patients who received phototherapy for their moderate to severe psoriasis while listening to tapes that initially provided guidance in mindfulness meditation and subsequently provided instructions on visualizing ultraviolet light slowing the growth and division of skin cells reached the "halfway clearing point" 50 percent sooner—again a significant difference—than did a control group who received only phototherapy.

Note that in all these studies, an organism was not whacked with a germ or a drug or subjected to a situation and then left to fend for itself. Instead, through instructions, suggestions, and encouragement, people were asked to use their internal powers to do something within their bodies, and to varying degrees, they did. All the studies provided a modest intervention—an implicit request of some sort, directed at what can reasonably be called the mind—and produced a clinically significant effect.

If one were compiling a list of the possible powers of the mind, one might tentatively conclude from these studies that the mind can move blood as an aid to surgeons, the mind can alter bodily conditions to make breech conversion more likely, the mind through meditation and visualization can quicken the results of the standard therapy for a skin disease.

---

*For a discussion of Bennett's study, see Dreher, 1998[4]; for a discussion of Mehl's study, see Dreher, 1996[5].

(One might ask: Does the mind follow the pattern of germ theory research and move along a different pathway in each instance, or is something else going on here?)

But there is considerably more that one can conclude about what the mind has the power to accomplish in the body, and it is itemized in the findings reported in a paper by Theodore X. Barber,[6] a prominent figure in the study of hypnosis and in the once-vigorous effort to study the capacity of people to affect their health through self-regulation (a term and an effort that may be undergoing a small revival). Barber's paper—called with careful precision *Changing "Unchangeable" Bodily Processes by (Hypnotic) Suggestions: A New Look at Hypnosis, Cognitions, Imagining and the Mind-Body Problem* (in this title every word and punctuation mark counts)—was published in 1984 (a slightly edited version appeared the same year in the second regular issue of *Advances*, Spring 1984), and it is, I believe, the foremost source of studies whose manifest purpose is to explore just how widely the mind can affect the health and, in one instance, a physical dimension of the body.

The paper is a sweeping collection of more than fifty studies that together illustrate both the extraordinary capacity of the mind to reach into the body and the extraordinary variety of the mind's powers. There are studies of women who increase the size of their breasts under hypnotic suggestion by seeing themselves on a beach, with the sun warming their breasts. (If women can increase the dimensions of their breasts through visualization, why could men not use visualization to shrink their swollen prostates, as a leading practitioner of treating physical ills with imagery, Gerald Epstein [1989],[7] claims is entirely possible.) There are studies of a small group of Japanese adolescents who are allergic to the Japanese equivalent of poison ivy but who, despite their allergy, mostly do not develop an allergic reaction when doctors rub their arms with poisonous leaves that the doctors declare are benign elm leaves but who do develop an allergic reaction when the doctors rub their arms with benign elm leaves that the doctors declare are poison ivy. (Anyone with a skin allergy has something to think about here.) Antedating the blood-shunting study of Bennett, there are studies of patients about to undergo dental surgery who are told under hypnotic suggestion that they can reduce the usual blood loss by moving the blood elsewhere and who, as in Bennett's study, lose less blood than the patients who do not receive the hypnotic suggestion.

To my thinking, the most powerful material in this collection, the material that simultaneously illustrates the farthest reach of the mind's powers and also perhaps a limitation of its powers, are five case histories of people with congenital ichthyosiform erythrodermis. Commonly called "fish-skin disease," this is a distressing, sometimes tormenting skin disorder, a scalelike hardening of the skin that can cover much of the body. Biological medicine does not know the cause of this disease and offers no cure. In Barber's terminology, the disease represents an "unchangeable" bodily process.

But it can be changed or, more precisely, substantially reduced by the mind. In each of Barber's five case histories, an assortment of doctors treat their patients with fish-skin disease using hypnosis, complemented in some cases by psychotherapy. Under hypnosis, patients are told things like "Focus on your arm. See your skin becoming normal." In a matter of weeks, all the patients cleared around 80 percent of their skin disorder. The cleared skin was smooth and healthy, entirely normal. The remaining 20 percent remained intractable. No additional hypnosis or psychotherapy made any difference. I like to put it this way: After the mind did what it could, it could not do more.

There seem to me at least two lessons that we might draw from these fish-skin disease cases. First, apparently the mind does not need to know the cause of fish-skin disease to act on it. Perhaps I am presuming too much. Perhaps the mind, having seen the disease develop, does know its cause and for this reason can act on it. The lesson might be better formulated this way, that we do not need to know the cause of fish-skin disease to involve the mind in its treatment. The question that follows is obvious: Can this situation be generalized to other disorders and to disorders that so far remain beyond medicine's prescriptive ken? Can we learn to use the mind as an aid in treatment whatever the state of our own collective knowledge about a particular disease?

The second lesson I see concerns the mind's possible limits. Apparently the mind does not rule sovereign over the body, at least in the instance of fish-skin disease. In none of the case histories that Barber presents—I assume he was exhaustive in his hunt for such cases—did the mind, responding to hypnotic suggestion complemented in some instances by psychotherapy, remove all of the disease. Put another way, in the mind's treatment of fish-skin disease, mind and body each reached a boundary line that neither could cross. It would seem, then, that the body has its powers too, which is comforting news for anyone who does not believe that the body is a figment of the imagination. The key question again is, How generalizable to other conditions is the existence of a balance between the powers of the mind and the powers of the body?

More broadly, given the fish-skin disease case histories, given the poison-ivy allergy studies, given the blood-flow diminution studies, given the full sweep of the findings that Barber presents in his really rather startling paper, how robust, extensive, and available are the treatment powers of the mind? This question, it seems to me, ought to have equal priority with any other question that now absorbs mind-body researchers.

Perhaps some answers can be elicited from the second source of material that I would point to as a basis for investigating the mind and its treatment powers. I refer to the well-known, presumably inexplicable phenomenon of the placebo effect, specifically as it is seen in drug studies.

To repeat what everyone knows, in the testing of every drug some percentage of the participants in the placebo-treated control group (30 percent on average) produce the same results that the drug under investigation is designed to produce. Consider what this means—that no matter what the purpose of a drug being tested, whether it treats stomach distress, arthritis, depression, allergies, hay fever, erectile dysfunction, or anything else, some percent of people get the same results from a placebo. That is, they give themselves, somehow, the same results. That is, the mind does. The long and short of the placebo phenomenon in drug studies is that the mind has an apparently limitless capacity to duplicate the results of whatever chemists concoct to relieve or resolve human ills and discomforts.

I hope this is clear. There is as yet no bottom to the well of the mind's capacity to do in the body (some bodies) what any newly invented drug can do. The problem the drug is treating does not matter. The mind is expansive enough to treat the problem. Put it this way: The mind so far can do (for some people) what all the pharmaceutical labs of the world together have been able to do.

I do not know why the bald facts of the placebo phenomenon in drug studies have not launched a thousand inquiries into the mind's treatment powers. Is the placebo phenomenon like a learned skill, which some have never learned and at which some inevitably are better than others? Or is it like the trait of hypnotizability, which is distributed through the population in the shape of a bell curve? Do the varying percentages of people who transform a placebo into the equivalent of a drug have anything to do with the mind-body boundary line that appears to exist in fish-skin disease? In terms of medical problems in general, could not the mere listing of the ills that are treated by drugs, the effects of which have all been duplicated in some percent of the placebo-treated group, provide a rough sense of the scope of the ills that the mind can help resolve?

In the movie *All the President's Men*, the two reporters trying to find out who broke into the Watergate Hotel and why are told, "Follow the money." Why is no one following the placebo?

The mind as a source of medicine is waiting to be explored. I do not pretend to know the royal road to mind-body medicine. In the case I have laid out here, all, ultimately, that I am asking, as the Beatles did not quite put it, is to give the mind a chance.

References for this essay are located on the DVD accompanying this book.

The Psychosomatic Network: Foundations of Mind-Body Medicine

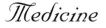

CANDACE B. PERT
HENRY E. DREHER
MICHAEL R. RUFF

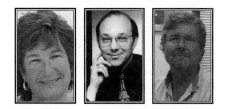

F̲OR NEARLY THREE DECADES, the mind-body field has gradually moved beyond the notion of segmented biological systems, even beyond the notion of interconnected systems. The provable connections between the mind-brain, nervous, endocrine, gastrointestinal, cardiovascular, reproductive, and immune systems inform but no longer accurately reflect the emergent understanding of the human organism. In the form of neuropeptides and their corresponding cellular receptors, our biological systems (the body) are literally flooded by our cognitions and emotions (the mind). Furthermore, our mind is created anew on a moment-to-moment basis by the interplay of ligands and receptors previously associated with only the "body." In illuminating the nature of mind (i.e., subjective experience, consciousness, feeling), the noetic sciences have contributed to a richer, more expansive, and more humanistic mind-body science. *Noetic* is derived from the Greek word *nous*, which may be translated as mind or direct ways of knowing. Noetic sciences seek to further the explorations of conventional science through rigorous inquiry into aspects of reality— mind, consciousness, spirit—that include yet potentially transcend physical phenomena. A guiding premise of the noetic sciences is that the interface of inner experience and the outer world may provide the greatest opportunity for breakthroughs in our understanding of health and healing. To more fully understand this point of view, it may be helpful to consider it in relation to two distinct perspectives: materialist science as it relates to biomedicine, and the writings of postmodern deconstructionism as they influence our models of health and healing.

Noetic investigations have set the stage for a profound integration in which disparate physical systems are no longer viewed as interconnected but as inseparable components of a dynamical mind-body system. This vision is consistent with Brendan O'Regan's conceptualization of a "healing system": a unified body-mind network designed to foster homeostasis, informational flow, and psychophysical regeneration.[1]

In the 1980s, Pert and colleagues[2,3] elaborated the concept of a psychosomatic network composed of neuropeptides, short chains of amino acids present in the brain as well as nonneural tissues, and their corresponding receptors. This psychosomatic network, extending to every molecular corner of the body, functions as a living processor of information—a means to transmit meaningful messages across organs, tissues, cells, and DNA. Moreover, the 70 to 80 neuropeptides identified to date can be viewed as the biochemical substrates of emotion. In brain-mapping studies, Pert and colleagues[2] found that core limbic brain structures, including the hippocampus and amygdala, long considered emotional centers of the brain, are infused with receptors not only for opioids but for the majority of known neuropeptides as well.

Our conceptualization broadened as it became clear that the biochemical substrates of emotion carry information across systems, from those traditionally associated with "mind" (i.e., the brain and autonomic nervous systems) to those traditionally associated with "body" (i.e., the endocrine, cardiovascular, digestive, and immune systems), and back again. Neuropeptide receptors are not limited to the brain; they are present on cells in tissues throughout the body. Emotions are therefore a bridge between mind and body. Research from allied fields of behavioral medicine has verified that our state of disease or health is inextricable from emotional experience. The ubiquity of the neuropeptide receptor network has provided the physiological basis for observations, from the age of Hippocrates to the modern age, that conscious and unconscious feelings are root factors in health and healing.

In the past decade the concept of a psychosomatic network comprising biochemical substrates of emotion has been affirmed and elaborated by research from widely differing fields with divergent designs. But a broad integrative view is needed to envision the big picture: the interlacing of mind-body systems, the inseparability of emotions and physiological processes, and the overarching purposes of such a unified system.

THE PSYCHOSOMATIC NETWORK REVISITED

An early impetus for investigation of bodymind communication was the recognition that for every mood-modifying drug there must be an endogenous neuropeptide ligand that binds to identical target receptor molecules.[2]

During the 1970s, Pert and Snyder[4] at Johns Hopkins identified the first brain drug receptor—the opiate receptor—a cell-surface molecule bound by both exogenous opiate drugs and their analogs, the endogenous opioids, neuropeptides with powerful pain- and mood-modifying properties.

Herkenham and Pert[5] developed sophisticated techniques to map neuropeptide receptor distribution throughout the brain and body. Using these methods, researchers in another study found that the amygdala, hypothalamus, and other limbic structures of the emotional brain were highly enriched with opiate receptors.[6] Later maps showing distribution of other neuropeptide receptors (e.g., substance P, bombesin, cholecystokinin, neurotensin, insulin, and transferrin) revealed the same pattern of enrichment in brain structures associated with emotional experience.[2]

It now appears that the emotional centers of the brain are flush with receptors for most neuropeptides.

Molecular neurobiology dictates that once bound in lock-and-key fashion by their corresponding ligands, cell-surface receptors are structurally modified to transduce "messages" to the cell nucleus, resulting in altered production of cellular proteins and functional activities. Put simply, the presence of these receptors means that cells "receive" messages from matching neuropeptide carriers of biochemical "information."

The boundaries of the classical central nervous system (CNS) were vastly expanded with the discovery of nodal points rich in neuropeptide receptors not just in the brain but throughout the body. The entire gastrointestinal tract, from the esophagus to the large intestine, is lined with cells that contain neuropeptides and their receptors, prompting the insight that the phrase "gut feelings" is more than a metaphor.[7] It seems probable that we experience emotions in our gut because of the richness of its receptors. Specific neuropeptides and their receptors also were found in the kidney, testis, and pancreas, as well as in immune system organs and cells, a point to which we will return shortly.

These and other related findings spurred a re-evaluation of traditional notions of synaptic neurotransmission. Until then, every aspect of mental activity, including perception, integration, and performance, was thought to be determined by synaptic networks and the neurotransmitters that convey information across these junctures in bursts of electrochemical discharge. The neuropeptide-receptor network revealed that it was not necessary for biochemical substrates of thought and emotion to pass along linear, hard-wired channels of neurotransmission. Neuropeptides flow throughout brain and body, finding their respective receptors and altering cell function through transduction of messages to the cell nucleus.[3] They act at great distances without linear connections to their cellular targets; it is the specificity of the receptors that allows for such far-flung bodymind communication.

The purposes and functional capabilities of the neuropeptide-receptor network are manifold, but one overriding function is transmission of information. Neuroscientist Francis O. Schmitt first suggested that the vast variety of neuropeptides, neurohormones (most of which are peptides), steroid hormones, neurotransmitters, growth factors, cytokines, and protein ligands communicate across alleged barriers between biological systems, and they all transmit information.[8] Moreover, many of these substances have feedback loops and receptors in emotion-mediating brain structures.[9] Schmitt termed these molecules "informational substances." He proposed the existence of a parasynaptic (parallel) system in which these information-bearing substances circulate throughout extracellular fluids to reach specific target-cell receptors.

Schmitt's model suggests that the bodymind can no longer be wholly characterized as a hierarchical system of hard-wired connections that descend from a putative ruling station (the brain) but rather as an expansive network of free-flowing information transmitted by molecules that enter at any nodal point and move rapidly to any other point.[2,10] Moreover, the fact that many of these molecular messengers are biochemical substrates of emotion underscores the role of mind—both conscious and unconscious—in linking and coordinating the major systems and their organs.

Perhaps the strongest support for informational substances was research by Carr and Blalock[11] at the University of Texas, showing that immunocytes also synthesize, store, and secrete neuropeptides. In other words, the cellular agents of healing—immune cells—produce the same chemical messengers we conceive as regulating mood and emotion. Because these cells also receive input from neuropeptides, there can be no doubt regarding bidirectional communication between brain and body. Furthermore, we have recently discovered that nerve cells can produce immune cell products, such as IL-1, and in the brain express receptors for $CD4^8$ as well as many of classical "immunopeptides."[12]

During the 1980s, the emergent field of psychoneuroimmunology yielded copious findings regarding brain-body interactions relevant to healing processes. Through the hypothalamic-pituitary-adrenal axis, stress and emotional responses were found to influence levels of corticosteroid hormones; these in turn were shown to modulate immune cell functions, most notably inflammatory responses.[13,14] But co-existent with this hierarchy is the circulating network of informational substances that interact with cell-surface receptors, all to regulate immune cells as they travel the body performing tasks associated with host resistance and healing.

THE PSYCHOSOMATIC NETWORK: CURRENT FINDINGS

Since the 1980s, psychoneuroimmunology and its allied fields (e.g., neuro-immunomodulation, psychoneuroendocrinology, behavioral medicine) have continued to produce findings that dismantle previously erected barriers between biological subsystems, bringing mental and emotional processes into the healing equation by showing bidirectional relationships with immune components. Often classified as part of this endeavor, research on neuropeptides as informational substances continues to substantiate and elaborate the construct of an integrative psychosomatic network.

The number and types of ligands that influence immune cell functions via receptor-binding patterns have expanded beyond the cate-cholamine neurotransmitters, neurohormones such as corticotropin-releasing factor, the corticosteroids, and opioid neuropeptides. The following are now included as immunoregulators: hormones such as insulin, melatonin, and prolactin; sex hormones including both estrogens and androgens; thymic hormones; human growth hormone[15]; and a vast variety of neuropeptide messengers such as β-endorphin, enkephalins, substance P, bombesin, corticotropin (ACTH), gastrin-releasing peptide, vasoactive intestinal polypeptide (VIP), somatostatin, calcitonin gene-related peptide, peptide histidine isoleucine, and peptide histidine methionine.[16]

Consider the immunological influence of one such peptide, VIP. VIP was first described as a vasodilator and is present in both the central and peripheral nervous systems, where it functions as a classical neurotransmitter. But VIP-secreting cells and receptors also line the entire gastrointestinal tract, suggesting that they are possible mediators of so-called "gut feelings." Scores of recent investigations further confirm that VIP is "a potent immunoregulatory signal which can influence a variety of lymphoid cells around which immune responses pivot."[17-19] The interplay of emotional and immune responses is arguably typified by the protean properties of VIP.

Such findings have radically altered the landscape of basic immunology research, which as recently as 10 years ago embraced the idea that the immune system was regulated only by immune substances—cytokines, lymphokines, chemokines, and growth factors. It is now clear that many immune cell products also are produced by nerve cells and that nerve cell products are pivotal regulators of immunity.

Now we have strong evidence that immune cells actually produce neuropeptide molecules. This line of inquiry began with the observation by Smith and Blalock[20] that leukocytes secrete ACTH- and endorphin-like molecules after injury of the immune system in the form of viral or bacterial infection. After further study, these molecules were shown to be more than similar to pituitary ACTH and endorphin—they were identical. Later research[10] demonstrated that immunocytes produce the following: thyrotropin, a glycoprotein secreted by thyrotropes of the anterior lobe of the pituitary gland; chorionic gonadotropin; and growth hormone. Immunocytes also were found to contain and probably synthesize VIP, somatostatin, substance P, oxytocin, and neurophysin.

Completing the reversal of prior theoretical constructs about the nervous and immune systems is the discovery that nerve cells also synthesize immune cell products. Purified and enriched cultures of astrocytes and microglia secrete IL-1, IL-6, and tumor necrosis factor (TNF).[21,22] Microglia also secrete IL-10,[23] and Schwann cells produce TNF-α.[24]

Importantly, the shifting roles of immune and nerve cells occur conspicuously when our bodies are challenged by pathogens and other foreign entities. Under these conditions, immunocytes make neuropeptides, and nerve cells make immune cell products (cytokines), suggesting that the dynamic interplay among systems occurs in response to microbial threats. The informational substances are messengers engaged in continuous feedback loops among these systems, the purpose of which is ongoing self-regulation of defensive responses to external challenges. Because it has been shown that neuroimmune modulation is clearly responsive to stress and emotional factors, there is no question that psychological traits and states influence immunity, and vice versa—that immune activity can influence psychophysical states.

From an evolutionary psychobiological perspective, it makes sense that social/environmental conditions and concomitant emotional states— fear, anxiety, sadness, anger, joy—should have immunological correlates, because these conditions and emotions necessitate a more or less vigorous defense of the integrity of the self.

EMOTIONS, NEUROPEPTIDES, AND THE HEALING SYSTEM

The interlacing of the nervous, endocrine, and immune systems surely suggests a unified healing system. But what of the emotions? The fact that biochemical substrates of emotion are intimately involved in immune regulation does not, in itself, help us to understand how and why states of mind are integral aspects of the healing system, or what kind of interventions will strengthen that system.

Among the most compelling studies of the influence of emotional states and the immune or healing system involves not stress, but rather lack of control in the face of stress. A series of animal studies by Shavit and colleagues showed that animals exposed to inescapable or unpredictable stress—experimental conditions that put subjects into positions of helplessness—experienced chronic elevations in endogenous opioids, which in turn depressed natural killer cell functions.[25,26] Further, rats exposed to this sort of "opioid stress" (to use Shavit's term for any type of stress that simultaneously yields a sense of helplessness and boosts endogenous opioids) were more susceptible to the development of tumors after being injected with carcinoma cells.[27]

But the human analogs of helplessness are certainly more complex. One partial analog is repression, or the nonexpression of emotions. Jamner et al[28] conducted psychological evaluations of 312 patients seen at their medical clinic and found that those who exhibited repressive or "defensive high anxious" coping styles, as measured by combination of the Marlowe-Crown Social Desirability and Taylor Manifest Anxiety scales, had significantly decreased monocyte counts, a sign of relative immunological weakness. (Defensive highly anxious persons have been theorized by Schwartz and others to be repressors whose defenses have become ineffective, leaving them in a state of chronic distress.[28]) These individuals also had elevated serum glucose levels, which coincides with research showing β-endorphin to be a potent hyperglycemic stimulus when delivered intracerebrally[29] and demonstrating the reduction of stress-induced hyperglycemia by centrally active opiate antagonists.[30,31] The investigators concluded that their behavioral, immunological, and endocrine profile was consistent with the "opioid peptide hypothesis of repression."[28] The theory implies that habitual repression of strong emotions results in chronically high levels of endogenous opioids, which in turn cause immune deficits that reduce resistance to infectious and neoplastic disease.

Although Jamner and associates did not link their patients' immune decrements to disease, other studies have correlated repression, immune dysfunction, and poor health. A longitudinal study of 100 HIV-positive patients showed that patients who developed symptoms over the course of 1 year were significantly more likely to exhibit psychological defenses of repression or denial, whereas those who remained asymptomatic evidenced fighting spirit.[32] In research with 58 melanoma patients, Temoshok[33] demonstrated that repressors—persons who evidenced nonexpression of emotions in videotaped structured interviews coded by independent raters—had thicker and more aggressive lesions and fewer lymphocytes infiltrating the site of the tumor to stem the tide of malignant growth. In a related series of studies, Temoshok[34] found that melanoma patients who did not express emotions exhibited other related coping characteristics, including appeasement, extreme self-sacrifice, and a pleasant facade, a constellation referred to as "type C behavior."

Human beings experience helplessness under chronic stress, which is often interpreted to mean that no expression of emotion or active behavioral response will change inescapably unpleasant circumstances or alleviate the pain of loss or separation. Indeed, in many social settings (e.g., family, school, work), the message received is that expression of strong emotion—anger, fear, grief—will exacerbate interpersonal tensions and hasten rejection or opprobrium. The response is often helplessness, and the long-term coping strategy is often repression. (Genetic and early environmental factors may play a role in the evolution of habitual coping styles.) From a psychobiological perspective, the release of opioid peptides is an organismic attempt to quell pain or at least to establish the bliss and/or "bonding" associated with interpersonal closeness. If emotional pain or "loss" is repressed and never resolved, the continuing synthesis and release of endogenous opiates is a possible result, with unintended injurious consequences for the health of the individual.

Are the disorders of a compromised bodymind system—the infections, chronic pains, autoimmune diseases, even the cancers—in part messages to the chronic repressor that his or her defense is no longer serving his well-being? Can illness be a macrocosmic variant of the microscopic molecular feedback loops that govern the workings of the internal healing system? Is it simply another signifier in the language of mind-body distress?

If so, illness is a signifier that must be properly interpreted. Disease is never a punishment, because the etiology of most illnesses involves complex biopsychosocial factors, and the psychological components—including both affective states and personality traits—are unconscious, unintentional contributors to host vulnerability.[34] "Blaming the victim" should be expunged from any scientifically and ethically sound model of biopsychosocial medicine. Although disease is no indicator of insufficiency of character, many one-time patients insist that it can be a wake-up call. From their perspective, illness is a signifier that imbalance—psychosocial, emotional, nutritional, physiological—reigns in the body-mind system, and that efforts made to restore balance will yield benefits in both psychospiritual and physical realms, even when "cure" is not a likely or possible outcome.

EMOTIONAL EXPRESSION: FLOW IN THE PSYCHOSOMATIC NETWORK

What are the clinical ramifications of research on the biochemical substrates of emotion, the psychosomatic network, and the healing system? In some quarters, the simplistic answer is to promote "positive" emotions while discouraging "negative" feelings. But refined research in the mind-body field suggests that the variety of emotions, though associated with different biochemical substrates and unique immunological correlates, are not intrinsically maladaptive, immunosuppressive, or deleterious to health. Primary emotions such as anger, sadness, grief, fear, and joy are essential elements of the repertoire of human experience, and each emotion serves adaptive psychobiological and evolutionary functions.[35] By contrast, long-term states of distress (e.g., helplessness, hopelessness, depression, despair) often result from inescapable or overwhelming stress, rigidly repressive psychic defenses, anger turned against the self, unresolved grief, and ineffective coping styles. These chronic states are frequently cited correlates of serious perturbations of the healing system.

Schwartz[36] and Temoshok and Dreher[34] explicate the linkages among repressive defenses, chronic helplessness/hopelessness, and dysfunction of the healing system. Over time, the inability to express emotion reinforces unconscious hopelessness, because the person unable to experience or communicate emotions may be unable to alter stressful social conditions or assert legitimate needs or rights. He or she also may lack contact with primary psychospiritual sources of creative energy and relatedness to others. Viewed from an existential perspective, the repressive coper is missing essential components for an authentic selfhood, having unconsciously sacrificed access to emotions that form the foundation of a mature identity. The sacrifice was usually made in childhood to maintain self-integrity, but in later adulthood, this sacrifice becomes an unconscious impediment to self-actualization.

This line of reasoning leads inevitably to the hypothesis that emotional expression, disinhibition, and self-actualization would strengthen the healing system. There is now experimental, longitudinal, and clinical evidence to support this hypothesis.

Steve Cole and his colleagues at the University of California, Los Angeles, analyzed data from a longitudinal psychosocial study including 80 HIV-positive gay men who were otherwise healthy from the outset and who were examined at 6-month intervals for 9 years.[37] The investigators sought to evaluate whether the extent to which these gay men were "closeted" had any influence over their disease course. Homosexual identity was measured by an index in which respondents were asked to rate themselves as being "definitely in the closet," "in the closet most of the time," "half in and half out," "out most of the time," or "completely out of the closet." HIV progression was measured from entry to the study to the following: the time it took to reach a critically low CD4 lymphocyte count (15% of total peripheral blood lymphocytes), time to AIDS diagnosis, and time to AIDS mortality. On all measures, HIV infection advanced more rapidly in direct proportion to the extent participants concealed their gay identity.[37] The investigators successfully ruled out explanations based on demographic characteristics, health practices, sexual behavior, and antiretroviral therapy.

Relative to participants who reported being "mostly" or "completely" out of the closet, those who reported being "half" or more "in the closet" experienced a 40% reduction in time to reach a critically low CD4 count, a 38% reduction in time to AIDS diagnosis, and a 21% reduction in time to death—faster progression of disease at statistically significant levels in each instance.[37] Viewed from another angle, the HIV-positive men who were relatively more "out of the closet" did not experience the more rapid disease progression experienced by their counterparts. These results were consistent with data from another study of 222 HIV-seronegative gay men that showed that men who concealed expression of their homosexual identity experienced a significantly higher incidence of cancer (odds ratio = 3.18) and several infectious diseases (pneumonia, bronchitis, sinusitis, and tuberculosis; odds ratio = 2.91) during a 5-year follow-up period.[38] These effects could not be attributed to health behaviors, socioeconomic factors, anxiety, depression, or reporting biases.

The findings of Cole et al[38] are consistent with prior research linking psychological inhibition to physical illness, and these results suggest that concealing one's identity, which certainly encompasses a whole gamut of emotions, personality traits, and proclivities (e.g., insight, humor, self-expression, honest communication with others) can compromise the healing system. By contrast, being able to fully accept and acknowledge one's identity may be interpreted to mean that one is freed from the physiological "work" of repression or inhibition, with its deleterious effects on immunity and health.

An extensive body of research by Pennebaker[39] has shown that disinhibition—emotional expression and processing—has a salutary influence on immune functions and resistance to illness. In experimental studies, subjects who wrote their deepest thoughts and feelings about past traumas experienced enhanced T-cell responsivity[40] and improved overall health[39,41] compared with control subjects who wrote about trivial events. Pennebaker has shown that for disinhibition to foster health or healing, previously blocked emotions must not only be expressed but also cognitively processed—understood and resolved over three or four 20-minute writing sessions on successive days. Moreover, the degree to which subjects disclosed previously inhibited painful memories and emotions was associated with better health outcomes.[41]

The data linking emotional disclosure (or expression) with improved immune functioning continue to build. The relevance of these findings to disease and health has been questioned, because it is not certain that the observed immunological fluctuations are sufficient to affect health outcomes. A few studies, however, have demonstrated the clinical relevance of immunological outcomes. Temoshok's study showing correlations between emotional expression and levels of tumor-infiltrating lymphocytes in melanoma is clinically relevant, because these infiltrates have been associated with tumor regression and, in several reports, improved prognosis.[42,43] In addition, in Temoshok's study, patients with fewer infiltrating lymphocytes also tended to have thicker tumors consisting of melanoma cells with a higher mitotic rate, both of which indicate a poor prognosis.[33]

One of the most intriguing lines of inquiry involves the long-term health effects of early physical and sexual abuse, traumas that are typically suppressed or repressed. The best studies of the long-term pathophysiological effects of early abuse involve gastrointestinal diseases, most notably irritable bowel syndrome and inflammatory bowel disease.[44-46] The potential influence of biochemical substrates of repressed emotion should therefore be strongly considered in gastrointestinal disorders. Neuropeptide receptors line the entire gastrointestinal tract, and a recent study[47] showed that three of these neuropeptides—VIP, somatostatin, and substance P—have profound stimulatory (and occasionally inhibitory) effects on T-lymphocyte populations present throughout the mucosal lining of intestines. One hypothesis worthy of investigation is whether the inhibition of emotions and memories of early abuse results in overactivation of immunoregulatory intestinal peptides and subsequent chronic inflammatory bowel disease.

Experimental studies of disinhibition are building blocks for intervention research that evaluates whether a psychosocial treatment that facilitates emotional expression and active coping strengthens host defenses sufficiently to promote healing of disease. Several such studies have been conducted, and the results well documented and publicized. In a decade-long study of 86 women with metastatic breast cancer, Spiegel et al[48] found that patients who participated in "supportive/expressive therapy," a group psychosocial intervention, lived twice as long (mean of 36.6 versus 18.9 months) as control subjects who did not participate. Spiegel has emphasized that the intervention was designed to encourage emotional expression—sharing and processing the most difficult emotional states associated with a life-threatening condition. We await results from his current replications, which will include analyses of neuroendocrine and immunological mediators.

Fawzy et al,[49] who conducted a similar randomized controlled trial with 68 patients with melanoma, found that participation in a 6-week structured psychosocial intervention was associated with a reduction in the risk of recurrence and a statistically significant threefold reduction in the risk of mortality over 6 years. Although the finding received little attention, Fawzy's study also found that patients who expressed more distress at the outset of the study, and who evidenced an increase in active-behavioral coping, were significantly less likely to experience a recurrence or die of their disease.

These intervention studies support the proposition that the healing system, in all its multilayered complexity, is strengthened and balanced not simply by "good" emotions but by the experience, expression, and cognitive resolution of all emotions. Indeed, we propose that emotional expression/resolution is the psychospiritual correlate of a properly balanced flow of neuropeptides throughout the bodymind system. This appropriately balanced flow, in turn, generates a functional healing system, which also involves a balanced flow of endocrine secretions, a vigorous but finely tuned immune system, perhaps even the minimization or control of cellular abnormalities caused by inappropriate gene expression.

MIND-BODY MEDICINE AND THE HEALING SYSTEM

Research on the biochemical substrates of emotion, emphasizing the pivotal role of neuropeptides and receptors in the psychosomatic network, has enhanced our understanding of the healing network as explicated by O'Regan, which includes but is not limited to the immune system. It encompasses the integral activities of virtually all biological subsystems, including those associated with "mind" and "emotion."

Research on the nature of the healing system should also now focus on what Rossi[50] calls "the mind-gene connection." Informational substances—especially neuropeptides—that interact with receptors can modify gene expression through the transduction of messages from the cell surface. A remarkable series of studies by immunovirologist Ronald Glaser, psychologist Janice Kiecolt-Glaser, and their colleagues have shown the influence of stress and emotional factors on gene expression. In one study, 17 first-year medical students were tested for levels of messenger RNA expression of the proto-oncogenes c-myc and c-myb in peripheral blood leukocytes at the time of academic examinations and at a baseline period approximately 1 month before the examinations. It was shown that during the stressful period of examinations, subjects evidenced increased levels of messenger RNA expression of c-myc and c-myb in peripheral blood leukocytes.[51] The increased expression of c-myc and c-myb proto-oncogenes was consistent with previous data demonstrating down-regulation of these immune cells during stress.

In other words, gene expression is altered during stress, and this alteration changes cellular functions, with consequences for the health of the individual. If stress can increase expression of proto-oncogenes, presumably through the intermediary effect of neuropeptides interacting with receptors and causing transduction of messages to cellular DNA, it raises a critical question: Can stress (and related emotional factors) transform proto-oncogenes into active oncogenes? Can a fundamental oncogenic process be influenced by the psychosocial realm?

The theories of Rossi and the research of Kiecolt-Glaser and Glaser, among others, suggest that the healing system must be broadened to include dialectic relationships among emotions, neuropeptides, endocrine products, immune system components, and the influence of this entire cascade on gene expression and the regulation of gene products within the cell.

In an attempt to grapple with the question of why psychological traits and states should be so fully intertwined with biological systems of defense and healing, molecular biologists Roger Booth and Kevin Ashbridge developed a model of the psychoneuroimmune system.[52] They propose that the immune system, commonly viewed as a defense network, is engaged in a broader process of self-determination. Our psychological, neurological, and immmunological subsystems share a common goal: establishing and maintaining self-identity. They refer to this unifying principle as "teleological coherence" and argue that biological subsystems overlap due to their common purposes: to maintain harmony within and without the organism, to distinguish "self" from "nonself," to uphold organismic integrity.

Booth and Ashbridge's model is reinforced by the many conspicuous metaphors between the mind-brain and immune-healing systems, long ago postulated by psychoimmunology pioneer George Solomon.[53] Both systems have the capacity for memory; both are designed for adaptation to environmental stressors; both serve functions of defense; both are harmed by inadequate defenses; both are harmed by excessive defenses; and both develop either tolerance or sensitivity to "noxious" (i.e., stressful, antigenic) agents.

But here is a central question regarding this model: At what level in the bodymind "system" can we identify the interpolation of awareness? To what extent do we consciously participate in self-determination at the psychological, immunological, or even the genetic level?

One speculative approach, consistent with Booth and Ashbridge's model, suggests that the mind is a nonphysical substrate that holds together the flowing psychosomatic network of informational substances and cells, linking and coordinating the major systems and their molecular constituents in an intelligently orchestrated symphony of life processes. Although this network appears to operate below the level of consciousness, it is impinged upon by biochemical substrates of unconscious mental processes. Moreover, therapeutic interventions can bring unconscious mental processes into awareness, and psychosocial and behavioral changes can again be transduced down through the network, resulting in concomitant physiological changes. Interventions designed to facilitate emotional expression are prime examples of the interpolation of consciousness into otherwise autonomic (unconscious) psychobiological processes, resulting in beneficial health outcomes.

Interventions that encourage conscious efforts toward identity formation, self-assertion, and self-expression may indeed generate comparable qualities in the healing system. Teleological coherence is an organismic reality, but for the human animal, consciousness can intervene in seemingly involuntary processes.

Deeper questions concern the nature of mind—that presumably nonmaterial, nonphysical substrate of observable processes characterized by the flow of information throughout the bodymind. The word "soul" is still assiduously avoided by academic scientists. But what animates the neuropeptides in their flow patterns through the body? What animates the receptors? These flexible cell-surface molecules vibrate, shimmy, and even hum as they change shapes, awaiting arrival of their matching ligands. The entire healing system is propelled by chemical energies, but to reverse the usual question: What is the immaterial substrate of these ceaseless biochemical reactions? Rachel Naomi Remen refers to the "life force," heretical psychoanalyst Wilhem Reich spoke of "life energy," and poets and theologians conjure an *élan vital* and "spirit."

These questions may be largely unanswerable by the current methods of mainstream science, though researchers have sought to explain how varieties of energy medicine,[54] prayer,[55] and other spiritual practices[56] support the healing system. But research on healing energies, whether delineated in Western terms (bioelectromagnetism, nonlocal consciousness) or Eastern spiritual or medical terms (e.g., *qi*, *kundalini*, *prana*) may shed light on the immaterial substrates of the molecules of emotion. Levin,[56] who has uncovered more than 250 published empirical studies on the largely beneficial health effects of religious or spiritual practice, has developed a series of hypotheses for these effects, including behavioral and social factors as well as the psychodynamics of belief systems and religious rites. He also includes as an alternative hypothesis the role of a "superempirical force," an energetic phenomena that is tapped or accessed through spiritual or religious practice, a pantheistic, discarnate force or power.[56] Levin emphasizes that, in the near future, this force may no longer be considered superempirical but empirical; some scientists are claiming success in measuring bioenergy fields.[54,57]

A point of intersection between efforts to explicate the psychosomatic network and efforts to explicate biological energies is the concept of information. Rubik[54] has endeavored to shift the emphasis in studies of bioelectromagnetic fields, which are relevant to energy-medicine applications such as healer interventions, acupuncture, and homeopathy, from a strictly energetic model to an information-based paradigm. In her view, energy-medicine applications may involve bioinformation that interacts with endogenous electromagnetic biofields or at the level of membrane receptors in the organism.[54] Thus, information can be viewed as a unifying concept that spans many levels of organization of living systems, including emotional, energetic, biochemical, molecular, and genetic levels.

The integration of energy-based models with neuropeptide-receptor–based models under the rubric of an informational paradigm goes beyond the scope of this chapter. But the translation of meaning on both energetic and molecular levels should be considered, as Dossey[58] has emphasized. For instance, psychospiritual states of "hopelessness" or "joy" have specific energetic and molecular correlates; the organismic experience of such states cannot be reduced to either level but appears to be translated on both levels, simultaneously and indivisibly. One can best "read" such meanings and their multileveled correlates by evaluating the whole person, combining the clinician's art with the biologist's technological probes. Perhaps that is why we have emphasized the pivotal role of emotional expression in the healing system: It may be the best available marker for a psychospiritual vitalization of the life force, however one defines such a phenomenon. The forms of mind-body medicine that awaken our healing potential are those that rouse emotion and generate spirit, which could be defined in terms once used by Rollo May[59]: "Spirit is that which gives vivacity, energy, liveliness, courage, and ardor to life."

References for this essay are located on the DVD accompanying this book.

Psychological Aspects of Mind-Body Medicine: Promises and Pitfalls from Research with Cancer Patients[*]

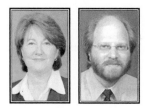

STEPHANIE SIMONTON-ATCHLEY
ALLEN C. SHERMAN

THE PSYCHOSOCIAL DIMENsions of cancer have long been an important focus of attention in the expansive field of mind-body medicine and will be significant in the emerging field of integral medicine. The possible role of psychosocial factors in contributing to disease progression—and, conversely, the potential value of psychosocial interventions to enhance disease outcome—are topics of great interest and debate for

[*]Adapted from Simonton S, Sherman A: Psychological Aspects of Mind-Body Medicine: Promises and Pitfalls From Research with Cancer Patients, *Altern Ther Health Med* 4(4):50-64, 1998.

researchers and clinicians. This article considers the impact of psychosocial or mind-body interventions on immune function and disease outcome in the cancer experience. We begin with a discussion concerning which patients might be most at risk for adverse outcomes or most likely to benefit from mind-body interventions. We conclude with comments about clinical applications and neglected areas or promising directions for further research. It is our intent to offer a panoramic update about interesting advances and notable gaps in our understanding of this area. How these findings might relate to the broader arena of behavioral medicine is also noted. Because the focus of this article is on established disease, interventions geared toward cancer prevention and detection are not considered.

Research in psychosocial oncology has been marked by several notable methodological advances over the past two decades. Studies have become more specific concerning site, stage, and histology of disease, with greater deference to the enormous heterogeneity of neoplastic diseases (cancer is compromised by scores of distinct disease entities). Psychosocial research has begun to include more adequate controls for confounding medical and demographic factors. Psychological measures are better validated and less idiosyncratic, and research designs are more apt to include appropriate multivariate analyses.

Often, however, studies are compromised by small sample sizes that eclipse the prospect of finding positive results, as well as by incomplete controls for prognostic factors, which sometimes make it difficult to interpret results that do emerge. There is less exclusive reliance on measures developed for psychiatric patients, though assessments of adjustment are often confounded by somatic items so results are spuriously affected by degree of medical illness. Finally, whereas many areas reviewed in this article have a broad base of research, most have narrow foundations in theory. Many of these challenges and triumphs will sound familiar to those who are familiar with behavioral medicine research concerning other chronic illnesses.

IMMUNE FUNCTION AND DISEASE OUTCOME
Psychosocial Factors Contributing to Disease Progression
One of the most intriguing questions in psycho-oncology concerns whether psychosocial factors contribute to disease onset or progression

for certain malignancies through alteration of health behaviors or disruption of biological regulatory mechanisms. Unfortunately, the allure of this question is counterbalanced by prodigious methodological and theoretical complexities. Most research has focused on disease progression (i.e., recurrence, metastases, survival) rather than onset, because progression can be more definitively operationalized and measured within a circumscribed time frame. The following discussion is therefore restricted to psychosocial correlates of tumor progression, highlighting findings from longitudinal studies. Our intention is to share how research in this area is evolving. Among the multiple variables investigated have been transient state characteristics such as mood, psychiatric distress, and coping; trait measures such as locus of control, extroversion, and dispositional pessimism; and situational or contextual factors such as stress and social support.

Growing evidence suggests that social isolation, which long has been associated with all-cause mortality after controlling for traditional risk factors,[1,2] may be associated with cancer mortality as well. Higher levels of social support have predicted significantly longer survival in several studies of patients with localized or regional breast cancer,[3-5] acute leukemia,[6] and in heterogeneous samples of patients with mixed disease sites[7-9] after adjusting for medical prognostic factors. However, negative findings also have been reported,[9,10] and thus the "medicinal" value of cohesive relationships remains to be elaborated.

Consistent with findings in other areas of behavioral medicine, social support may have differential effects on survival among men and women[6] and among different age groups.[7,11] Social support is a complex, multilayered phenomenon. Marital status often has been used as a crude proxy for support in clinical and epidemiological studies. Unlike heart disease research, in which studies with predominantly male samples indicate that marriage may lower risk of recurrence and mortality,[12] cancer studies, which include greater proportions of women, have not produced consistent findings associated with marital status.[5,11,13-17] In a few studies,[5,11] being single has predicted longer rather than shorter survival.

Almost all oncology research exploring the survival value of relationships has focused on structural or quantitative aspects of social support (e.g., marital status, number of friends and relatives, organizational involvement). (For an exception, see Ell et al.[18]) Qualitative or emotional dimensions of support rarely have been investigated for their potential relevance to disease outcome, which is striking because emotional support has been consistently associated with better quality of life.[19] Qualitative aspects of supportive as well as strained relationships should be further explored.

The impact of emotional distress (e.g., depression, anxiety) on recurrence and survival also has been the subject of many prospective studies. Most of these investigations have focused on breast cancer,[20,21] but hematological malignancies[17,22,23] and heterogeneous samples of cancer patients[24, 25] have been studied as well. There is little evidence that clinical or subclinical depression or distress predicts tumor progression.[17,20-25] This should be reassuring to patients who believe that if they fail to maintain a "positive attitude," they will be more vulnerable to medical decline. The fact that depression seems unrelated to tumor promotion mirrors the equivocal findings that have emerged in studies with HIV patients,[26-28] but contrasts with recent findings[29,30] in coronary heart disease studies that associate depression with greater mortality.

On the other hand, a number of studies of cancer patients have reported associations between poorer disease outcome and lower levels of self-reported distress.[31-35] These results often have been interpreted as reflecting the deleterious effects of a repressive, avoidant coping style, in which situationally appropriate emotional discomfort is unrecognized or disavowed. Such findings are consistent with an older, methodologically limited literature dating back to the 1950s,[36,37] in which patients with rapid tumor progression were characterized as highly passive, compliant, accommodating, and unable to express negative emotions. However, research on mood and distress has yielded mixed results, with most studies[*] reporting no significant relationships and a few studies[3,6,15,39] reporting the opposite pattern: higher expressions of negative affect correlated with poorer disease outcome.

The concept of repressive or avoidant coping has a long history in cancer research, but is clouded by conceptual and methodological difficulties. On its own, self-reported negative affect seems a poor proxy for measuring this variable. More direct measures of this construct

---

[*]References 9,10,15,17,20-23,38.

are required, though the use of related trait and state measures such as "alexithymia," "repression-sensitization," "defensiveness," "emotional control," and "passive coping" is not without limitations. The few studies that have attempted to assess emotional suppression or avoidance more directly have reported significant relationships with disease progression. Positive findings have emerged in prospective and cross-sectional studies of patients with breast cancer,[40] malignant melanoma,[41] premalignant cervical dysplasia and early-stage cervical cancer,[42-46] and in more heterogeneous samples of cancer patients.[38] (See Gross[47] for a review, and Razavi and colleagues[48] for negative findings concerning repression-sensitization.) The potential importance of repressive coping requires further investigation.

Research also has explored other aspects of coping and disease progression. Studies have evolved from those that focus on coping styles, which are construed as relatively global attitudes toward disease and recovery, to those that focus on coping strategies, which represent more dynamic, situationally specific thoughts and behaviors that shift over time as the demands of the illness evolve.[49] In a well-known series of studies concerning coping style, Greer and colleagues[50,51] and Pettingale and colleagues[52] reported that early-stage breast cancer patients who reacted to their illness with "fighting spirit" (an attitude of beating or overcoming the illness) or "denial" (rejecting the significance of the illness), as assessed at 3 months after diagnosis, had longer recurrence-free survival at 5-, 10-, and 15-year follow-up than did those who were rated as "stoic" or "helpless." Although these studies controlled for a number of prognostic factors, controls for nodal involvement were incomplete and hormone receptor status was not measured.

In a subsequent prospective study of younger women with operable breast cancer, Dean and Surtees[15] found that increased "denial" predicted significantly longer recurrence-free survival and marginally longer survival at 6- to 8-year follow-up after controlling for prognostic factors. Andrykowski and colleagues[53] reported that "anxious preoccupation" about the illness predicted shorter survival among leukemia patients who had received allogeneic bone marrow transplants. However, other teams have found no relationships with disease outcome in studies of bone marrow transplant patients[23] and of breast cancer patients with localized or regional disease.[54] Negative results may have been influenced by the shorter follow-up intervals of these later studies. Overall, whereas initial findings regarding "fighting spirit" sparked considerable attention, they generally have not been replicated. Findings concerning denial also are inconsistent. A related concept, avoidant coping, generally has been associated with poorer quality of life[55-57] and perhaps poorer survival as well.[38] Among heart disease patients, denial has been associated with positive short-term effects on disease end points[58-60] but negative long-term effects.[58] Among patients with HIV disease, denial has foreshadowed more rapid disease progression.[61]

Researchers also have begun examining the potential effects of coping strategies on disease outcome. In one study it was found that active-behavioral coping strategies (e.g., exercise, consultation with medical staff, relaxation practice), as opposed to more passive responses, predicted significantly lower recurrence and mortality rates for stage I melanoma patients.[32] Other studies reported no significant relationships for patients with hematological, rectal,[17] or advanced breast cancer.[62] Inconsistent findings may in part reflect the different measures that have been used with different populations. However, it is also likely that any relationship between coping and survival is moderated by other important variables such as stress, personality, age, and disease severity, and that multivariate research models may prove more illuminating.

Several investigators have pursued the possible links between various personality traits and disease progression. Positive findings have emerged from a few of these explorations, but there has been little replication. (See Temoshok's work on the multidimensional type C personality style.[63,64]) One of the most interesting results concerns the impact of dispositional (i.e., trait) pessimism, because this concept has long been of theoretical interest inside and outside oncology, and because these results echo earlier findings regarding coronary heart disease[65] and HIV disease.[66]

In a recent study[67] of patients with advanced disease who received palliative radiation treatment for diverse types of cancer, a pessimistic orientation predicted higher mortality among younger subjects (those aged 30 to 59 years). Although the investigators controlled for disease site and physical symptomatology in their analyses, other potentially important prognostic factors, such as time since diagnosis and number or site of metastases, were not controlled. Scheier and Bridges[68] speculate that individuals with generally pessimistic expectations about outcomes in life are more prone to withdraw and disengage in the face of adversity, rather than to reestablish alternate, more appropriate life goals. A pessimistic predisposition may therefore set the stage for a range of unhealthy reactions to illness, such as stoic fatalism, helplessness, "vital exhaustion," or depression, each of which has been associated with poorer outcomes among patients with cancer[50-52,69] or coronary heart disease.[29,30,70-72]

The relationships between psychosocial factors and disease progression remain murky, and sweeping conclusions regarding psychological prognostic factors are not justified by current data. However, promising findings support the potential importance of a number of variables, including social support, emotional suppression, coping patterns, and dispositional pessimism. Although no comparable database exists in oncology concerning the effects of spirituality, this is another variable worthy of further investigation. Studies that examine these variables using prospective, multivariate designs among patients selected for specific sites and stages of disease, with appropriate controls for medical and demographic covariates (particularly age), would help to move the field forward. Psychosocial correlates of established biological indicators, such as hormone receptor status in breast cancer patients[48,73,74] or lymphocyte infiltration in malignant melanoma patients,[41] are also worthy of further study.

The selection of more refined psychosocial measures would be helpful as well. More specific, targeted measures geared toward particular constructs may yield more promising returns than either the simplistic, one- to two-item indices often used in epidemiological studies, or the global, omnibus assessment instruments sometimes employed in clinical research.[38,67] In particular, positive and negative aspects of qualitative social support merit further investigation, as do clearer, more focused measures of repressive coping.

Underlying Mechanisms

The potential impact of psychosocial factors on disease outcome remains a fertile area for further research and theory building. Although mechanisms underlying these relationships are not well understood, researchers[61,75] have pointed to behavioral, psychoneuroimmunological, and neuroendocrine changes as potential pathways. Psychological factors such as stress, pessimism, or isolation might affect the medical treatment that patients receive by reducing compliance or undermining self-advocacy for more aggressive or experimental treatment protocols.

Stress and psychological factors also influence health behaviors, contributing to poor diet, diminished appetite, disrupted sleep, limited exercise, increased cigarette smoking, or intensified substance abuse. These adverse changes in functional status might reduce the patient's capacity to endure optimal doses of toxic, debilitating treatments. Stress-induced changes in coping and self-care (e.g., poor nutrition, inadequate sleep, substance abuse) also are known to affect immune functioning,[76-78] possibly increasing the risk for infectious complications[79] or altering the course of disease.

Apart from contributing to unhealthy behavior, psychological factors also can have more direct effects on neuroendocrine activity[80] and immune functioning.[81-83] Advances in basic immunology, molecular biology, and stress research over the past 20 years have uncovered connections linking the central nervous, neuroendocrine, and immune systems.[84] Although few studies have been conducted with cancer patients, research with other populations in the growing field of psychoneuroimmunology has demonstrated an array of immune parameters that appear responsive to psychosocial influences, including alterations in natural killer (NK) cell activity, proliferative response to mitogens, numbers and percentages of T-cell subpopulations, and antibody titers to latent infections.[81,82] Situational challenges such as stressful events and disrupted relationships, as well as personal characteristics such as loneliness, depressed mood, or repressive coping, are among aspects of psychosocial experience that seem to resonate within the immune system.[84] There is great interest in observing whether these changes could affect host resistance to tumor progression, particularly among patients with malignancies more closely associated with immune monitoring, and among those whose immune systems are already compromised (e.g., the elderly, bone marrow transplant recipients, those with nutritional deficits).[85]

Given the enormous complexity of the immune system, the optimal measures, normative ranges, and clinical relevance of immune changes are not always clear. Nevertheless, research in psychoneuroimmunology is becoming more sophisticated. Descriptive studies in oncology have been limited. However, a number of prospective and cross-sectional investigations have begun to uncover relationships between psychosocial factors (e.g., mood, social support, coping) and cellular immunity, particularly NK cell activity, which plays a role in host defense against metastatic spread.[86-91] For example, in a cross-sectional study of women with stage I and stage III breast cancer, higher levels of stress were associated with significantly lower NK cell lysis, decreased response of NK cells to recombinant interferon-γ, and reduced lymphoproliferative response to mitogens and T3 MAb, after controlling for a number of confounding variables.[92] Similarly, among patients with malignant melanoma, the level of emotional expression has been tied to the degree of lymphocyte infiltration of the base of the tumor[41]—an important prognostic factor. Other researchers have offered theoretical models concerning potential psychoneuroimmunological influences on progression from premalignant cervical dysplasia to invasive cervical cancer.[93]

The immune system has been a focal point for investigators seeking links between psychological functioning and disease outcome. Other pathways through which psychological experience might alter tumor progression—such as through hormonal effects on angiogenesis, growth factor production, apoptosis, or desmoplasia—have received little exploration.[94] (See Temoshok[41] for an exception.) Some researchers have wondered whether the fascination with NK cells has rendered research a bit myopic.[94]

Psychological Interventions to Enhance Immune Function

Research concerning the adverse effects of psychosocial disequilibrium on immune function has generated interest in whether psychological interventions might enhance immune activity (for a review, see Ironson et al[61]). Only a handful of controlled studies with cancer patients have explored this possibility. As with HIV research, however, there is much activity in this area and additional work is under way. Published studies have centered on brief interventions. Whereas some emphasize self-regulation training (e.g., imagery, biofeedback), others focus on group psychotherapy. In a study mentioned earlier, Fawzy and colleagues[86] examined the effects of participation in a 6-week psychotherapy group, which involved health education, relaxation training, problem-solving skills, and interpersonal support for 61 patients with stage I or II melanoma. Those who participated in the group demonstrated reduced psychological distress, increased NK cell cytotoxic activity, increased percentage of large granular lymphocytes (the NK cell phenotype), and a small reduction in percentage of helper-inducer T cells. Most of these changes did not emerge until 6 months after the intervention.

Other studies focus on breast cancer patients. Gruber and colleagues[95] examined the effectiveness of 9 weeks of biofeedback–assisted relaxation and imagery practice for 13 premenopausal, lymph–node–negative patients, all of whom had received modified radical mastectomies. Following treatment, the experimental group demonstrated increased mixed lymphocyte responsiveness, increased lymphoproliferative responsiveness to concanavalin A, and differences in numbers of circulating white blood cells, lymphocytes, and plasma immunoglobulin G (IgG) relative to wait-list controls. When the wait-listed subjects received the same treatment, they showed comparable increases in mixed lymphocyte responsiveness and concanavalin A responsiveness, as well as increases in interleukin-2 (IL-2) and plasma IgM relative to pretreatment levels. No changes were found in psychological measures as a result of treatment. Consistent with the study by Fawzy and coworkers,[86] several weeks to several months were required for most immune changes to reach statistical significance.

Similarly, in an ongoing, large-scale study of breast cancer patients, preliminary data indicated that women enrolled in a structured therapy group showed significant changes in NK cell activity compared with controls.[96]

Our work in this area also has been promising. In a study sponsored in part by the Institute of Noetic Sciences, Simonton[97] employed a within-subjects research design to assess the immune effects of 3 weeks of imagery and relaxation training for a mixed group of 17 patients who had completed radiation therapy for head and neck, breast, or lung cancer. Following the behavioral intervention, a significant increase was found in in vitro lymphocyte stimulation by varicella-zoster (VZ) viral antigen, with 12 of 17 patients demonstrating changes in the expected direction. However, no change was found in lymphoproliferative response to mitogen. Change in VZ measures correlated significantly with the amount of imagery practice. Immune outcome was not associated with elapsed time following completion of radiation therapy. Nevertheless, to determine whether these results were an artifact of recovery from radiation therapy, a subset of the original patients were re-enrolled in the intervention 1 year later. All patients had discontinued imagery practice at the completion of the previous study, and all VZ assays had returned to previous baseline levels or lower. Following a second administration of relaxation and imagery training, there was an average increase of 93% in VZ levels across subjects, though the small sample size precluded statistical analysis.

On the other hand, a more recent study of breast cancer patients yielded more negative results. Richardson and colleagues[98] compared the effects of a 6-week imagery group with a support group and a control condition for women with localized or regional disease who had completed medical treatment an average of 11 months earlier. The imagery group was quite broad in scope, focusing on issues such as coping with anxiety, goal setting, and finding purpose in life, as well as immune-related imagery. Relative to controls, women in both intervention groups reported significant improvements on a number of psychological measures, but no differential improvements in mood. Differential effects were not found on measures of cellular immune function or cytokine levels, including NK cell activity, neopterin, interferon-g, IL-1 and IL-2, or beta endorphin, after controlling for age, stage of disease, and time since cessation of medical treatment. However, as in the Simonton study,[97] frequency of imagery practice was associated with altered immune activity; specifically, greater practice was correlated with increased NK cell activity.

These results support the possibility that mind-body approaches can alter aspects of cellular immunity among a diverse range of cancer patients. Immune changes often show delayed effects (i.e., requiring time after completion of the intervention before becoming salient) consistent with the delayed effects sometimes noted for psychological outcomes. Whether the immune changes observed in these studies have any clinical meaning remains to be determined. In studies with HIV patients, interventions have sometimes led to a number of interesting alterations in immune function, but significant effects on markers of disease promotion have been elusive.[61]

Psychological Interventions to Enhance Disease Outcome

If mind-body interventions can alter various immune parameters, what about their potential impact on recurrence or survival? Does enhanced quality of life serve as a stepping-stone to enhanced quantity of life? Positive findings have emerged from two studies. Although highly preliminary, these results have generated intense interest, and multiple attempts at replication are now under way. In a pioneering study by Spiegel and colleagues,[62] women with metastatic breast cancer were randomly assigned to a long-term psychological intervention or a control condition. The intervention consisted of participation for 1 year in a weekly supportive-expressive psychotherapy group, which included discussion of adjusting to life-threatening illness, processing of existential concerns, and self-hypnosis for pain control. Those who received the therapy group fared better psychologically than did control subjects.

At 10-year follow-up, however, it was found that these women on average had survived twice as long (an average of 1 ½ years longer) than those in the control group, with the difference in survival time beginning 8 months after the intervention ended. No measures of health behaviors, immunity, or endocrine functioning were included in this study, and it is unclear what mediated these differences in survival time.

Another controlled study reporting significant effects on disease outcome was conducted by Fawzy and colleagues,[32] which was mentioned earlier. A 5- to 6-year follow-up of patients initially diagnosed with stage I melanoma revealed that those who participated in the brief therapy group survived significantly longer and experienced marginally fewer recurrences than did control subjects after controlling for established medical risk factors (i.e., Breslow depth). With respect to immune parameters, the changes in NK cell activity that occurred following group treatment were not predictive of disease outcome, though high baseline levels of NK cell activity were associated with lower recurrence rates.

Not all results have been confirmatory of mind-body approaches. A nonrandomized follow-up study by Gellert and colleagues[99] found no differences in survival (relative to matched control patients with comparable disease) for a group of 34 breast cancer patients who participated in a support group, individual and family counseling, and imagery practice.

Clinical Implications and Directions for Further Research

Initial studies offer evidence that psychological interventions may not only enhance quality of life (an increasingly well-established finding), but may also alter immune functioning and perhaps survival. Further exploration is needed to confirm whether psychological approaches can contribute to improved disease outcome, and, if so, to clarify the behavioral, immune, and neuroendocrine mechanisms involved. This work is under way.

Questions that await further study include whether changes in cellular immune function associated with psychosocial interventions[86,95-97] can be replicated in other patients, and whether different patterns of response emerge for different age groups or for individuals with different types and stages of disease. Patients at greatest risk for compromised immune function (e.g., the elderly, those undergoing immunosuppressive treatments) and patients with tumors thought to be influenced by immune or endocrine changes (e.g., malignant melanoma, hematological malignancies, estrogen-receptor–positive breast cancer) may be the most promising candidates for research in mind-body therapies.

The most important question is whether any of the immune changes generated by these interventions are sufficiently robust to alter clinical status (e.g., infectious complications, metastases, recurrence, survival). Other pathways through which psychological experience might affect disease progression, such as hormonal modulation of tumor angiogenesis,[100,101] apoptosis,[102] growth factor formation, or DNA repair,[94,103] await further investigation.

CONCLUSION

Over the past two decades, considerable advances have been made in our understanding of the relationships between psychosocial functioning and disease outcome. Questions have become more specific, and inquiries better controlled. Continuing movements in this direction are apt to be illuminating as research shifts toward greater specificity in constructs assessed, measures used, sites and stages of disease examined, and phases of recovery explored. Provocative findings have emerged from a first wave of controlled studies concerning the impact of mind-body interventions on immune parameters and disease end points. Within the next few years, it is anticipated that this database will expand considerably as new research initiatives come to fruition.

ACKNOWLEDGMENTS

A grant from the Institute of Noetic Sciences was instrumental in helping Dr. Simonton to explore the immunological effects of mind-body interventions for cancer patients at a time when such an approach was rarely evaluated. Through the dynamic work of such institutions, the foundation is being laid for a more comprehensive and multifactorial understanding of cancer.

References for this essay are located on the DVD accompanying this book.

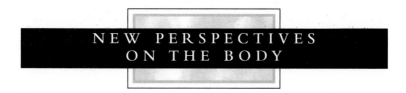

NEW PERSPECTIVES ON THE BODY

Meaning and the History of the Body: Toward a Postmodern Medicine *

DAVID MICHAEL LEVIN

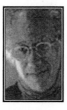

THE HUMAN BODY IS AN evolutionary biological entity, but it is more than that. It is also an ongoing achievement of socialization and acculturation. As these social processes interact and communicate with the body's biological nature, they shape and transform it. Human beings are sociable from the very beginning—that is to say, our bodies are biologically organized and ordered for social interaction and communication. Consequently, it is not possible to draw the boundary between the body of nature and the body of culture with any precision, certainty, and finality.

---

*1990 Adapted from The Discursive Formation of the Body in the History of Medicine by Levin DM, Solomon GF. Reproduced by permission of Taylor & Francis, Inc., http://www.taylorandfrancis.com

The boundary has, in fact, been continually redrawn, especially in this century, as the science of medicine accumulates knowledge that incorporates the body into ever more subtle and more intricate models and analyses.

In other words, what we interpret as the human body—its development and processes—is formed by communication networks extending within, through, and beyond the visible organism.[1]

More specifically, the point I want to emphasize in this article is that the human body is also formed within the context of the history of medicine. That is, as the interpretations and images of the human body changed historically, these changes were intimately related to the historical development of medicine itself.

CHANGING INTERPRETATIONS OF THE BODY

A concern for the nature of the body is at the very heart of medicine—consequently, the history of medicine calls for an interpretation that sheds light on the history of the body. Such an interpretation, ideally, would bring out essential correspondences between evolving conceptions of the body and progressive conceptions of disease and healing.

This article presents six parameters for interpreting the history of the body as it figured in the history of medical research. I shall concentrate on the advances that distinguish the medicine of the "classical age" from the medicine that began, broadly speaking, in the seventeenth century, and that I call "early modern." But as well as highlighting the limitations of late-modern medicine, I will also touch on some very recent advances—new ways of thinking that begin to define what could be called a "postmodern" medicine.

The following parameters represent not so much dichotomies or dualities but something more like a dialectic or stages of a spiraling progression. As the meaning of the body changes through time, the movement of understanding in each case is toward integration and a transcending synthesis of each pair of parameters. In each case, a new perspective is emerging, forming the basis for a new, postmodern discourse in medicine.

(1) From abstraction to concreteness. The body recognized by medicine in the Middle Ages and early Renaissance was an abstract construct, an

idealized projection of speculative reason, an entity the nature of which was reduced to the logic of an intelligible form. During this period "classical medicine" did not directly look at, nor did it really see, concrete, individual bodies. What it saw, in fact, were confirmations or deviations from disease classifications described in its authoritative texts. It is as if medicine looked at bodies "sideways," making only occasional glances that turned away from the established texts.

However, in the seventeenth century, at the beginning of the modem age, medicine began to think of itself as an empirical science, and it began to insist on the need to understand disease concretely by examining individual bodies. But in the final analysis, what we take to be "concreteness" is only a product of interpretation. Today, as we near the end of the twentieth century (late modernity), medicine is beginning to realize that the "concreteness" of its mechanistic paradigm is not an ultimate truth and that, just as classical medicine projected an interpretive abstraction onto the concrete, lived-in, body, so, analogously, has late modern medicine.

Postmodern medicine is consequently groping toward a new, more adequate concreteness—consistent with the fact that the patient's body is always the site of meaningful experience.

(2) From exteriority to interiority. The body of classical medicine was a very subtle body of humors and dispositions, but the perception of its "nature" conformed more to pre-established classifications than to the truth of its observable condition. By contrast, when, in the early modern period, physicians started really to look at the body, what at first they saw was a gross mechanical body, dense and opaque. The body of early modern medicine was seen as an extremely intricate machine, and it was examined, for the most part, from a very detached, external standpoint. The opening up of cadavers for research and learning was therefore emblematic of a revolutionary change in the way medicine began to look at the body. The once sacred body, surrounded by cultural taboos, suddenly became a worldly machine, a matter of interiority, a profane flesh to be seen into and seen through, a presence conceived as if its mechanisms would eventually be transparent for technological knowledge.

However, late modern medicine has penetrated so deeply into the invisible interiority of the flesh that it has begun to abolish the notion of a boundary separating the body's exterior and interior reality. Body and environment are not only inseparable, they are in continuous interaction and in continuous interdependence. Current research into the logic of the body's immune processes has already signaled the beginning of a postmodern discourse.

(3) From qualities to causalities. Classical medicine (influenced by early Greek philosopher-physicians such as Hippocrates in the fourth century BCE) thought of the body as an association of qualities, a substance timelessly qualified by its various states and conditions. By contrast, anatomical pathology initially promised the possibility of penetrating the density of the flesh and finding "first causes" for all diseases. However, as late modern medicine has strictly followed out the logic of its explanatory models, it has increasingly found them inadequate. The very precision of its principle of causal agency, the very power of its explanatory work— and, subsequently, the very successes it celebrated in understanding and controlling diseases caused by bacterial infections—has enabled it to continue revising the simple concept of agency. Now this principle can be given up. Medical knowledge has advanced far enough to conceive a postmodern alternative.

Better models were eventually found. In responding to virus epidemiology, late modern medicine has finally been able to reconceptualize the principle of simple agency in the language of host environments, communicative systems, interactive fields, local economies, and planetary ecologies.[2] Ultimately, the infectious cultures of biology and epidemiology cannot be isolated from their larger social and political cultures, and so causal explanations cannot be confined to the activities of isolated agents. For modern medicine, the body exists in time and space, a continuous succession of physical states, conditions medicine has long attempted to explain by a causality of spatiotemporal proximities.

But late modern medicine is increasingly finding itself compelled to abandon its model of simple causes and to work out a new model of multifactoral influence: a model for which the network, rather than the straight arrow, might be an appropriate symbol.

(4) From states to processes. Early modern medicine abolished the old Aristotelian logic of qualities and set out to understand how the body it was looking at actually works. In its earliest phase, it saw structures and it submitted the body to structural differentiation, concentrating on

describing its structural complexity (for example, the layout of the organs). This structuralism may be characterized by saying that late modern medicine increasingly attended to the body's functional complexity and differentiation. By pushing this mechanistic research program to its limits, however, late modern medicine has recently begun to move to a postmodern discourse (a way of thinking and talking about medicine) that can recognize both states and systemic processes. Even so, it should be noted that such a discourse has not yet abandoned an essentially mechanistic way of thinking—and that, in point of fact, very little systems-theoretical thinking in medicine has as yet been driven by the logic of its research to give up the powerful resources of mechanism.

I am not proposing here the total abandonment of mechanistic thinking. However, (a) we must take care not to blur the essential distinction between mechanistic and nonmechanistic models, and (b) we must acknowledge that almost all systems-theory discourse today is still operating within the mechanistic paradigm that has prevailed since the beginning of modernity in the seventeenth century. Moreover, (c) we should continue to work with this paradigm, pushing it to its limits and seeing how far we can proceed by its light. This is the only way we have to get beyond it.

Nevertheless, (d) we should also at the same time hold ourselves open to alternative possibilities, exploring, in particular, the possibility of systems-models that are not based on mechanistic principles.

(5) From analysis to holism. Whereas classical medicine conceptualized the body as an organic whole, but only abstractly and only in terms of a pre-established system of categories, modern medicine (in both its early and its late phases) has conceptualized the body more concretely and empirically, but also more mechanistically and more analytically, as a totality of discretely functioning parts.

However, finally able to take up the organicism circulating in cultural discourse since the late nineteenth century, recent medicine has been laboring to use its analytic knowledge as a basis for understanding the body, once again, in more systemic terms and as an organic whole. The age of postmodern medicine may be said to begin with a theoretical and clinical commitment to the process-holism of systemic understanding.

(6) From mechanical isolation to systemic integration. Whereas classical medicine thought of the body as an instance of the sacred whole, a register of the cosmological order, early modern medicine could only begin to understand the body empirically and concretely by making it totally profane—reducing it to a mechanism isolated from the surrounding world: something essentially, or virtually, self-contained and self-sufficient. Recently, however, late modern medicine has begun to restore the body to the larger world-order. With increasing success, it has tried to see the body as a self-regulatory system whose functioning is dependent on, and inseparable from, the larger world and that consequently can exist only in continuous, psychologically mediated interaction with a complex field of social, cultural, historical, and environmental conditions. Working with this model of the body, late modern medicine has increasingly recognized diseases as meaningful epidemiological processes belonging to distinctive life-world "economies."

Thus, research programs in epidemiology are now coming together with research programs in the logic of endocrine and immune processes to establish the need for a postmodern medicine capable of understanding the body in all the dimensions of its systemic integration.

SEVEN MODELS OF THE BODY

Each of the previous parameters can serve as guides for assessing how conceptions of the body have progressively changed through time. This progression demonstrates the historically indisputable power of mechanistic and analytic thinking. But the evolutionary implications of mechanistic models and analytic logic have now been followed out to a point where their inherent limitations are finally becoming apparent. Present research suggests that the future of medicine requires a different logic: a new direction in thinking that is more organic and integrative.

The historical progression points in the direction of a fundamental paradigm-shift.[3] To understand the significance of this change and to sense the new direction it implies, the history of medicine may usefully be conceptualized by reference to a succession of "bodies." If it is possible to speak of an evolutionary logic, a history marked along the way by paradigm-shifts in models of the body, perhaps the seven models proposed in the remainder of this article will contribute to our understanding of the history of modern and contemporary medicine.

(i) The rational body. The body we find represented in the discourse of classical medicine was essentially a rational body, a body pictured in conformity to an aesthetic of rational intelligibility, a sacred and universal body replicating the larger cosmology.

(ii) The anatomical body. By contrast, the body that emerged in the clinical and discursive practices of early modern medicine was essentially an anatomical body, a body understood in purely structural terms, a body of organs, displaying the sites for the ancient theory of humours.

(iii) The physiological body. Increasingly, though, as knowledge dared to penetrate the veil of the skin and explore the interior it conceals, the body that figured in medical discourse was a physiological body, a body-machine whose structures were seen as mechanisms and required mechanical explanations of their functions.

(iv) The biochemical body of cells and molecules. Making use of old and new technology, analytic medicine began to invade the invisible nature of the flesh, looking with a microscopic eye into the most minute structures of the skin, the musculature, and the organs and accordingly representing the body as an intricate network of tissues. Yielding to even deeper, even more analytic, more atomic methods of probing, the body of tissues disclosed itself to be a differentiated cellular body, ultimately analyzable into molecular interactions. Because late modern medicine has faithfully and relentlessly followed out the logic of its analytic, atomic method, and new techniques of research have made possible even more subtle forms of analysis, the body of cells was in its turn disclosed as a gross body, concealing a body of much more subtle nature: a body of biochemical processes. The breakthrough to this dimension brings us into the present. It represents a great achievement—and discloses the latest implications—of analytical medicine, the research program whose mechanistic logic has governed medicine ever since the seventeenth century.

(v) The psychosomatic body. In the early years of this century, however, psychosomatic medicine, encouraged by the contributions of psychoanalysis to our understanding of hysterical conversions, introduced a representation of the body that, for the first time, attempted—albeit with

only limited conceptual resources—to break away from the analytic methodology, to break out of mechanism, to break through the ontology of distinct minds and bodies, and to think of the body of medicine in a radically new way.

However, one limitation that has hobbled psychosomatic discourse comes from the fact that, while advocating the unity of mind and body, it has failed to overcome the dualism that isolated this unity from its environment, nature, society, and culture. There is also a second and more fundamental limitation, which comes from the fact that it has not sustained the courage of its original intuitive conviction: It talks boldly about a psychosomatic whole, but it limits the conceptual reference of "psychosomatic" to a very small range of cases and instances. If what we have been calling "mind" and "body" are really one, then all diseases, without exception, are and must be "psychosomatic." But the discourse of psychosomatic medicine has never been prepared to support such a radical and consequential thesis. It has required a new generation and a new discursive formation to conceptualize and demonstrate this point. Only now, with the development of psychoneuroimmunology, can the science of medicine begin to represent the body as a psychosomatic unity integrated into its environments and begin to articulate the networks of causal correlations implied by this representation.

(vi) The body of psychoneuroimmunology. Now, as we approach the beginning of a new century, revolutionary research into the logic of immunocompetence is realizing the vision inaugurated by psychosomatic medicine, making visible a body of extraordinarily subtle functions and processes. This dynamic, synergic body is seen as a system functioning in a larger system, a multifactoral network of causes and effects, in which effects can also become causes. This body cannot be represented as a "substance." It has become necessary to represent it, rather, as a system of organized processes, intercommunicating and functioning at different levels of differentiation and integration.

A growing body of evidence supports a new concept of disease and a much broadened understanding of epidemiology, according to which diseases do not take place in an environment conditioned only by the forces of nature, but occur, rather, in a field of communication—a world of social, cultural, and historical influences and meanings. Thus, epidemiologists and immunologists are beginning to understand that the individual body is also a social body and is therefore inseparable from the social and cultural life of populations.

(vii) The body of experienced meaning. Psychoneuroimmunological research represents a growing body of evidence pointing to the day when medicine will be able to understand how the diseases afflicting us, as well as the body's processes of healing, are sensitive to the effects of bodily experienced meaning, and how, more generally, processes of disease and healing are correlated with experienced meanings. The body that would correspond to this achievement is the body of psychoneuroendocrinology: the body now being brought to light by neurological, immunological, and epidemiological research—the first medical body subtle enough to promise the possibility of testable correlations with the phenomenological body of experienced meanings.

For the first time, medicine is equipped with a discourse capable of formulating very specific correlations between (a) the patient's bodily experienced meanings and (b) conditions or states of the medical body, the body that figures in the research and clinical practices of medicine.

However, it must be noted that medicine's success in making such correlations does not depend only on advances in medical knowledge. It also depends on the ability of patients to fine-tune their embodied awareness, their sensitivity to processes of bodily experiencing, and their skillfulness in carrying those processes forward into more articulate, more discriminating meanings. For many centuries, Western culture has denied recognition to this ability and consequently made it very difficult for people to enjoy contacting and working with their body's felt meanings the intricate meanings carried by their bodies in co-responsiveness to particular situations and circumstances. At long last, however, our culture has begun to recognize, to legitimate, and to facilitate this natural skill. As experienced-meaning processes become more subtle, more intricate, more discerning, it is reasonable to expect that there will be an increasing convergence between the body of medicine and the body of lived experience, due as much to the learning of this skillfulness in articulating bodily-felt meanings as to the achievements of systemic, postmodern medicine.

THE BODY OF LIVED EXPERIENCE

To sum up: The convergence between the body of medicine and the body of experience will be greatly enhanced by a recognition that the human body is more than a biological organism, more than a physical substance—that is, it is also, in short, a "discursive formation." It is inherently organized in terms of intercommunicating processes, and it is shaped or formed by the evolving historical interpretations with which it interacts.

For medicine, the recognition of the body as a "discursive formation" means (a) that it relinquishes the epistemological assumption of naive realism (the assumption that its concepts are observer-neutral and correspond to a totally independent, objective reality); (b) that it comes to terms with its status as a hermeneutical (an interpretive) science; and (c) that its relation to the entity it calls "the body" is mediated by a network of historical assumptions and representations that are never more than provisional and tentative and remain always open to reassessment.

By the same token, insofar as patients themselves begin to understand their bodies in this new way, they too will be freed from counterproductive conceptions of the body and may begin to realize the extent to which the body that they present to medicine for diagnosis and treatment is a body of meaningful experience, a body of significant intelligence, inherently informed about itself, a body the very nature of which can be profoundly changed by virtue of each patient's sensitivity and embodied awareness, and his/her own skillfulness in articulating the body's carried meanings.[4]

NOTES

1. The human body, therefore, may be considered a "discursive formation" (to borrow terminology from postmodern philosopher Michel Foucault). Essentially, this term means that what in fact we call "the body" is in part a product of social discourse—it is formed or shaped by the interaction of the biological organism with socialization processes. (See *The Order of Things: An Archaeology of the Human Sciences* [Pantheon, 1971] and *The Archaeology of Knowledge* [Harper & Row, 1976].) Foucault succumbed to AIDS in 1984. At the time of his death, he occupied a chair in the History of Systems of Thought at the prestigious Collège de France.

2. See Roger Levin, "Cancer and the Self. How Illness Constellates Meaning," in David M. Levin (editor), *Pathologies of the Modern Self: Postmodern Studies on Narcissism,*

Schizophrenia and Depression (New York University Press, 1987). I want to acknowledge Roger Levin's crucial collaboration in the preparation of this paper, and to thank my friend Wayne Hening, now doing research in the neurology of motor disorders at the Veterans Administration Hospital in Lyons, New Jersey, for his very helpful comments. I also want to give thanks to Don Johnson, Director of the Somatic Psychology Program at the California Institute of Integral Studies, San Francisco, and of the Somatic Research and Education Programs at Esalen Institute, Big Sur. The collaboration on this paper began in June 1988 with George Solomon, thanks to a seminar that Don Johnson organized at Esalen.

3. The shift from structural accounts to functional explanations was an important development, but these functional explanations are still conceived in mechanistic terms; they do not call the mechanistic paradigm into question. In this sense, structural and functional approaches are not as different as they have commonly been thought to be. Although even research programs formulated in terms of processes, systems, and energy can be—and indeed have been—conceived in such a way that they, too, continue the mechanistic paradigm, some current research seems to indicate the need for a genuinely new paradigm, formulated in terms of systems and processes that would be understood nonmechanistically.

4. For a more specific, more concrete formulation of what I mean by a call for self-developing practices and learning processes that work with the body as a "discursive formation," see Eugene Gendlin, *Focusing* (Bantam, 1981); "A Philosophical Critique of the Concept of Narcissism," in David M. Levin (editor), *Pathologies of the Modern Self* (New York University Press, 1987); "Experiential Psychotherapy," in Raymond Corsini (editor), *Current Psychotherapies* (F. E. Peacock, 1973), 1st edition only; and "Experiential Phenomenology," in Maurice Natanson (editor), *Phenomenology and the Social Sciences* (Northwestern University Press, 1973).

Breathing, Moving, Sensing, and Feeling: Somatics and Integral Medicine

DON HANLON JOHNSON

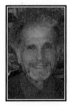

THE EDITORS OF THIS COL-
lection rightly argue that a truly
Integral Medicine needs to include subjective experience. And yet, we are
surrounded by sobering contemporary and historical instances where
subjective experiences—personal and social—are misleading and often in
serious error. What we feel is "just right," what we hunger for, see clearly
in front of us, and fervently value are shaped within a matrix of an impoverished and often perverted education of sensibility. F. Matthias Alexander,
creator of the Alexander Technique, put the problem in stark relief, arguing that "trusting the body" is impossible when we have been brought up
in a culture of distorted bodily experiences. The unreliability of subjective experience becomes even more problematic in the face of serious

illness, where disorientation combined with a desire for cure cuts even deeper into the reliability of our individualistic experience. And yet, without the ancient and wise knowing of the situation that is carried by the body, objectivist analysis alone leaves behind the most important healing factors.

It is within this context of providing a more rational basis for dealing with subjective experience that the wide variety of works, which many now call "Somatics," has particular relevance.

SOMATICS IN HISTORY

"Somatics" was a word coined by the late Thomas Hanna, playing on its classical Greek origins in *soma*, used to signify the whole person, the term used by Paul, who argued that the essence of Christianity lay in the transformation of a raw secular body, *sarx*, into the immortal body, *soma*, of the Christian community.[1] Hanna, by profession a philosopher, was particularly inspired in that definition by the vision proposed by the founder of phenomenology, Edmund Husserl, in the early years of the twentieth century. Seeing the deleterious effects of the Western intellectual removal of subjective experience from the realm of science, Husserl proposed a "somatology," a new science that would integrate a methodical study of subjective experiences of the body with the objectivist sciences.[2] To do that, he argued, required a discipline that would face the rigors of sorting through bodily experience in such a way that one would gain some degree of trust in outer and inner sensations and bodily feelings based on a cultivated discernment between relatively clear experiences of the world and the cloud of obsessions, addictions, and other sensible confusions.

Hanna's earlier, groundbreaking *Bodies in Revolt*[3] was a reflection on a series of thinkers who represented an organized resistance to the mind-body dualism infecting Western thought—Darwin, Freud, Konrad Lorenz, Piaget, Wilhelm Reich, Kierkegaard, Marx, Ernst Cassirer, Albert Camus, and Maurice Merleau-Ponty. Hanna argued that the complex of ideas set in motion by these figures set the stage for a radical revolution in the way our culture thinks about bodily existence, and shapes institutions rooted in that thinking. He went on to link these theoretical analyses with the practical works of people like Moshe Feldenkrais and Charlotte Selver in his new journal *Somatics*, the first public forum in which practitioners of individual schools could engage in a public dialogue. He wrote a seminal series of essays on the unity of the field, using the neologism "Somatics" in contrast to the more common usage "somatic" (an adjective synonymous with "physical" or, more technically, "the musculoskeletal frame of the body") to define the field as the study of first-person bodily experience, in distinction to biomedical sciences of third person, object-bodies.[4]

Hanna's journal and neologism were the first steps in making it clear that there was already in place an old and widespread movement whose focus was on the systematic exploration of bodily experience: methods of breathing, moving, touching, and directing awareness to specific bodily parts and processes.

From the mid-nineteenth century until the beginnings of World War II, there was a vibrant counterculture of the experiential body widespread throughout Western Europe and the Eastern seaboard of the United States. It was set in motion by a number of teachers who traveled back and forth between Northern Europe and the Eastern Seaboard of the United States: François Delsarte, Genevieve Stebbins, Bess Mensendieck, Leo Kofler, and Emile Jacques-Dalcroze, to name a few.[5] These people shared a new vision of embodiment that was at odds with the dominant models found in classical ballet, physical education, religion and biomedicine. Instead of training dancers and athletes to shape their bodies to fit a preconceived highly defined classical form, they encouraged individual expressiveness and a return to a more "natural" body. Rejecting biomedicine's and religion's separation of the human spirit from a mechanistically conceived body, they envisioned an intimate unity among moving, breathing, sensing, health, and spiritual consciousness. At a time when medical doctors were still practicing the crudest uses of surgery and medication, the practitioners of various branches of gymnastics were engaged in sophisticated healing work using expressive movement, sensory awareness, sound, music, and touch.

An early pioneer of this movement was François Delsarte, born in 1811, a Parisian actor and director of a school of drama. Under the pressure of his job teaching actors, he became fascinated with how certain movements could be expressive and others inexpressive. He gradually developed a method that emphasized the relationship between movement and breathing. He was such a failure in Paris that he decided to emigrate to New York around 1860, where he soon gained a number of students, including Steele McKay and Genevieve Stebbins. In the last years of his life, Delsarte returned to Paris, where he died in 1871, forgotten and alone.[6] Stebbins, meanwhile had managed to gain such wide acceptance for the work that two German women, Hede Kallmeyer and Bess Mensendieck, heard about it and came to New York to study with Stebbins. They took the work back to Germany, where they developed their own systems. Mensendieck's work once again crossed the Atlantic where it eventually became the basis for the widely influential posture training method used in East Coast prep schools and private universities. (For some three decades, before-and-after-photos of upper-class boys and girls in the buff were taken and subjected to analysis by William Sheldon for his visual studies of the human form. They were also widely traded among the Ivy League schools, until the salacious underground activity reached the news media and was stopped.)

Leo Kofler emigrated from Switzerland to Kansas in the late 1800s, where he contracted tuberculosis of the larynx. When he gained a position as organist and choirmaster at St. Paul's Chapel, Trinity Parish, in New York in 1877, he consulted a throat specialist, who inspired him to immerse himself in studies of the anatomy and physiology of the larynx, the voice, and respiration. Out of those studies he healed himself and developed a system for exploring the relationships between what he identified as "natural" breathing and voice. He described this system in his work *The Art of Breathing*, translated into German in 1897 by Clara Schlaffhorst and Hedwig Andersen, who used it as the inspiration for their Rotenburger School.[7] That translation has persisted through 36 editions, and the School still flourishes in Germany. Significant for what it indicates about American intellectual interest in this kind of serious bodily exploration is the fact that the book rapidly passed out of print in English. A third major figure in the early stages of this movement was Émile Jacques-Dalcroze, a musician who lived in Geneva and developed a method of education based on combining rhythmic movements with music. In his Hellerau School, he counted among his students Rudolf von

Laban and Mary Wigman, who were among the principal creators of movement therapy and modern dance.[8]

The World Wars loom large in the shaping of this movement. Before and between the two wars, Western Europe had witnessed the origins of a widespread practical and theoretical critique of the concretization of body-mind dualism in medicine, education, philosophy, and the bodily practices of dance, exercise, and sports. The first war rent the international and interdisciplinary community of dancers, physical therapists, craftspeople, artists, and scientists, leaving various schools of body-teaching intact but more isolated. The rise of Hitler and Stalin had a devastating impact on this movement. In addition to their racist ideologies, which took the lives of many innovators in this movement and radically displaced others, the two engineered severely puritanical measures against the sensuality of the expressive body practices. Many of the pioneers had to flee from their homelands, dispersing throughout the Americas and Australia. The public collaborations were finished for the time. Refugees like Charlotte Selver, Carola Speads, Wilhelm Reich, Fritz Perls, and Marion Rosen went from being active participants in a vital cultural movement to practicing their work in isolation with handfuls of students, while trying to gain a financial foothold in their new and unfamiliar homes by practicing what looked like physical rehabilitation or psychotherapy.

In addition to the scars left by Fascism and Communism, there was another unforeseen by-product of the wars that accounts for the dramatic decline in the intellectual and scientific value placed on first-person experiential knowledge of the body. The enormous stores of money and intellectual talent brought to bear on the creation of weaponry and detection devices had the unforeseen results of electronic technologies that would revolutionize biomedical research. New possibilities of exploring the submicroscopic interstices of the living body by advances in electronic imaging devices enabled researchers to produce a practical science of the object body to an extent unimaginable before the wars. While the increase in knowledge of the object-body, supported by rapidly growing funding and institutional culture, provided one of the most dramatic stories of the postwar era, practices for furthering the experienced body remained on the sidelines.[9] There was indeed a vital subculture of dance, massage, and exercise, but they had little effect on the intellectual climate.[10]

In the 1960s the proliferation of growth centers, such as Esalen Institute in Big Sur and Omega in New York, and a counter-culture exploring different states of consciousness provided the opportunity for re-gathering the lineages that had been dissipated in the violence of the wars. A new cooperative venture began to form. Some of the old pioneers, like Charlotte Selver,[11] Alexander Lowen,[12] Moshe Feldenkrais,[13] and Ida Rolf,[14] traveled westward from the East Coast and Europe, gathered large numbers of students, established formal trainings and certification programs, and often eventually brought their teaching back to its sources in Europe where it had been forgotten. (I remember a revealing moment about this circular trajectory when I was teaching at a growth center in Berlin in the 1980s and mentioned Ilsa Middendorf to the local participants. She had been teaching a sophisticated breathing work there for over 50 years. Her technique is well-known in San Francisco, where she has a popular training center and annually gives well-attended public workshops, with her writings published in English. None of the Berliners in my workshop had ever heard of her.)

Although the United States was a politically safe refuge, mainstream scientists and intellectuals were not so receptive to the work of these scattered teachers. Until the early 1920s, the medical climate of the United States included a robust variety of healing modalities associated with the founding democratic ideals combined with a rejection of European intellectual formalism. Old World folk practices brought here by immigrants, Native American healing methods, midwifery, homegrown osteopathy and chiropractic, and herbalism were among the few modalities that flourished here. At that time, John D. Rockefeller and Andrew Carnegie commissioned Frederick Gates and Abraham Flexner to purify the protean medical practices and establish the hegemony of the single model of European academic medicine based on a mechanistic view of the body conceived as separate from the soul. State by state, Flexner and Gates went about lobbying for the passing of laws outlawing those practices that were judged to be at odds with this imported biomedicine. Under constant threat of persecution for practicing medicine without a license, the many teachers of body practices were confined to quiet teaching and work in anonymous offices and studios far from the public dialogue, often living for years within blocks of one another without any contact. In this environment, somewhat like an alchemical alembic, the various works did indeed simmer quietly, with skills being honed, goals purified. But they had little, if any, effects on the larger culture.

The 1960s saw the beginnings of a regathering of the fragments dispersed by the war. Charlotte Selver, who died in 2003 at the age of 102, is a clear example of how this happened. As a young woman teaching in Heidelberg, she had been an active participant at the height of the gymnastic movement between the wars. She had gone to the summer rallies of the Wandervogel where she encountered the Sensory Awareness work of Elsa Gindler, who became her teacher. She taught at the Bauhaus during the fertile Weimar period and finally left Germany for New York in 1938, when her university required her to wear the Jewish star. Supporting herself by cleaning apartments, she slowly worked her way into the intellectual community of New York and began teaching her work more publicly, attracting the support of better-known refugees like Erich Fromm. Alan Watts, then on his houseboat in Sausalito, heard of her work, invited her to California, and introduced her to the fledgling Zen community and to Esalen Institute, where she became the first in a long series of teachers of body practices who would offer regular workshops there: Moshe Feldenkrais, Ida Rolf, Alexander Lowen, Anna Halprin, Gabrielle Roth, Ilana Rubenfeld, Judith Aston, Bonnie Bainbridge Cohen, Emilie Conrad, Fritz Smith, and a host of others. In the final decades of her life, she was warmly welcomed back to Germany, where she once again took up the broken lineage of Gindler's teaching.

During the 1960s and '70s, the scars resulting from the postwar fragmentation of these various schools brought about a cultish attitude, which was redolent of the theological disputes of the late Middle Ages, almost surreal in specificity about body parts. Ida Rolf dismissed F.M. Alexander as having the third lumbar and third cervical vertebrae move back too far from an imaginary vertical plumb line through the body; Moshe Feldenkrais argued that it was futile to work on body structure, which could only be changed through changing function, and jokingly characterized Rolfers and Aston-Patterners as people who were devoid of imagination about all the possible ways one might move. Rolf and Aston countered that functional changes were trivial and evanescent. Reichians argued that Rolfers and Alexander teachers were like crazed arborists crashing into forests to straighten out the redwood trees. Charlotte Selver disdained them all as vulgar and insensitive louts. Most of them argued that psychotherapy and spiritual teaching were made irrelevant by their practices, since emotional health and enlightenment could now be attained by improving the flow of cerebrospinous fluid, aligning the body with gravity, indulging in better sex, introducing more flexibility into the joints, or just paying attention to the sensations of a banana in one's mouth. Ida Rolf often said, "There ain't no psychology; just biology." The claims of each bordered on a megalomania bred of isolation. Not only did they reject the methods of their peers, they also disdained older practices from other cultures, such as hatha yoga and tai chi, which they considered anachronistic. It was a collection of body churches, each arguing dogmatic superiority.

At the same time, members of the more unified and mainstream biomedical community were publicly dismissing these works as modern instances of quackery and predicting their rapid demise.

What happened in the late 1960s and throughout the 1970s was something akin to the contemporaneous ecumenical movement among the world religions, with its weakening of dogma by biblical hermeneutics, cultural anthropology, and frank dialogue. This collection of idiosyncratic inventors suddenly found themselves in the same dining rooms at growth centers and conferences, sometimes crowded around tables with undesirables of a competitive school. When they were relaxed and away from their teaching roles, eating and drinking, they found that other very creative and courageous people had ideas about the body that were not all that different from their own and that they too had something important to offer a damaged world. Even when the major figures did not directly interact, they could not avoid thinking about each other because their students were always interacting and posing questions that arose from the different teachings. The primacy of physical structure or function? The need for catharsis or not? Does direct work with the body displace the need for depth psychoanalysis? Is touch inherently intrusive? And like embattled Christians in an increasingly secular world, they began to realize that their differences were trivial in light of the radical gap between their shared vision of the human body and the dominant paradigm.

At this stage, which lasted throughout the 1970s, there was only an inchoate community organized around these practices, formed by students who were cross-training and raising questions about apparent theoretical and practical conflicts among the methods they were studying. But there was little conceptual work moving towards an understanding of what the various works shared. Esalen Institute played a crucial role in bringing together senior teachers and practitioners of the various schools for study seminars, dialogues with humanistic scholars, biomedical researchers, and social scientists. These events led to the publishing of historical and theoretical essays about the field.

With Thomas Hanna's journal, his philosophical essays, and my own work,[15] in addition to the ongoing proliferation of skill-development in different methods of body practice, the conditions were set for the marriage of the two prongs of this movement, practice and theory, issuing in a new field of inquiry.

In 1983, Michael Kahn and I founded the first graduate studies program in the field, which is now located at the California Institute of Integral Study, a fully accredited graduate school in San Francisco. I was invited by State Assemblyman John Vasconcellos to be a member of a three-person task force of the California State legislature charged with revising the laws governing the practice of counseling. That appointment enabled me to make legal space for the incorporation of body practices within the scope of practice of counseling psychology. In 1987, I organized at Esalen Institute the first of many ecumenical seminars in the field, inviting scholars and scientists in many fields to interact with the creators of the major schools of Somatics. Out of the seminars have come an ongoing series of books on the field, co-published by CIIS and North Atlantic Books.[16] The journal, the graduate program, the ongoing study seminars, and the Somatics book series have issued in a dramatic change in the collection of these schools. It is now commonplace for teachers and practitioners to consider themselves as specialists in a more generalized field and to engage in collaborative activities involving shared needs for education and research. There are now a handful of graduate programs in the field, yearly national and international congresses, a professional organization, and a growing body of books and articles.[17]

SOMATICS AND BIOMEDICAL RESEARCH

At this juncture in the history both of Integral Medicine and Somatics, a major challenge is to develop models of research that do justice to the integrity of the methods being investigated, not simply to Somatics methods but to ancient medicines of China and India, classical homeopathy, and other approaches to healing that do not share the mechanistic, dualistic model of the body at the basis of biomedicine. Up to this point, the tendency within the research community has been to take a particular strategy used by practitioners of a school of body practices and subject it to double-blind efficacy studies. For example, a Rolfing pelvic lift or a Feldenkrais sequence are applied to patients with chronic back pain, and the results might be compared to those receiving standard medical treatment, acupuncture, and hatha yoga. The problem with this approach, as seasoned practitioners know, is that any one of such moves taken out of context does not represent the method; it could just as well be a physical therapy intervention or massage. The method of touching the pelvis or shoulder, the time in the process at which it is used, and the qualities of human contact between the therapist and patient are all central factors in the Somatics methods, left behind in empirical studies as currently conceived.

On the side of the Somatics community, until recently there has been a lack of systematized documentation of the works and of organized field notes describing in careful detail the people with whom the works are done, their problems, what happened over time, and exactly what the practitioner did. Only very slowly have such documents been accumulated and organized in such a manner that outside researchers might use them.[18] Another problem is that the dominance of the empiricist mentality in popular culture tempts Somatics practitioners to account for the efficacy of their works in the jargon of laboratory operational concepts, a language that is foreign to them.

What is at issue here is a classic instance of phenomena not yet fully accessible to empirical investigation as it is now modeled but potentially accessible to ingenious methods of research design. The Somatics strategies are widely repeated observable activities that have been embedded in the pedagogical methods of many training schools for 50 years or more, utilized to judge the successful training of thousands of practitioners and to evaluate the efficacy of working with particular kinds of human problems. These learned bodily skills are not in essence psychic, immaterial, or mental. They are empirical realities, involving physical movements, susceptible—in principle at least, if not by currently accessible technologies—to instrumental detection. Although current methods of research design may not be adequate to investigate the full effects of these works, the existence of such repetitive and widely recognized empirical realities holds out the promise of breakthroughs in research methodology, as has always been the case in the history of science, where new phenomena were originally resistant to the old methods.[19]

FINAL REFLECTIONS

Somatics practitioners encourage people to "listen" to the messages of their flesh, to "embrace" their breathing patterns, to "follow" their styles of moving, and to pay attention to the insights that emerge within the movement itself. Frequently, the language of other alternative healing practices—hypnosis, meditation, prayer, relaxation techniques, and guided imagery—reveals a belief that "meaning" or "healing thoughts" come from somewhere other than the depths of the flesh. These modalities do not require a radical—and sometimes uncomfortable—attitude-shift toward the body. Yet it is precisely this radical shift in viewpoint, embracing the body as a repository of wisdom and meaning, that constitutes the heart of the various Somatics methods.

In that profound descent of consciousness into breathing, moving, and sensing, Somatics is similar to Indian, Japanese, and Chinese traditions. The great meditation traditions of Asia, many of which occupy essays in this collection, address the problem of experiential ambiguity by sophisticated methods of sorting through complex states of consciousness to the point where the practitioner begins to gain facility in navigating through various kinds of specific illusion toward glimpses of the real. In these traditions, the emphasis is on purging experience and desire from images, thoughts, inner conversations, and distorted values. They view flesh, blood, and lungs as the raw material to be cultivated by meditation, the martial arts, ethical behavior, and other aesthetic practices to bring about a flowering of intelligence and hopefully wisdom.[20]

Despite differences in method and style among the thousands of today's Somatics practitioners, they share a vision of reality more akin to older, indigenous ideas than to modernist European scientific models. That vision includes an awareness of the significance of natural forms and processes and of the human spirit's interaction with its environment. Although bioenergeticists, Rolfers, and Feldenkrais practitioners may differ as to the effectiveness of specific procedures, they all share the assumption that sensing, feeling, breathing, moving, postural changes, and excitation are crucial factors in the human search for meaning. Whether a client is being probed by a Rolfer's elbow, vibrating under a Reichean's palm, or trying to concentrate on the sensual effects of the disorienting Feldenkrais movements, he or she is constantly reminded that the realities categorized under "body" or "mind" are experiential: aching muscles and frayed nerves at one extreme, love and cosmic intuition at the other. Healing takes place in creative interweaving of these extremes.

This practiced intimacy with the body cultivates an intimacy with the cosmos itself, the natural world, the great works of evolution. In that sense, Somatics practitioners have something precious to contribute to those who are joined in resisting the enormous forces afoot that make little of material reality, even to the point of supporting social measures that are destroying the environment, eliminating species, and endangering health.

References for this essay are located on the DVD accompanying this book.

Transformational Surgery: Symbol, Ritual, and Initiation in Contemporary Cosmetic Surgery

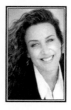

LOREN ESKENAZI

The ultimate goal of human life is accomplished through a series of ordeals of the initiatory type.[1]

MIRCEA ELIADE

THE CONTEXT OF COSMETIC SURGERY

Rites of beauty and rites of passage have been connected throughout the whole of human history. Understanding the larger context of body modification, ancient and modern, and its relationship to humanity's individual and collective growth and spiritual longing provides a backdrop for understanding "cosmetic" surgery and its real and symbolic meaning.

The use of body manipulation as a rite of initiation is recorded as early as 450 BCE by Japanese clay figures with tattoos, piercings in 400 BCE, and plastic surgery as early as 200 BCE. In all cultures at all times in history, humans have sought to alter or enhance their bodies, with virtually no part of the anatomical canvas escaping the creative attention. But at no previous time in human history has the power to recreate our image been what it is today. Early practitioners, wielding blades and brushes, performing piercing, tattooing, molding, binding and scarification upon their peers, never dreamed of the array of possibilities available to the contemporary plastic surgeon.

At the beginning of the twenty-first century, the number of cosmetic surgeries performed continues to grow exponentially and shows no sign of abating. 6.6 million people had cosmetic surgery in 2002; 85% were women, 24% between the ages of 19-30.[2] How are we to understand this phenomenon, which crosses economic, racial and gender boundaries? The rising popularity of such procedures is a phenomenon that we don't understand but are nonetheless quick to judge.

For a country passionately and single-mindedly devoted to self-improvement in all of its forms, our cultural attitudes toward cosmetic procedures are usually hostile or ambivalent, a river fed by many streams. The ways in which we disapprove of cosmetic surgery have historical roots and may indeed prevent us from seeing the larger context in which it belongs. I see those attitudes reflected in the waiting room of my practice, where half of my patients are women who are facing breast cancer and now look forward to restoring their bodies and moving on with their lives as healthy women. The others are women in search of something our culture decrees is more elusive, less necessary, more compromising—the benefits bestowed by less cumbersome breasts, a more shapely body, and a straighter nose. More than half of my patients consciously and freely choose to have their bodies altered.

Because our culture's ideas about self and selfhood locate the essence of what we are on the inside, we tend to ignore the profound transformative power of body alteration. Our western perspective is influenced by the Cartesian divide; we talk about mind, soul, and spirit, identifying them wholly as separate from the corporeal. We primarily locate our identity on the inside and see the body as no more than an envelope or a surface that presents itself to the world. Cosmetic changes, whether surgical or nonsurgical, are thought to deal only with surface, leaving the essence or "self" unaffected. In addition, our society tends to believe that only inner work can lead to true transformation; thus, internal or spiritual change cannot be driven by exterior or superficial alterations.

All of these ideas have historical roots and give rise to a number of beliefs, which marginalize the importance of changes to the surface of the body. Among those ideas are:

- Anything good is worth working for
- Natural is always preferable over man-made
- Any alteration of the body betrays self-love
- The mind is superior to the body (intelligence over instinct)
- The highest spiritual attainment (enlightenment) involves gradually leaving the body behind.

But these ideas shed little light on why millions of Americans each year undergo cosmetic procedures, which entail real risk. Are we to believe they are driven by vanity alone?

The ideas we have about cosmetic alteration create an invisible divide in my waiting room, even though everyone sitting there is in search of transformation and some measure of healing for herself and on her own terms. Half of the women (many with wigs and turbans) have not sought out surgery but have been drawn into it involuntarily by their "disease." These women are on a journey of healing and find themselves suspended between the two worlds of life and health or sickness and death. Our society understands and validates why these women seek out restoration of their bodies as a path to healing their souls. As for the other women who are there by choice and who are apparently healthy, society is far more critical, keeping us from acknowledging, much less accepting, the fact that the surgery offers them "healing" as well.

NOT JUST SKIN DEEP

As a physician and healer schooled in the Western paradigm, my own training defined "healing" within a strict set of confines. My own surgical training encouraged a disconnection between my mind and body in order to perform optimally under arduous and difficult circumstances. As a surgical resident, I learned to shield myself systematically against the impact of the forces I was both responding to and putting into motion. It was virtually impossible to become technically proficient if one reacted to the emotional and spiritual aspects of each case. According to the medical model I was taught, curing and healing are the same and meant the eradication of symptoms of disease. Medical behavior repeatedly reinforced the notion that a cure should be pursued no matter what the cost. I couldn't have been more misguided.

It was only after my 12 years of medical training, when I had my own surgical practice, that the true nature of healing began to unfold before me. I realized that "curing" entails the eradication of specific symptoms, whereas healing involves the entire individual, socially and spiritually, as well as the physical body. I believe that *healing* means to be made whole, to connect with source, essence, or purpose.

One of my first lessons came unexpectedly, when I treated a patient with Botox, an inert toxin, which temporarily paralyzes the muscles it is injected into. Most people, including myself, view it as an insignificant procedure, a lunchtime dunk into cosmetic surgery, done on a regular basis by people seeking facial rejuvenation. 1.1 million people used it in 2002.[3] It is a body modification of such small proportions and such low risk that I barely considered it to be one at all. But early in my career the experience of one woman illustrated that the internal changes brought about by the smallest of physical changes can be dramatic and important.

Some years ago, a woman in her 30s wearing glasses walked into my office. She complained of the deep furrows between her eyes, which came from years of poor vision and squinting. Although she felt as if it were vain on her part, she did want to know if Botox could help. She had just finished her PhD, and she was about to get married.

I gave her an injection, and when she came back 8 days later, her eyes were puffy and red and she appeared miserable. I was afraid I had inadvertently caused some damage to her eyes. She said that as soon as that muscle became paralyzed many old memories from her childhood started flooding up. She recalled how her parents used to say "quit frowning— you are such a pretty girl when you aren't frowning." These and other memories caused her to cry for 3 days. Her whole body went into an energetic release from the paralysis of this one tiny little muscle—a muscle no bigger than a piece of steak caught in your teeth.

I was astonished and began to wonder: If there is that much memory in one little muscle, what information does the rest of the body hold? My curiosity led me to explore the vast field of somatic psychology and to work with my own body. Slowly, I came to realize that the history of our lives, our joys and sorrows, has been inscribed upon our bodies. Our bodies remember everything from our first breath to our last dream. Many scientific studies have proven that our thoughts can transform our body's chemistry and structure. For example, if we imagine the color "red," our blood pressure and heart rate go up; on the other hand, if we imagine the color "blue," the reverse effect takes place. The idea that thoughts can predictably and reliably change measurable physical variables is the basis of the field of biofeedback. The placebo effect, well-documented in Western medicine, suggests that simply thinking that a medication is working enables the physical response without any medicine being given at all. The intricate connections between aspects of mind and properties of matter, something Western scientists are just beginning to substantiate, have been appreciated in other cultures for centuries. If the mind can change the body, doesn't it seem reasonable to assume that restructuring the body can transform our thoughts and thus affect who we are?

In search of answers to these questions, I began to try to understand the impulses, which existed just below the desire to "look better." Was there a deeper, more profound need that motivated my patients to modify their body, and could "healing" proceed from this type of surgery as well? One simple question revealed a surprising pattern.

I have always asked my patients, "How long have you wanted to make this change in your body?" Most of them will say "several years" or "all my life." It has almost always been at least a year. Then I ask the most important question, "Why now?" Most people have an easy, superficial answer, such as, "Now I can afford it." Yet virtually everyone, on further questioning, is within a year of a major life-transforming event. Face-lifts after divorces, breast reductions before marriage, augmentations after the birth of a child or the accidental death of a husband are just a few of the procedures I perform at the request of my patients. I began to notice that there are few exceptions to this rule, even when the patient may herself not be fully aware of the life change she is undergoing. For example, a woman in her 60s came in for a breast reduction, which she had wanted most of her life. She was in a stable marriage, enjoyed good health, and had a satisfying job; her life was smooth, seemingly without recent or upcoming transition or change. I was baffled until I went to schedule her surgery. She called us back and told us she could not have surgery on the date we chose because her first grandchild was about to be born the same week. This story is typical of the pattern I have noted in most of my patient's lives. The pattern began to suggest a widespread need to celebrate, validate, or authenticate a life change with a mark on the body.

SHEDDING SKIN: INITIATION AND SURGERY

Modern man no longer has any initiations of the traditional type.....thus initiatory themes and urges remain alive chiefly in the unconscious. Initiation remains at the core of any genuine human life... crises, ordeals and suffering, loss and reconquest of the self, "death and resurrection." The hope and dream of these moments is to obtain a definitive and total renewal, capable of transmuting life.[4]

MIRCEA ELIADE

According to the anthropological and psychological literature, human beings have used rites of passage to mark times of major transformations, such as the birth or death of a loved one, marriage or divorce, a major birthday (40, 50, 60, etc.), a major biological change such as the onset or cessation of menses or a serious physical challenge such as an illness or injury. From Navajo baby-naming ceremonies to Burmese coming-of-age rites, from the warrior initiations in Ghana to Egyptian ritual circumcisions, all over the globe and throughout history there are commonalties to these ceremonies. According to Carl Jung, they are part of the collective unconscious, shared by all of humanity.

The psyche is not of today, its ancestry goes back millions of years—individual consciousness is only the flower and the fruit of the season sprung from the perennial root beneath the earth.[5]

CARL JUNG

What are we doing in our modern Western society to mark these times? In America we are gradually becoming bereft of meaningful rituals and collective celebrations. Almost everything has become an excuse for greater materialism. We are substituting possessions for connections, and most of us no longer live in stable larger communities that affirm our identities. Most life passages go virtually unrecognized and unwitnessed by all but the few individuals in the inner circle of immediate family and friends, a small, sometimes non-existent group. Seen in this context, my patients' decisions to alter their bodies in conjunction with major life changes—whether they consciously acknowledged the connection or not—opened my mind to new understanding. As I learned more about how humanity culturally and historically venerated and revealed the meaning of these passages through ritual, I had another remarkable realization.

Many years into my daily practice of surgery, I realized that the steps used in the enactment of a surgical operation mirror in pattern and sequence those used in rites of passage, which the anthropologist Mircea Eliade and others have delineated. The parallels between the two sequences, both on the literal and symbolic level, are indeed remarkable.

Summary of the Initiatory Sequence (Rites of Passage)
- A crisis, social or individual
- Fasting and contemplation (separation)
- Purification and stripping off outer life
- Voluntary entrance into sacred space
- Death/rebirth sequence
- Blood or sacrifice ritual
- Regeneration/rebirth

Surgical Sequence
- An illness, accident, or other potential life-changing event
- Fasting (NPO—nothing by mouth the night before)
- Purification and cleansing
- Remove garments of outer life
- Enter an inner sanctum (operating room)
- Lay down on an altar (operating table)

- Undergo a death/rebirth (soma/anesthesia)
- Healing /rejuvenation

Just as in an initiation rite, wherein the initiate is removed from outer life and is cleansed with smoke, water, blood or other means, we ask our patients to fast and to cleanse themselves with antibacterial soap the night before. The initiate is stripped naked and redressed in ritual garments, and our patients must take off their street garments and wear a special, albeit humiliating, hospital gown. Initiates often engage in an elaborate procession to the temple, church, or sacred ground where the ceremony occurs, and surgical patients kiss their loved ones goodbye and walk down a long hallway and enter the sacred space of the "operating theater." Like the initiate, they willingly lie down on a table, which is the altar upon which the transformation occurs. As most cultures use trance dancing, drumming, or soma (mind-altering drugs) to induce altered states, surgical patients surrender to anesthesia, where they are unconscious and without any control. Often, people are more nervous about the anesthesia than the surgery itself because they are afraid they may not wake up. Certainly unconsciously, they are undergoing a symbolic death and rebirth upon awakening. Surgery is a modern blood ritual enacted for the purpose of healing. After an operation, the community witnesses the scar and knows that the individual has been forever changed.

Victor Turner's perspective, as explained in *Ritual Process,* offers a fascinating description of this sequence. He defines what is called *liminal* space as a moment out of time and social structure in which the neophyte is passive, is helpless, is basically like a tabula rasa.[6] These spaces are identifiable by their otherworldly or dreamlike quality. Examples of such spaces are found in churches, temples or mosques, Aboriginal dreamtime, the shamanic journey states, drug-induced altered states of consciousness. Dramatic theater and the "theater of war" are also cited as examples of liminal space. According to Turner, within liminal space individuals experience an absence of status and a sense of merging with all of humanity. There is humility as the initiate is stripped of everything and learns to accept what is in the present moment, including ecstasy and pain.

One cannot help but remark upon the ritualistic type of behavior involved in the practice of modern surgery in the "operating theater."

I believe this is also a modern version of liminal space. My patients all comment on the eerie feeling they have when entering the operating room. The lights are bright and suspended above the central table (altar). There are many mysterious people dressed in blue, and there are sounds, sights, and smells that are totally unfamiliar. The patient (initiate) finds himself or herself totally vulnerable and exposed in every sense of the word.

For some of my patients, the process they have experienced remains unconscious; others, though, have wanted to pursue the aspect of surgery as a rite of passage on a more fully realized level. To that end, I work as a team with psychotherapists, art and movement therapists, and others to design an individual ritual to perform in the operating theater at the time of surgery. We have adopted our methods from the design of these rituals in different cultures and religions. Since we can't sequester someone for 6 months or call up all his or her elders, we work with the patient's internal landscape, validating it all, including social censure for wanting a "vain" procedure. Depending on what comes out of patients' artwork or dream work, we determine what aspects of their individual lives they are trying to transform. It is my belief that this process is already taking place unconsciously, or the patient would not be seeking elective surgery. Once patients re-frame their surgeries in this context, the process can become truly healing. We have observed that patients bleed less, need less pain medicine, and are much less likely to come back for more procedures. They have a totally different experience because they are less fearful and rejecting of the path they have chosen.

> *It's good to remember these rites of passage mark*
> *the end of who we were and the beginning of who*
> *we will become, and the images that supported us*
> *in our crossing.*[7]

MARION WOODMAN

Although the motivation for seeking surgical transformation is highly individual, often the patient seeking surgery feels stuck in her life. She may want to leave her job or her relationship, or she may be grieving a loss. Sometimes she is trying to move from one role to another—for example, from mother to an elder wise woman, or from wife to seductress or goddess. She feels as if the manifestation of the internal change is not in accord with the representation of her external self.

As a surgeon, I try to see myself like a highly trained shaman or guide. I explain to selected patients that I am simply going to open the door and that they can choose whether to walk through it. Working with my patients in this manner encourages humility about my role in the surgical process because it is obvious to me that the patients choose the healing themselves. The hard work is theirs; I can only encourage them to make the conscious decision to grow and heal.

The forces, which are part of this type of healing, are timeless and profound. Like some unstoppable force of nature, the sheer tenacity of the initiatory drives I have witnessed in my patients leaves me in awe. As Peter Matthiessen has written, "We die and are reborn many times. The passage from one state of being to another occurs not just at birth and death but over and over throughout life.... Rites of passage lift us above our petty existence and make us pay attention to the human transformations that bind us together, link us to the natural world and to the wonder of it all."[8]

LIFE IS DESTINED TO GROW AND TRANSFORM

I believe human beings are longing for connection and that some turn to cosmetic surgery as a way of making their inner transformation concrete and visible. On a simple level, perhaps we feel bigger breasts or a more youthful face will help us to achieve the connection we seek. On another level, I believe this connection is not with a specific individual or object of desire but with the divine essence, independent of how one conceives of it. True healing is the realization of oneself as a being connected to all of life, no longer isolated and alone. Through illness, crisis, and surgery, as well as many other of life's initiations, this universal noetic experience is revealed.

Just as birth and death take us from down the often-painful path from spirit into matter and back again, rituals serve to remind us whence we come and of what we are made. We are no longer constricted in form and separated from God (the One). We are part of it once more, for an interval between dying and being reborn.

For out of nothingness we are not born, and into nothingness we do not die. Existence is a circle, and we err when we assign to it for measurement the limits of the cradle and the grave.[9]

MANUEL ACUNA

References for this essay are located on the DVD accompanying this book.

Healing and Transformation Through Expressive Arts *

ANNA HALPRIN
MICHAEL SAMUELS

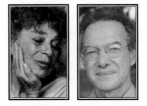

DANCE AS INTEGRAL THERAPY

Anna Halprin

Movement has the capacity to take us to the home of the soul, the world within for which we have no names. Movement reaches our deepest nature, and dance creatively expresses it. Through dance, we can gain new insights into the mystery of our inner lives. When brought forth from inside and forged by the desire to create personal change, dance has the

---

*"Dance as Integral Therapy" is excerpted from Halprin A: *Returning to Health: With Dance, Movement, and Imagery,* Mendocino, CA, 2002, LifeRhythm. "Dance as a Healing Force" is adapted from the chapter by Michael Samuels in Halprin A: *Returning to Health: With Dance, Movement, and Imagery,* Mendocino, CA, 2002, LifeRhythm.

profound power to heal the body, psyche, and soul. Our journey through illness and health, and the power of dance to illuminate the way, is a passionate aspect of my life's work.

I have been using a combination of drawing images, writing about them, and dancing them with children since 1945 as a method for generating creativity in my children's dance classes. I found the process so intriguing that I began to use it with adults. In 1972, I did a drawing of myself in one of my classes and drew a round gray mass in my pelvic region. Partly because I resisted dancing this image, it struck me that there might be something wrong. It turned out that I had drawn my own malignant tumor. I had an operation, and 3 years later a recurrence. This time, I drew a self-portrait to heal myself, and I danced the drawing. Afterwards, I went into spontaneous remission. This may sound strange and unbelievable, but in recent years more and more doctors and therapists acknowledge this phenomenon. The late Dr. Brendan O'Regan, who did his research through the Institute of Noetic Sciences, reported 800 cases of spontaneous remission.[1] It can and does happen; I do not believe anyone knows exactly how.

The new acceptance of the mind-body connection in the healing process builds a bridge between the fields of expressive arts therapy and Western medicine. This bodes well for an integration of both our intuitive and rational knowledge about healing. It is also a way for expressive arts therapies to become more widely accepted and used by people in this culture, who have mostly been conditioned to believe that the mind and body are separate entities that do not reflect upon one another. The history of cancer research reminds us to appreciate the immensity of what we have yet to learn about the impact of the mind-body connection on the course of illness. The next frontier is to begin to explore the impact of expressive arts therapies, especially dance, in the treatment of illness. Dance seems particularly important because it can engage all the arts: movement, drawing, writing, music, and drama. Dance has a highly integrative nature. Exploring this expressive art modality is a beginning step toward reclaiming the healing power of dance.

There is a distinction between "curing" and "healing," which is useful when we approach dance, or any of the arts, as a healing modality. To "cure" is to physically eliminate a disease. In the case of cancer, this is usually done through surgery, chemotherapy, radiation, or other treatments aimed at the physical body. To "heal" is to operate on many dimensions simultaneously, by aiming at attaining a state of emotional, mental, spiritual, and physical health. Healing also addresses the psychological dimension and works with belief systems, whether they are life-enhancing or destructive. It is possible, therefore, that a person with a terminal diagnosis may not be cured but can be healed and, inversely, that someone can be cured but not healed. Taken together, the healing process and the curative efforts of standard medicine support both the expansion and extension of life.

It is, of course, our greatest ideal to be both cured and healed. I recall how, after my operation for cancer, my doctor said to me, "You're just fine now. You are cured of cancer. You can live a normal life as before," and I answered him by saying, "That's funny because I don't feel just fine. I'm scared. I don't know why I was stricken with cancer, or what kind of life I can live right now." I had been cured, perhaps, but not healed. For this reason, I personally encourage people to follow an integrated approach to health that is inclusive of Western and so-called "alternative" medicine. I am very careful to make no claim that expressive arts be used as one's sole treatment for cancer, or even that it extends life. I am certain, on the other hand, that it does expand or transform the quality of life. There is also intriguing evidence that, in some cases, people who undertake healing processes that make sense to them can extend their lives as well as expand them.

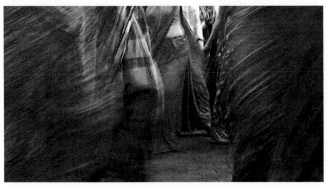

"Saris Dancing." (Courtesy David "Dudi" Shmueli.)

As I began to teach dance sessions in a number of venues, for varying lengths of time and to different sorts of people at various stages of wellness, I noticed that in spite of the differences, a common thread ran through the classes. I was able to identify the four components I believe are intrinsic to this approach to movement, which were included in each session I taught. These are the realms of sensation, movement, feelings/emotions, and imagery. They cannot, in truth, be separated. Movement affects the way we feel; the way we feel affects the way we move. This in turn feeds the images evoked. In working with dance, a holistic art form, our intention is to help the participant understand herself in an integral manner.

DEFINING TERMS

I make a distinction between the words "sensing," "feeling," and "emotion." The dictionary gives a broad definition of "sensation," including "sentiment, emotion, and passion." It also refers to sensation as a way to think of feeling. You might say "feel" this and mean "touch" this. The interchangeability of these words can be confusing. For our purposes, I would like to define the words as follows:

> "Sensing" refers to the physical sensations of the body.

For example, you might ask questions like these to help people bring awareness to their bodies: What do you sense at this moment? Do you sense any tightness anywhere? Do you sense heat or cold in any part of your body? Do you sense your eyelids trembling when you close them? Do you sense your shoulders lifting? Do you sense the difference when you let go and drop them?

> "Feelings" refers to moods, such as grumpy, romantic, upset, impatient, or vulnerable.

> "Emotions" rest behind "Feelings."

They are deeper layers of feelings, such as love, hate, fear, grief, ecstasy, etc. They are the deepest responses we have to our life experiences.

Life/Art Process

A direct type of movement that anyone can do is the basis of this approach. Therefore, the material in each of my classes is accessible to everyone. A larger purpose of this work is to use simple movements that will generate immediate and personal responses. This direct approach to movement enables each person to connect to her or his own creative experience, rather than trying to imitate someone else's. It is the purpose of this work to integrate physical movement with feelings, emotions, personal images, and spirit. It is, in essence, a holistic and integral approach.

When our dances are connected to our real-life issues in this manner, it is called the Life/Art Process. This method of working with dance seeks to access the life story of each person and then use this life story as the ground for creating art. This is based upon the principle that as life experience deepens, personal art expression expands, and as art expression expands, life experiences deepen. I have found this interactive process to be especially effective when applied to people living with cancer. This work is about a way that everyone can discover a healing dance of his or her own though this Life/Art Process.

Sensations

Dance is a medium of the body and our instrument of expression. It helps us become present in many ways. Our first step with this work is to enter and inhabit our bodies. We do this through our senses. Our sensations are the pathway leading us into the body. Before you read further, make a list of the senses.

They are sight, sound, touch, smell, and taste. There are also motor and kinesthetic senses. Invariably, people tend to forget these last two. Did you remember them? If you did, you are the exception. Most people do not, although the kinesthetic and motor senses occupy the largest part of our brains. Perhaps we forget this because these senses have been dulled by the way most of us live. Our lives are dominated by sitting in cars and driving, sitting and watching TV, sitting and working at desks or drafting boards. Sitting, sitting, sitting.... When we walk, it is usually on cement. We wear confining shoes for protection and lose the touch of the earth and the sensations of our feet. In urban centers we must protect ourselves by shutting out the overload of the noise and smells that surround us.

Almost everything in our modern industrialized society denies the life of the body and rewards the life of the mind. Fritz Perls, innovator of Gestalt therapy, had this well-known saying: "Lose your mind and come to your senses."[2] Our usual response to the overstimulation in our lives is to tune out our senses. When we do this, we leave our bodies, and in a way, we leave home, set adrift from the rich world within us. This inner world houses our feelings, our emotions, and our spirit. It holds the memories of our ancestors, our past, our present, and our future. Each of us lives in a body that has taken millions of years to evolve and that will continue to evolve as we pass from one generation to the next. Each of us has a unique body; there is not another one like it anywhere in the universe. And this body is intricately designed to survive. It has wisdom, wonder, and magic in it to perform the great dance of life. Our personal and cultural abandonment of our bodies can create illness and a void in understanding how to regain our health. When we become ill, we may feel that our body, which we have taken for granted, has suddenly betrayed us. At this time, it is crucial to return to our bodies, to return home and reawaken our senses, so that the natural healer within can renew its strength and power.

Movement

When you think of dance and movement, do you think of ballet, a modern or jazz dance, or some other form of stylized movement? Many people are shy about dance because of this association. This is not the way I think of dance movement at all. Dance can be approached as a direct and natural way to move without any personalized aesthetics imposed from an outside authority. Dance is not necessarily graceful, pretty, or spectacular. Dance can be grotesque, ugly, clumsy, funny, frightening, and conflicted. It can stomp, fall, attack, clutch, and reach. It can open, close, tip-toe, crawl, twist, turn, pound, jump, run, or skip. We can move together or alone. We can move backwards, sideways, up and down. Movement is happening everywhere all the time. It is the motion of our cells, the pulse of our blood, the rhythm of our breath. It is, as well, the ocean waves rising and falling and the alternating patterns of night and day. Movement is life, and movement is the source of dance. Any body, no matter how old or young, in whatever physical condition, has a capacity to move, even if it is just your little finger or a movement carried as an image in your mind's eye. No matter what physical condition a person is in, it is important to remember that there is still a possible connection to movement.

THE FEEDBACK PROCESS BETWEEN MOVEMENT AND FEELING

When movement is liberated from the constricting armor of stylized, pre-conceived gestures, an innate feedback process between movement and feelings is generated. For example, try throwing your arms into the air above your head with vigor and say out loud, "I'm so depressed." Now cross your arms over your chest and double over, saying, "I feel so happy." The movement and the emotional feedback between these two things are so incongruous as to seem absurd. Throwing your arms in the air is uplift-ing. It can inspire a feeling of victory and celebration. Doubling over is more congruent to pain or fear.

This feedback process between movement and feelings is an essential ingredient of expressive movement. When you understand this, move-ment becomes a vehicle for releasing feelings that are essential in the heal-ing process. Repressed or incongruent emotions shut down the immune system, causing pain and illness. We are working toward expression and congruency, and understanding movement and feelings in a constantly circulating feedback loop facilitates this process.

Since so much of our ability to experience and express ourselves fully lies in this relationship between movement and feelings, as teachers we need to be careful to offer a broad spectrum of movement possibili-ties. Remember that it works the other way as well: As we develop a broad vocabulary of movement, we have greater freedom to express the way we feel. It is important to keep in mind that in this work, movement is the key player. Our feelings and emotions are channeled into movement.

Imagery

"One of the things about people who are sick is that they have no control of physical reality. Their body is changing without them doing it. So taking a blank piece of paper and putting the image down is the first step towards con-trolling the rest of their life. They are controlling the outer-world."

MICHAEL SAMUELS, MD

The feedback process between movement, feelings, and images operates on a level below words. It is not always possible to understand the content of what we feel, where our feelings come from, or how to apply the feelings that arise to our personal lives. In trying to understand the messages our body is giving us, rather than analyzing or interpreting in a cognitive way, participants make drawings of the images in their mind's eye in response to their movements and feelings. When we draw these images on paper or canvas, they are called *visualizations*. When we connect these images to our movements and feelings/emotions through dance, I call them *Psychokinetic Visualizations.*

The Psychokinetic Visualization Process has three parts. We go inside to find our personal image; we draw it on a piece of paper; and then we take this image into movement, or we "dance" it. When doing this process, participants draw on a piece of paper that is 18" by 22", big enough for them to draw freely, but not so big that the empty space is intimidating. It's amazing how easily people draw in spite of their initial hesitation and lack of confidence. It is as natural to draw as it is to move. A professional, skilled ability as a visual artist is not necessary in this work. In fact, it can sometimes be a barrier to a more spontaneous and real expression. Sometimes, while activating this process, an image may come first and then the embodiment will follow.

Dance

We have looked at movement, feelings and emotions, and imagery under three separate headings. This is misleading because actually the three levels of awareness just described cannot be separated. They function together, though we can focus on one aspect over another when we are teaching. This artificial separation helps us cultivate a larger range in each level of awareness. Ultimately, however, these aspects are integrated. When the three levels of awareness unite in our bodies and through movement, we will make dances with the power to heal. These dances will be special because they are uniquely our own. They come from our direct movements, feelings/emotions, and images, and because of this, they are unique and representative of our lives.

This integration of the three levels of awareness is a process that generates creativity, through the act of dancing. Dance and the creative act are stunning in their application to healing for many reasons:

- Cancer cells are manufactured in our bodies; they are not a foreign invasion from the outside. Just as there are no two people in the world exactly alike, no two bodies are exactly alike. Because of this, cancer cells are also unique to our bodies. This makes cancer difficult to treat: There is no one treatment which works for everyone. Treatment needs to be targeted to the specific needs of the individual. This is a powerful indication that the dance experience needs to be approached as a creative process enabling each participant to express herself, rather than following a preconceived formula or pattern imposed from the outside. When we do our dances and they come from ourselves, they are unique and will adapt to our needs. We can create dances that work for us because they come from our bodies and our particular illness. Dance that is approached creatively allows for and encourages this perfect adaptability.

- Dance as a creative act reaches an important state of objectivity. Over and over, I hear the pain and suffering that participants arrive with when they come to class. When they leave, there has been a great transformation. Something has changed. Through an experience of our creativity, we have the opportunity to break the chain of identifying ourselves with our suffering. We are often released from our identification with our suffering by the creative act of a dance that reveals, externalizes, and clarifies our experience for others to witness. This does not imply denial; it implies a new perspective. I like to think of the act of creation as giving birth to a myth—a primary, life-giving act. Since in creation myths we are all created in the image of God, the great spirit, Allah, Buddha, Shiva, the stars, the earth, the life force— whatever that great mystery is that connects us all to each other, all living creatures and the earth herself—when we dance, we are the mystery and the creative principle.

- Dance engages our whole being. It is, in my opinion, the most powerful of the arts because it is holistic in its very nature. Our body is our instrument. It is immediate and accessible, holding our wisdom and truth. We use all of our senses when we dance.

We move, make sounds, sing, chant, draw, write. Perhaps this is why the anthropologist Kurt Sachs said, "Dance is the mother of the arts."[3] In dance, all the arts are engaged. By experiencing this integration through dance, we can also experience the artist as a whole, integrated person. We are all artists by nature and do not need years of specialized training to be dance-artists. We all move, respond, feel, and create. This is the basic belief in this approach to expressive movement: It is inclusive. Everyone can do it.

SUMMARY

> *"God guard me from the thoughts men think in the mind alone.*
> *He that sings a lasting song*
> *Thinks in a marrow bone."*

WILLIAM BUTLER YEATS

This approach to movement and teaching movement is based on the belief that when we begin to use the language of movement rather than the language of words, a different kind of image and emotion arises, which bypasses the controlling and censoring mind. Words label what we already know; expressive movement reveals the unknown. Sensations, feelings, emotions, and images that have been long buried in our bodies are revealed through movement. This is also useful for shifting old patterns, habits, and destructive belief systems.

At the time of this publication, it is 19 years since I walked into the Cancer Support and Education Center to explore the ways dance and healing are connected. I have learned much from listening to those who have participated; by responding to their fears and terror through dance; by witnessing their anguish and tears through dance; by supporting their confusion and anxiety through dance; by experiencing their grief and loss through dance; and by rejoicing in their courage and victories through dance. I have learned much about the power of groups where everyone coaches and urges a member who falters or is depressed, where each person shares his or her story and, by doing so, adds to each of our stories. There is power in community when people take great risks to show themselves and their illness, and the community responds with loving support. I have done my own dances when I felt saddened by the death of another person in my life or the excruciating joy of one more person's triumphant survival. Through it all, I have always remembered to return to dance as an affirmation of my will to live. I believe this is the strongest lesson I have to impart to people who participate in this work: Dance, and renew your life force.

Teacher or Student

"If I can stop one heart from breaking
If I can ease one life the aching I shall not live my life in vain"

EMILY DICKINSON

Teachers, and therapists of all kinds, we need you. People in the art world—dancers, musicians, painters, sculptors, actors, poets, writers, performance artists—we need you. We need you to turn your practices of art and the imagination into tools for healing. And I believe you need us. Those who have lived through the trauma of facing death gain insight into life. The courage, dignity, and commitment of people who have cancer and other life-threatening illnesses are an inspiration and a lesson to all of us. You may well find yourself as much the student as the teacher.

DANCE AS A HEALING FORCE

Michael Samuels

When I refer to "art" in this essay, I am referring to all of the arts: dance, music, painting, sculpture, story-telling, poetry, architecture, and environment. All of these forms are art.

Art, prayer, and healing: All come from the same source—the human soul. The energy that fuels these processes is the basic force of life, of creativity, of love. Deep within us we have memory of a beautiful place where our spirits were given breath. We are connected to the soul of God in the deepest marrow of our being. By traveling inside ourselves, we can glimpse the deep spaces of our lives, feel them, live in them. We can bring back their memory and their spirit, through art and ritual.

I believe that the voices of the inner world speak to us in a language most similar to art. It is below words, above silence, and close to poetry.

It is God singing and dancing. It is our soul listening. It is the voice of the life force, of expansion and love within us. When we pray, when we travel inward and heal, we can bring back traces of pure spirit. Art and ritual are the voices of the spirit. They are the energy of healing. Art and healing are lovers, tied together with a silver thread and bound irreversibly through time. Today the artist and the healer are feeling the rebirth of this ancient connection. In an age where art has become decorative and lost its spiritual meaning, in an age where medicine has lost its connection to the heart and the intuitive spirit, art and healing can be reunited through ritual to become one again.

If the force is love, and the voice is the soul, its language art and ritual, and its product healing, where are we going? How is ritual coming into the medical center, or healing coming into the artist's studio? Art and ritual are the doorways into the realm of the heart, the tool for transformation we now seek. They are what opens and what changes. When a patient in a cancer ward is visited by an artist, lets herself move into the land of spirit, then lets a piece of art come out into the world and cries and is touched for the first time since she has been in the hospital, a healing has taken place. She has opened her heart to love. Ritual as the vehicle through which an open heart can enter medicine is very real. In love we need a lover and a loved one; in healing we need a healer and a person who needs healing. Here the bridge is art and ritual, the language of love. How do art and ritual heal? How can an image change reality? How does experiencing an image or moving through a dance ritual actually change our body's physiology? We are just beginning to understand the answers to these questions. Let me describe how the body physically and physiologically deals with the phenomena of imagery and movement.

Thoughts, emotions, and images form in different areas of the brain and involve different neurotransmitters. Images of movement and dance are held in areas of the brain responsible for instigating muscle movement. A discharge of neurons comes from both an instigation of movement and its memory. This is experienced by the person as an image of movement coming from her imagination or memory. Since dance involves so many proprioceptive sensory and motor pathways, both imagining and remembering a movement is very real and intense when experienced. The movements are reflected as discharges in areas of the brain that send messages to muscles. Even though the dancer does not move, the proper muscles will respond microscopically. The place where the images of movement are held send nerve messages to the hypothalamus that go out to the rest of the body. Likewise, the movement itself is picked up by the brain and sends messages to the hypothalamus. A dancer sends out messages to her whole body when she moves or remembers a movement. In the areas of the brain that control movement and the memory of movement, nerve cells discharge and images come to life.

The hypothalamus activates the autonomic nervous systems, resulting in the arousal or realization of a "double balancing" system that reaches out to the whole body, touching virtually every cell. The sympathetic branch is the branch of the fight or flight reaction. An image in the big brain of a threat alerts the hypothalamus to cause sympathetic arousal. This speeds up the heartbeat, increases breathing, sends blood to the large muscles, floods the body with adrenaline and hormones, and creates a state of alertness. The memory of moving away from a threat, or facing it and fighting, releases tension and puts the person in a state of release. The stimulation of the parasympathetic nervous system results in relaxation, healing, and maintenance. Heartbeat and blood pressure slows, breathing slows, blood goes to the intestines.

This oversimplified model gives an idea of how the mind is connected to the body, and how muscle movements stimulate the whole body. When a person dances or imagines dancing, the area of the cerebrum that holds images of muscle movement is stimulated and sends messages to the hypothalamus. This allows us to respond to the dance imagery. If the dance image is one of deep joy or release, the body is put in a healing state through the hypothalamic pathways. If it is one of persistent fear or tension, the body remains tense and in the physiology of stress. In addition, the body can bathe every cell in the body with a hormonal flood as the imagery of threat or love lights up the neural nets in the brain. As this flashes through us, the hypothalamus sends messages to the adrenal glands to release epinephrine, adrenaline, and other hormones that go throughout the body and are picked up by receptors in our cells, causing some cells to contract, others to relax, some to act, others to rest. Our entire physiology is changed a second time by an image or dance movement held in our consciousness, and to it we respond.

Another realm is that of the neurotransmitter. Images cause specific areas of the brain itself to release endorphins and other neurotransmitters that affect brain cells and the immune system. The neurotransmitters relieve pain and make the immune system function more efficiently. They make killer cells eat cancer cells, white blood cells attack the HIV virus, and generally change the body's ability to respond to illness. When a person dances, or imagines a dance movement that is freeing or that brings out inner healing images, the body actually changes its physiology in response. A person need not do anything; the body will do it just through the impetus of dancing or imagining movement.

How does healing occur? The resonating body-mind-spirit balances our physiology by the threefold path we mentioned above: thoughts in the brain; autonomic nervous system balance, hormonal balance and neurotransmitter balance; cellular change. What are images, and how do they relate to healing? I divide imagery into two basic types—receptive and programmed. Receptive imagery comes to you, bidden or unbidden, and rests in your mind's eye. It can come onto a blank screen and appear as itself, or it can come over your thoughts and appear mixed. Programmed imagery is different. You choose an image and hold it in your thoughts for a reason. The choice may be deliberate, or you may choose an image that comes to you from a receptive place. Either way, the image affects your world. How does this happen? The image affects your body by the three-fold path. Images affect your world by giving you ideas to plan from, emotional motivation to continue, and meaning. When a person gets an image of the future, then she can make it happen. Magic is the image becoming real in the outer world.

Healers work with imagery by having a patient picture her illness, her healing forces, and the healing process in her mind's eye. First, the patient imagines what the illness looks like in as much detail as she can. Next, she imagines how the body's resources could deal with the visualized illness. This is done as a process over time. Biologically based imagery is effective when it is anatomically accurate and detailed. Researchers have found that when imagery is very specific—a mental picture, for example, of one type of white blood cell—it alone is found to change. Next, patients are encouraged to allow metaphorical imagery to form. This is the state in which little men, dogs, or white light blast, eat, or dissolve blackness, mud, or other little men. This metaphorical imagery often takes place spontaneously after the biological imagery. Finally, patients can hold a programmed image in mind. They can picture themselves healed, surrounded by white light, as God, as a power animal, or being strong and secure.

Healing art can be used by a patient in two obvious ways. The images can be viewed and allowed to change a person's consciousness, or images can be used to help a person visualize the healing process or a healed state. Imagery is healing if it puts a person in an altered state, relaxes her, opens her heart, or gives her energy. Monet's "Water Lilies" paintings were so relaxing that patients would visit them in museums and sit and meditate in front of them for hours. The third way art heals a viewer is by showing patients images that move them. When patients with breast cancer see art, music, or dance made by other breast cancer patients, it opens them up to emotions they may have hidden. This allows them to discuss these emotions with their families, support people, and healers. Patients who have a particular illness are moved by art that portrays other people's experiences with the same illness. It makes them feel connected, relieves isolation, and releases deep emotions. This type of art can be very disturbing for other people to view. This imagery is not for relaxation or transcendence; it is for opening the heart.

All of these kinds of art work by changing consciousness, freeing energy, and awakening the spirit to resonate with the body-mind. They are technologies for using ritual as healing. Imagery can be most powerful when it comes from the inner world of the person who is ill. It is direct, meaningful, and sometimes more effective than other images. However, images made by artists can be so powerful that they can transform, even though they are not personal to the patient.

Throughout recorded history, artists have believed that their images have power in themselves. The shaman was the first artist and healer. The shaman traveled inward, glimpsed the spirits, acted, brought back the healing, and made art. He or she told the tale, crafted the masks, danced the song, and brought the inner world outward through ritual. Shamanic ritual was believed to actually have the power to change the physical world. What is going on now that has caused the growth of ritual and healing worldwide? Why are you reading this book and doing dance ritual as a healing art? Art and ritual as a healing force is being born as we speak. The concept is catching fire, awakening people's spirits. The idea is being born in the world of the artist and the world of the healer. Art in the hospital, or art at the bedside of a person who is ill, is an electrifying experience. It becomes a doorway to the spirit, a vehicle for the opening of the heart. It is integral to healing. There are now artists making healing art purposely. It is a whole new field in art. This work, as I see it, heals the artist or the world. It works by freeing the artist's own healing energy and resonating with her body, mind, and spirit. The artist can also make art to heal another person or a group of people. This is a transpersonal healing, the art of interconnection that joins us at our centers. Thus art heals by releasing the energy of the viewer, relaxing her, allowing something within her to be freed, resonating with her body, mind, and spirit. Another type of art that heals the world is beautifully demonstrated in Anna Halprin's "Planetary Dance" rituals done in and by communities. The artist works with the energy of the whole system, whether it be a neighborhood, an ecosystem, or the planet itself. This art can be ceremonial, environmental, performative, or static. It involves the community, energy, and movement. It is truly shamanic; it balances the world.

The second category of healing art is the art patients create to heal themselves. Art at the bedside, dance with cancer patients, art workshops, art and dance therapy, exhibitions at hospitals, and environments created in healing centers all represent this type. It does not matter whether healing art is made by an artist or a patient. The cancer patient who dances frees her inner artist and her inner healer; the ancient movements allow her to change, physiologically, and spiritually. This is not a passive art form. Healing art is not meant to be watched. It is the life force. This art is made to change reality. It has the power to transform.

We are on the doorstep of a great journey. Anna Halprin's work is one of its first steps. Imagine where we can go from here. Imagine art, music, and dance in every hospital, art for anyone who is ill. Imagine lifting the spirits of someone who is about to die. Imagine being in love.

References for the Halprin essay are located on the DVD accompanying this book.

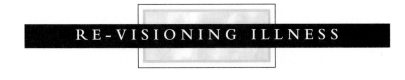

What Does Illness Mean?*

LARRY DOSSEY

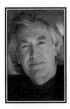

"CANCER IS THE BEST thing that ever happened to me!" This comment, which was not uncommon, never failed to irritate me as a young physician. Although the illness varied, the message was often the same: The disease led to an increase in wisdom and understanding, and held lessons that paradoxically made life better. The illness, it seemed, meant something.

I was not impressed. Humans will stop at nothing, I told myself, to rationalize their plight. When we face problems we can't control, we try to put the best face on them in order to preserve our self-esteem, dignity, and sense of self-worth. My patients were trying to make the best out of a terrible situation. The possibility that cancer could contain positive value seemed absurd.

In the no-nonsense world of internal medicine I inhabited, the concept of meaning seemed a philosophical nicety that could safely be

*From Dossey L: What Does Illness Mean? *Altern Ther Health Med* 1(3):6-10, 1995.

ignored. Meaning might have a place in the dreary libraries of philosophers, but not in coronary care units and oncology wards. Meanings belonged to the mind only; they floated safely above the clavicles and did not influence the rest of the body. If negative, they might cause anxiety or tension, but at most they were a nuisance with no bottom-line consequence. But what of the reports of patients that disease could send people back to the drawing boards of reality and transform their lives?

The meaning of illness is only one sense in which the question of meaning arises in medicine. There is also the issue of whether perceived meanings, once present, can influence health and illness. Are perceived meanings causal? Do positive meanings increase health, and are negative ones harmful? Again, the patients' stories were unambiguous. They were convinced that their perceived meanings, manifesting as thoughts, attitudes, and beliefs, figured heavily in their health.

MEANING AND SCIENCE

It has been difficult to ask these questions in contemporary medicine. Health and illness, we're told, are a function of what the atoms and molecules in our bodies happen to be doing at any given time. They follow the so-called blind laws of nature, which are inherently meaningless. This implies that meaning is something we read into nature, not something that can legitimately be read out of it. The molecular biologist Jacques Monod expressed this point of view in his influential book *Chance and Necessity,* which powerfully influenced a generation of scientists. "The cornerstone of scientific method," he confidently proclaimed, is "... the systematic denial that 'true' knowledge can be got at by interpreting phenomena in terms of final causes—that is to say, of 'purpose.' "[1] For Monod, purpose and the related concept of meaning do not belong in science because they do not exist in the natural world science studies. To believe otherwise, Monod implied, is scientific heresy.

I, like most physicians, accepted this point of view. In fact, I liked it very much. It was clean and unadorned, and it was courageous as well. It demonstrated the principle of parsimony, one of the cornerstones of modern science. It excluded anthropomorphism by refusing to project human qualities and feelings onto the natural world.

But after entering clinical practice, I discovered that it is much easier to hold this view if one is dealing with mitochondria in test tubes than if one is treating sick human beings. Mitochondria don't talk back. What would Monod have concluded, I have since wondered, if he had spent time in an intensive care unit instead of at a laboratory bench? What if he had heard a dozen patients a day tell their stories? Would meaning still have seemed silly? This is not a rhetorical question. Many of the scientists who have interpreted nature as meaningless and purposeless—particle physicists, molecular biologists, geneticists, even mathematicians and theorists—have approached nature at the remotest levels. They have never seen a patient; they have not heard "meaning stories" day after day. Shielded from this data, how can they confidently exclude a role for meaning and purpose at the human level?

'I DO IT WITH MEANING'

I once admitted a patient to the coronary care unit with excruciating chest pain I believed was caused by a heart attack. After his pain had subsided and he was all wired up, Frank, to relieve his boredom, positioned his bedside table in such a way that he could view the cardiac monitor behind him in the flip-up mirror. By the time I went by to see him on evening rounds, he had a trick up his sleeve. "Doc," he said, "keep your eye on the monitor. I want to show you something." Frank closed his eyes. The oscilloscope registered a steady rate of about 80 per minute. Then it fell gradually, settling in the 60s. "Now watch this," Frank said, his eyes still shut. The heart rate climbed slowly into the 90s. Frank beamed. He knew I didn't know what was going on. I checked to see whether he was holding his breath, clenching his fists, or maneuvering in some way to affect his heart rate, but he seemed perfectly placid and relaxed. In the next 24 hours I went to visit him several times. He became increasingly adroit at changing his heart rate, and he seemed delighted that I was perplexed. He was right. I knew that individuals could learn to control their heart rate in biofeedback laboratories, but I knew also that this usually requires a skilled instructor, several sessions, and a relaxed environment. Frank didn't fit this picture. He had learned his skill, without instruction, in one of the most stressful situations imaginable—being hospitalized for a possible heart attack.

Frank's tests were normal; he had not sustained a myocardial infarction. When I went by to discharge him, I said, "I give up. How do you do it?" This was the question he had been waiting for. "I do it with meaning," he said. "If I want my heart rate to fall, I close my eyes and focus on the chest pain. I let it mean to me that it's only indigestion or perhaps muscle pain. I know it's nothing; I'll be back to work tomorrow. If I want to increase the heart rate, I switch the meaning. I think the worst: I've had a real heart attack, I'll never get back to work, I'm just waiting around for the big one."

I was impressed. Frank had turned the cardiac monitor into a meaning meter, which was giving a direct readout of the impact of perceived meaning on a crucial indicator of cardiovascular function. He helped me understand that meanings are not ethereal entities confined to the mind. They are translated into the body and, as I was later to discover, they can make the difference in life and death.

WHAT DO YOU THINK ABOUT YOUR HEALTH?

"Is your health excellent, good, fair, or poor?" According to several studies done over the past few years, the answer people give to this simple question is a better predictor of who will live or die over the next decade than in-depth physical examinations and extensive laboratory tests. This question is a way of asking what our health means to us—what it represents or symbolizes in our thoughts and imagination.

A remarkable study on health perceptions and survival by sociologist Ellen L. Idler of Rutgers University and Stanislav Kasi of the Department of Epidemiology and Public Health at Yale Medical School was published in 1991.[2] Results of the study involving more than 2800 men and women aged 65 and older were consistent with the results of five other large studies taking in more than 23,000 people aged 19 to 94. All these studies lead to the same conclusion: Our own opinion about the state of our health is a better predictor than physical symptoms and objective factors, such as extensive exams and laboratory tests, or behaviors such as cigarette smoking. For instance, people who smoked were twice as likely to die over the next 12 years as people who did not, whereas those who said their health was "poor" were seven times more likely to die than those who said their health was "excellent."

These studies do not mean that physical symptoms and harmful behaviors should be ignored or that physical examinations and laboratory tests should be abandoned. They remain vitally important. The larger lesson is that they are not, of themselves, sufficient; our medical attention must also be trained on the issues of meaning, no matter how slippery we may consider them to be (Note 1).

'IS IT THE FOURTH?'

History is replete with stories of how perceived meanings have made life-and-death differences in health. George L. Engel of the University of Rochester School of Medicine investigated 170 cases of "emotional sudden death," which has been reported from ancient times to the present. Engel found that the emotions immediately preceding collapse and death were heavily tinged with perceived meanings. The three major categories were "personal danger or threat of injury, whether real or symbolic" (27%); "the collapse or death of a close person" (21%); and "during the period of acute grief (within 16 days)" (20%).[3]

Similar instances involve two founding fathers and presidents of the United States, John Adams and Thomas Jefferson. Both died on July 4th, 1826, the fiftieth anniversary of the signing of the Declaration of Independence. As recorded by his doctor, Jefferson's last words were, "Is it the Fourth?"[4] Jefferson's and Adams's deaths seem to mean something; they reach beyond the purely physical; they symbolize something greater than the blind play of atoms.

Skeptics are generally unmoved. Why shouldn't Jefferson and Adams die on July 4th? They have one in 365 chances of doing so. Nothing remarkable here!

MEANING IN ILLNESS: AN INEVITABILITY

It's no use, in my opinion, to argue that disease means nothing. One can insist that the illness should mean nothing, as Susan Sontag has eloquently done in her influential book *Illness as Metaphor*,[5] but this is a hopeless ideal. Anyone who is seriously ill will find or create meaning to explain what is happening. It is simply our nature to do so, and I have never seen an exception to this generalization. Even if we claim that our illness means nothing, as did Sontag in her experience with cancer, we are nonetheless creating and inserting meaning into the event. Here the meaning takes the form of denial of any underlying significance, purpose, or pattern, which is meaning of a negative kind. But negative meaning is not the same as no meaning. We may tell ourselves that our illness is nothing more than an accidental, purposeless, random event, that it is simply a matter of our atoms and molecules just being themselves. But this denial of meaning is meaning in disguise. It can assure us, for example, right or wrong, that the illness is not our fault, that we were not responsible for it, that it "just happened," which can be a great consolation. Thus, negative meaning can be extremely meaningful.

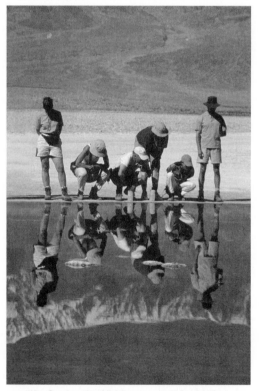

"Reflection Pool." (Courtesy Michael Eller.)

MEANING AND SCIENCE: ANOTHER VIEW

One gets the impression that the debate within science about meaning and purpose is final or is nearing completion and that all good scientists know that nature is blind, meaningless, and purposeless. However, first-rate scientists, many of Nobel caliber, who have inquired deeply into the place of meaning in nature have disagreed with the point of view expressed by Monod and others.

Sir Arthur Eddington (1882-1944), the English astronomer and astrophysicist, was such a person. He was one of the first theorists to fully grasp relativity theory, of which he became a leading exponent. He made important contributions to the theoretical physics of motion, evolution, and internal constitution of stellar systems. For his outstanding contributions he was knighted in 1930. Eddington was not only an outstanding scientist but an eloquent writer and accomplished philosopher as well, and he possessed a penetrating wit.[6] Eddington pointed to the practical impossibility and the absurdity of attempting to live one's life as if it were devoid of any meaning higher than the purely physical. He wryly observed,

> The materialist who is convinced that all phenomena arise from electrons and quanta and the like controlled by mathematical formulae, must presumably hold the belief that his wife is a rather elaborate differential equation, but he is probably tactful enough not to obtrude this opinion in domestic life. If this kind of scientific dissection is felt to be inadequate and irrelevant in ordinary personal relationships, it is surely out of place in the most personal relationship of all—that of the human soul to a divine spirit.[7]

The preference of scientists for a tidy, aseptic world without meaning and purpose is itself a meaning, one smuggled into science in the name of objectivity. This point of view is a preferred aesthetic, but it is not science.

In fact, it is a misconception to say that science has disproved meaning in nature. Nothing could be farther from the truth. The failure to prove meaning in nature is not the same thing as disproving it. It is more accurate to say that science has nothing to say about meaning and purpose, to acknowledge that these issues are a blank spot on the scientific map. Science can tell us that electrons and protons attract each other but not what this phenomenon means, whether there is a purpose behind it, or whether it is a good thing. That is why the proper response of the physical sciences to questions of meaning is, I believe, silence. And that is why science, properly understood, is more a friend than an enemy to questions of meaning.

This point of view is eloquently expressed by transpersonal psychologist Ken Wilber. Although speaking of the relationship of physics and religion, his observations apply equally to the relationship of science and meaning:

> ...[W]hereas classical physics was theoretically hostile to religion, modern physics is simply indifferent to it—it leaves so many theoretical holes in the universe that you may (or may not) fill them with religious substance, but if you do, it must be on philosophic or religious grounds. Physics cannot help you in the least, but it no longer objects to your efforts. Physics does not support mysticism, but it no longer denies it. ... Many people are . . .disappointed or let down by the apparently thin or weak nature of [this development], whereas, in fact, this view... is probably the strongest and most revolutionary conclusion vis a vis religion that has ever been "officially" advanced by theoretical science itself. It is a monumental and epochal turning point in science's stance towards religion; it seems highly unlikely that it will ever be reversed, since it is logical and not empirical in nature ... therefore, it, in all likelihood, marks final closure on that most nagging aspect of the age-old debate between the physical sciences and religion.... What more could one possibly want?[6]

A RELEASE FROM PATHOLOGY'S CURSE

"Cancer is the best thing that ever happened to me." Now I believe, many years later, that this comment often represents great wisdom and insight and can be a healing force. Psychologist C.G. Jung knew how the discovery of meaning could ease the burden of disease. He wrote about the domain of the numinous, that transcendent place where life's richest meanings are found:

> . . . the approach to the numinous is the real therapy and inasmuch as you attain to the numinous experiences you are released from the curse of pathology. Even the very disease takes on a numinous character.[8]

One of the most numinous meanings encountered by patients during severe illness is a belief in an afterlife. To the skeptical clinician these interpretations may seem jejune, desperate gropings in the face of impending death. But even though therapists may not share the beliefs of their patients that "something more" follows death, the most humane and compassionate response might be one of loving support. The most shameful behavior is to engage in a contest of meanings with a patient, denigrating or ridiculing what one does not agree with. Jung emphasized the extraordinarily sensitive nature of this meaning and the need for tolerance:

> If . . . from the needs of his own heart, or in accordance with the ancient lessons of human wisdom . . . anyone should [believe in] . . . what is inadequately and symbolically described as "eternity"—then critical reason could counter no other argument than the *non liquet* of science. Furthermore, he would have the inestimable advantage of conforming to a bias of the human psyche which has existed from time immemorial and is universal. Anyone who does not draw this conclusion ... has the indubitable certainty of coming into conflict with the truths of his own blood. . . . [T]his means the same thing as the conscious denial of the instincts—uprootedness, disorientation, meaninglessness. . . . Deviation from the truths of the blood begets neurotic meaninglessness, and the lack of meaning is a soul-sickness whose full extent and full import our age has not as yet begun to comprehend.[9]

Is it ethically and morally wrong to indulge a patient in his or her meanings if we are convinced they are erroneous or misplaced? If the patient's belief is destructive to health, we must intervene. But we must not be self-indulgent and must not burden the patient with our views. This is easy to do; patients may be vulnerable to anything said by someone in a white coat. If we disagree with the spiritual meanings our patients find during illness, perhaps we can find justification for remaining silent in science, recalling that, on questions of meaning and purpose, science itself is mute.

MEANING AND ALTERNATIVE MEDICINE

Meaning is often disregarded in modern life. Not only are we told (erroneously) that science has proved there is no meaning in nature, we are assured also that God is dead. As a result, we find ourselves a society that is spiritually malnourished and hungry for meaning. This understood, it becomes easier to see why alternative therapies are enjoying a renaissance.

Although I know of no data to support this observation, I believe generally that alternative therapy practitioners are much more cordial to questions of meaning in illness than physicians, psychiatrists, and psychologists. They are more willing to entertain the symbolic side of illness and to suppose that health and illness may reflect more than the blind play of atoms. Patients respond warmly to this point of view, because it feels good to have one's quest for meaning acknowledged or to have one's meanings affirmed. The immense popularity of alternative therapies and therapists may be due in large measure to the fact that they help people find meaning in their lives when they need it most.

MEANING: THE SHADOW SIDE

Making a place for meaning in medicine may cause problems. These have to do with extremism. "The pendulum of the mind oscillates between sense and nonsense, not between right and wrong," Jung said. "The numinosum is dangerous because it lures men to extremes...."[10]

If the pendulum was once completely in the physical corner of the atoms and molecules, it can also swing wildly to the side of meaning. Then we may regard illness as having no physical component whatever, and believe that it is caused only by negative perceptions, thoughts, attitudes, and beliefs. The idea that illness is totally a function of the various expressions of consciousness, including perceived meanings, is common in the New Age. Convinced that the mind is everything, people easily succumb to New Age guilt—a sense of failure, shame, and inadequacy—if they get sick. Meaning, then, can be the nose of the camel under the tent. It can supplant the physical altogether. The belief that mental factors, including perceived meanings, are the only cause of illness can lead to disastrous consequences such as the refusal to employ physical methods (e.g., drugs and surgical procedures) when they might be life-saving.

These excesses make it all too easy to criticize the search for meaning in illness. Because the search so often goes astray, many physicians want nothing to do with it. If the pendulum must swing, they say, better it swing toward the physical. This attitude is common. Even Eddington experienced a longing for the comforts of the physical view when he was painstakingly elucidating the connections between science and mysticism.

He acknowledged "a homesickness for the paths of physical science where there are more or less discernible handrails to keep us from the worst morasses of foolishness." But in spite of the intellectual queasiness he experienced, Eddington persevered in his search for meaning. And so, I believe, must we.

MEANING THERAPY

The reason we must persevere has largely to do with science. Many "meaning studies" are beginning to elucidate the considerable role of meaning in health—for example, the already-mentioned study by Idler and Kasi showing the potent effect of perceived meanings on longevity.[2] Studies also show that the meaning of the relationship with one's spouse is a major factor in the clinical expression of heart disease; that the meaning of a job and one's level of job dissatisfaction can be major predictors of heart attack; that attention to the meanings surrounding heart disease, when combined with dietary discretion, exercise, and stress management, can improve cardiac performance and reverse coronary artery obstructions[14]; that the bereavement and mourning following a spouse's death are associated with severe immune dysfunction[15]; that negative perceptions of one's daily job can increase the risk for heart attack[16,17]; and that for certain cancer patients, group therapy in which questions of meaning are addressed can double survival time following diagnosis.[18]

These studies represent the pendulum at mid-point. They show that attention to states of consciousness need not replace physical interventions but can be used effectively in conjunction with them.

These findings are about meaning therapy, in which therapists deliberately attempt to reshape negative meanings into positive ones. If we choose to call these attempts "psychology," "behavioral therapy," or some other psychologically oriented term, we should be careful that we do not assign them second-class status in the process. Meaning therapy is no stepchild of allopathic medicine. Its effects are as real as those of drugs and surgical procedures. The previously cited studies show that reforming meaning can elicit significant clinical responses and can make the difference, even, in life and death.

THE CHALLENGE OF MEANING

Contemporary physicians—I say this as someone who has been in the trenches of internal medicine for two decades—hear that modern medicine is too technical, remote, and cold; that we don't take enough time with our patients; that we focus on their bodies and avoid questions of meaning, leaving them to psychologists, ministers, and priests. Yet most physicians continue to rely on the physically based methods we know best, justifying this approach with evidence that they do work. But if orthodox methods are so effective—and they are sometimes fabulously successful—why is the public not more grateful? Why the concerted attempt to dismantle the profession and "manage" it differently?

Much of society's disillusionment with modern medicine lies in its failure to acknowledge the importance of meaning in their lives and illnesses. If physicians continue to minimize or ignore the role of meaning in health, we shall continue to lose influence. The contest between conventional and alternative therapies is not just about economics, efficacy, safety, and availability; it is about meaning as well. We are discovering a painful fact: No matter how technologically effective modern medicine may be, if it does not honor the place of meaning in illness, it may lose the allegiance of those it serves.

In the future, when historians dissect our age, they may be shocked that we in science chose to place such a high value on the "systematic denial" of purpose and meaning. I suspect they may elevate this idea to a high place in the Hall of Human Silliness, if it exists. They may wonder why we chose to ignore the visions of those such as physicist David Bohm, who said, "Meaning is being,"[19] and Jung, who saw the importance of meaning and who had the courage to speak about it: "Meaning makes a great many things endurable—perhaps everything.... [T]hrough the creation of meaning... a new cosmos arises."[20] "Meaninglessness... is... equivalent to illness."[10]

If they fulfill their promise, practitioners of alternative therapies will have to continue to honor the place of meaning in health and illness. We must resist the temptation to treat these therapies as the "new penicillin" or the latest surgical technique, which can be applied in a purely utilitarian way. In the rush to gain respectability, practitioners will feel immense pressure to minimize or denigrate expressions of consciousness such as meaning. This temptation must be resisted, or alternative therapies will deserve little more than a footnote in history. We already have therapies aplenty that deny meaning. We do not need more.

As a result of the numerous studies affirming the crucial role of meaning in medicine, making a space for meaning has never been more justifiable. Are we up to the challenge?

NOTE

For a discussion of the role of meaning in health and illness, and how healthcare professionals might address issues of meaning in clinical practice, see Larry Dossey, *Meaning & Medicine,* New York, 1991, Bantam.

References for this essay are located on the DVD accompanying this book.

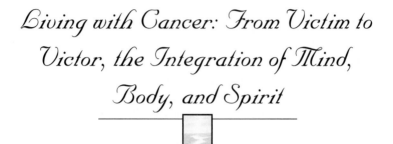

Living with Cancer: From Victim to Victor, the Integration of Mind, Body, and Spirit

CARYLE HIRSHBERG

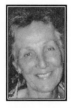

"**W**HAT WOULD YOU DO IF you were told, 'You have cancer?'" the dark-haired, dark-eyed woman asked me, while the other woman, fair, slight, skin almost transparent, looked on. I looked at the large philodendron draped behind them and tried hard to feel what that question meant to the women, both of whom had breast cancer, sitting across the table from me. I felt a mixture of sadness, embarrassment, guilt, fear, and "there but for the grace of God go I" feelings. I was flooded with emotions I couldn't easily explain. Hesitantly, I replied, "I honestly don't know. Part of me says that I would weigh the information, evaluate the treatments available, cry, deny, and then I think I would have to search inside myself to find the answers. What would

I do? How would I feel? I guess I don't know how I would react until I was faced with it." Both women nodded, with approval. It seemed they appreciated the honesty of my answer.

THE REMISSION PROJECT

At that time, I was the manager of The Remission Project, a project initiated by Brendan O'Regan, the director of research at the Institute of Noetic Sciences. We believed that if human beings possess usually untapped powers of self-repair that can affect the dissolution of a tumor, it is of vital importance that this capacity be investigated and understood. The goals of the project were to collect articles about spontaneous remission, both cases and research papers, reported in the medical literature; look for patterns; compile the material into a bibliography; and focus the medical community's attention on a subject that had no organized research agenda. The common view of the subject in medical circles at that time was that though it is highly interesting as a phenomenon, it was usually doubted that it could really be studied. There was no organized remission research program. There were no journals and few books devoted to remission—surprising considering the interest of both the medical community and the public in all aspects of cancer.

As people began to hear about the project, we received many phone calls and letters from people with cancer and cancer survivors. People wanted to know what we had found, but more than that they wanted a friendly and compassionate ear for their stories. Over and over I heard, "Can I tell you my story?" And what stories they were! The stories were filled with triumphs as well as defeats, and I realized that the work would have a greater impact on people with cancer than I thought.

We received a letter in 1989 from a woman who was diagnosed with lung cancer in 1983. Her letter began, "I'm so grateful that research is being done in the area of spontaneous remission.... Statistics gave me 6–8 months without treatment, but only 18 months with treatment. That was in January, 1983.... Even in your research in medical journals, you will still miss a lot of us who are surviving quite happily and with an insight that has to come when one looks death in the eye." Along with her letter she enclosed a letter she had written to her doctor: "I have decided not to pursue any treatment.... I have been interested and curious for a long time as to how a person accepts his own terminal diagnosis." Her doctor had replied, "I not only honored your decision but applauded [it].... I have always been rather surprised that patients, when presented with the reality of the situation, don't make this decision more frequently."[1]

Slowly over time, I realized that while spontaneous remission cases were the tip of the bell-shaped curve, the outliers, people who, while always hoping for a "miracle" and wishing the cancer would just go away and let them get on with their lives, mostly just wanted to survive, to live. So, from the point of view of the person with cancer, spontaneous remission and long-term survival mean the same thing.

One afternoon I receive a telephone call from a woman who, after telling her story, asked, "Do you know anyone who has survived the kind of cancer I have? Because if I knew just one person who had survived I would feel more like fighting."

CAN WE LEARN TO BE SURVIVORS?

Years later, sitting in the audience at a conference for women with cancer, thinking about the talk I was about to give, I looked over a sea of heads, many wearing wigs, some sick from treatment, some frightened by the prospect of dying, some hopeful about their prospects of living, I remembered that woman's words, and I asked myself, "Who are the people that survive? Can we learn how to be a survivor? Are survivors successful, happy people, enthusiastic about life, enjoying life, with some kind of built in belief in future success? Are there characteristics that survivors have in common, or traits that enhance survival and the ability to thrive? In a lifetime, we will all know people with cancer. We may be that someone with cancer. How will we react, what would we do?"

A diagnosis of cancer is unquestionably an overwhelming trauma, both the trauma of having cancer and the trauma of treating cancer. How we respond to the diagnosis, whether with shock and helplessness, with fear, or with relief that now our vague or not-so-vague feelings and internal messages are validated, may be predictive of the choices we make about this disease. Whether with defense or attack, each of us will respond in our own unique way.

People are different, so the approaches to dealing with cancer are different, and individual behaviors, beliefs, and attitudes combine in unique and essential ways to help a person decide how to approach this profound and life-changing time. Myriad factors have profound weight in the equation of cancer survival: genetics, extent of disease, availability of efficacious treatment, luck, timing, and socio-economics.

Cancer survival brings up some interesting questions. What percentage of medical cures may be instances of recovery that was mistakenly attributed to treatment? Why does one person benefit from chemotherapy and another doesn't? Since remission happens with unknown frequency, it can convincingly be argued that some of both conventional and unconventional therapies' "successes" are simply cases of remission and have nothing to do with the efficacy of either conventional or unconventional therapies.[2]

Cancer survivors, when asked to what they attribute their survival, will say they chose a variety of treatments, both conventional and complementary; self-directed activities (meditation, exercise, imagery, etc.); and treatments by others (chemotherapy, acupuncture, etc.).

Along with treatments and behavioral changes, most people report that psychospiritual factors played a key role in their recoveries. It is interesting that most survivors give greater weight to intangible factors—attitude changes; beliefs; new meaning in life; strong connections with mates, friends, and health practitioners; and expression of emotions—than to treatments they received.

Flexibility, a willingness to try anything that makes sense and to make changes when something doesn't seem to be working, a sense of adventure, challenge fraught with danger, commitment, and self-efficacy pervade the beliefs, behaviors, and attitudes of people who survive. For example, after being informed that he had a grave prognosis following a diagnosis of metastatic pancreatic cancer, one man—after a period of depression, fear, sorrow, and loss—rallied and exclaimed, "That's what they say; now let me see what I can do."

Dr. Johannes Schilder reports that prior to a spontaneous remission people get in touch with something "essential" to them. There is a precipitating crisis in which the life situation can no longer be tolerated; it goes "beyond the pale,"[3] and their subsequent behavior is aligned with their most deeply held beliefs, beliefs of which they may not be aware until the crisis. "You know," he says, "it's not what they do, I think, so much as who they are. But in these patients, the self who begins is a different self than the one who comes out of it."[4]

Self-evaluation and awakening realizations of a deep personal nature often occur in relationship to a crisis. The crisis of cancer and the realization of mortality awaken the desire to discover and understand who we really are, to take control of our lives, to believe we can influence the outcome. Often with the diagnosis of cancer comes an initial feeling of helplessness/hopelessness: "I am at the whims of others, the circumstances of my life are out of my control." Sometimes suddenly, often over time, those feelings transmute into the belief that "I can influence the outcome. I can show them I'm not a victim anymore."

If psychosocial factors can account for, for instance, even 5 percent of the equation of success, that 5 percent may be sufficient to make a difference between recovery and death. There isn't any one fixed set of behaviors, beliefs, or attitudes that promote survival, nor is there a specific "set" of personality characteristics that determine who survives and who does not, but the person can and does influence the outcome.

REMARKABLE RECOVERY: WHO ARE THE PEOPLE?

In the mid-'90s, I co-authored *Remarkable Recovery* with Marc Barasch. More than 60 people were interviewed. Each person's story was rich, told with emotion, humor, and compassion. Some people remembered their experiences in vivid detail, as if it were "happening to me all over again." Forty of the people interviewed agreed to participate in a pilot study.[5] More answers to "Who are the people?" began to emerge.

Some of the interviews were with people whose cases had been reported in the medical literature and included in *Spontaneous Remission: An Annotated Bibliography*.[6] People were referred by both allopathic and complementary health-care professionals and by psychosocial researchers and therapists. Some came through word of mouth, reports published in magazines and newspapers, cancer survivor groups, and letters and phone calls from survivors. Their stories were inspiring. One thing was certain: Many people recover.

Some people were diagnosed with cancer for which little or no treatment was available; in some remarkable cases, some refused treatment or recovered prior to treatment initiation. Surprisingly, after preparing to die, after "getting their affairs in order," they found themselves totally recovered.

One man, diagnosed with metastatic kidney cancer, sold his business, resolved his affairs, and waited. When, months later, x-rays revealed his cancer totally resolved, he said wryly, "It's as big a shock to find out that you're going to live as it is to face your death."[7] One woman, told she had terminal cancer, went home to reconcile herself to her imminent death and returned to the physician to discover the cancer gone. Instead of responding in joy, she was furious that she had been made to suffer, furious that the diagnosis could have been wrong, ready to sue the doctors and the hospitals for the anguish this diagnosis had caused. Another, faced with a similar situation, responded with joy.

Most people do not find themselves in that situation. Their recoveries are, as one person called them, "hard-working miracles," complex recoveries that require courses of chemotherapy or radiation, surgery, and a variety of complementary treatments over many months or years.

FROM VICTIM TO VICTOR: CHARACTERISTICS OF SURVIVORS

But the characteristics people considered important in their recovery were essentially the same. Seventy percent of the people in the pilot study reported that characteristics such as fighting spirit, seeing the disease as a challenge, realistic acceptance of the diagnosis without acceptance of the prognosis, caring relationships with family and practitioners, and belief in a positive outcome were significant in their recovery. Over 60 percent reported a renewed commitment to life, will to live, and a new sense of purpose, active changes in habits and behaviors, and the expression of emotions, both positive and negative.

It was surprising to find that almost 70 percent of the people had been married for over 20 years, considering the divorce rate (in the

United States) is nearly 50 percent. Many of the participants had been married for 30 or 40 years. The strong, supportive, and trusted relationship with one other person, a partner, was considered extremely significant.

People reported they no longer felt it was necessary to deny their feelings—one minute fearful, the next joyful; optimism and hope one minute, anger and tears the next. Suddenly, the full gamut of emotions was acceptable. No longer able to be tolerant or patient, with no time to "put off until later," they found that spontaneity developed, allowing them to be the children they used to be.

Cancer survivors frequently displayed increased appreciation for humor, more uninhibited laughter and release of emotions in their lives, and a greater connection with nature and the natural world. Moments of profound love for family, friends, nature, and a connection with a higher being all were reported with clarity. One man, whom his doctors believed was very close to death in his hospital bed, held his wife tightly in his arms and repeated "I love you, I love you, I love you," over and over again for 2 hours.

Love is an opening rather than a closing, an expansion rather than a contraction; it is the opposite of the constriction of fear. Perhaps along with this expansive emotional feeling, cells might also shift, relaxing the body, allowing more relaxed breathing, calmness of mind and body, a release of all that divides us from one another. Such shifts can alter the physiology of a person in a stressful state, a state most certainly precipitated by a diagnosis of a life-threatening disease. Feelings of connection rather than isolation may also cause this state of dilation and expansion, reducing the stressful states experienced with fear.

Therapeutic modalities can help a person feel expansive and loving, can transform stress to relaxation, and that can have a profound effect on the person's ability to heal. Biofeedback can help promote feelings of self confidence, help a person to relax, and provide the shift needed for feelings of connection, expansion, and empowerment that may help shift the physiological balance. For example, a 12-year-old boy with Ewing's sarcoma, introduced to self-hypnosis and biofeedback to control pain and nausea, gained self-confidence and recognition from others. Seeing the process of raising his finger temperature as a game, he said, "I thought it was a challenge to increase and decrease my temperature. I got good enough that they brought me to a neuropsychiatric institute and hooked me up to a more sophisticated machine. I showed I could raise my finger temperature from 90 to 106 degrees." He was very serious about his biofeedback and visualization since he "didn't want anything to interfere with my natural endorphins."[8]

Likewise, guided imagery can promote confidence and self-efficacy and relieve fear and anxiety. Many people have incorporated imagery into their self-treatment for cancer and report that the more unique, customized, detailed, movie-like, and personalized the imagery is, the more enjoyable it is.

For example, one man visualized "white-immune-cell bunny rabbits feasting on fields of orange cancer carrots." A particularly fascinating part of these elaborate imageries is that some of those who created them seemed to know prior to medical discovery that their cancer was gone. One morning the man with the immune-cell bunny rabbits "couldn't find enough carrots for all my rabbits." Shortly thereafter, his physician reported the cancer gone.[9]

The boy with Ewing's sarcoma knew before the doctors told him that his cancer was gone: "My white cells were actually coming to me at one point reporting they were cleaning up, and that was it. I could see them like watching a movie."[10]

THE POWER OF FAITH

Spiritual faith, religious conviction, belief in a higher power, and surrender are prominent in many survivors' stories. Many report that prayer, either their own or the prayers of others, contributed significantly to their recovery (67 percent). In some people, among them those with the "most remarkable" recoveries, was deep pervasive spiritual faith, a personal relationship with God, or the Divine Principle. For example, a woman diagnosed with liver cancer, a case reported in the medical literature,[11] said, when asked to what she attributed her remarkable recovery, that she "prayed to be forgiven, prayed for the return of health, prayed for the cancer to disappear and go away." Another woman, at the time of exploratory surgery for metastatic melanoma, remembered the last words of Jesus and repeated them to herself as she was wheeled into the operating theater: "Father, into your hands, I commend my spirit." Another woman, diagnosed with diffuse large-cell lymphoma whose case was reported in the journal *Cancer*,[12] attributed her recovery in large part to "Faith, Hope, Love, and Trust in God." In less than 6 weeks, every symptom of cancer was gone, a truly miraculous recovery.

When asked about religious beliefs, one woman wrote, "For me my spirituality is a part of my being, it is inside, so for me it is only logical that this spirituality influences my thought and acts in the world. To me God is the non-matter in the matter (the spirit of the matter). God is a force that is everywhere.... I never experienced God, I always know it is there, so I do not have to experience it.... My trust in the force is 100 percent. I have no doubt that it reacts to my cry for help." Another wrote, "I do not belong to any church or believe in any religion. I am aware of a great power in nature. When I feel peace in my body, harmony with the world, that is my religion. I feel good when I do 'what is right.' To cheat somebody would cost me my self-respect. I spend time in quiet meditation, I 'go to church' in my garden, watching the birds or the clouds, but I keep an open mind, anything is possible."

Belief in yourself; belief in something greater than yourself; taking a negative experience and turning it into a positive one; will and determination; enhancing intimacy; choosing activities and behaviors that promote self-efficacy, love, joy, playfulness, and satisfaction; a sense of purpose; support of others; and a bit of luck—these characteristics can have a profound effect on disease. But don't suppose that it is only positive states and emotions that play an important role in recovery. Facing the crisis; accepting and experiencing despair, sadness, and pain; and, through these experiences, discovering the inner power to find in the sorrow that life is meaningful and fulfilling are equally important.

A whole person is not 60 percent of one attribute and 70 percent of another but an indivisible combination of physical, spiritual, social, and emotional factors. Only by viewing the person in the context of their lives and experiences, their beliefs, attitudes, behaviors, loves, and fears, can we begin to see how the whole person, biology, psychology, and spirit, reacts to the crisis of cancer. Perhaps, in the end, the story of one person may tell us the most.

FRANK'S STORY

Frank Walker, "100 percent Irish" was born in the Bronx 2 days after Pearl Harbor. He remembers being 4 years old and sitting on his father's shoulders, watching as the liberty ships bringing the soldiers back from the war sailed into New York Harbor. "I was always fascinated by World War I," he recalled. "My heroes were all soldiers or cops; I wanted to be a marine when I grew up."

Frank learned survival on the streets of New York. "I was a tough kid, a street fighter," he said. "It was a New York thing; you had to fight; you couldn't be afraid; you had to be brave. I knew how to survive. Put me anywhere, and I'll survive."

Sitting in the living room, with a bright smile lighting up his face and the twinkling eyes of a leprechaun, a nose that looks like it might have been broken more than once, a balding scalp, and a slight middle-age paunch, Frank tells his story with a deep, gravelly voice, his words filled with images as he tells of his battle, the battle in which he had to make use of everything he was and everything he had learned on those long-ago streets of New York.

"In 1982, after many years as a radio and television news journalist," he begins, "I moved to Atlanta to work in documentary television." The job, along with challenging creative work, brought a great deal of responsibility, no acknowledgment, long working hours, a lot of travel, separation from his family, and great stress.

Five years later, he began to lose his voice and developed an intense pain in his shoulder, a pain so intense "it brought tears to my eyes." His diagnosis was bronchitis and overwork, and he was given antibiotics. The antibiotics didn't relieve the bronchitis, so he decided to stop smoking "for a while." That didn't seem to help either.

With no change in his condition and the pain remaining, he returned to his doctor for more tests. "I think it was on a Thursday," he remembered. "It's funny how some things just stick right in your head. Thursday morning." His condition being the same, he went back for more blood tests and a chest x-ray. After the tests his doctor asked him to come into his office. "That's when you get your lecture or there's something really wrong," he said. "So I did, and he opened his comments by saying, 'I may be wrong, so I don't want you to panic.' I said, 'You're talking cancer, aren't you?' and he showed me the x-ray and there was a dark dot. It wasn't very big, and it was close to the center of the chest. A biopsy was scheduled for the next week.

"When I left his office, I said, 'Jesus Christ, cancer. It's probably smoking.' I said to myself 'Was it worth it?' I went over to the 7-11 or one of those places across the street and bought a back of Luckies, jumped in my car, drove down to a little park about a half-mile down from the hospital where there was a creek running through; it's a beautiful, peaceful little spot, Civil War battle site and all that. I sat down next to the creek, opened the pack of cigarettes, and lit up. I was asking myself, 'Is this worth it?' And I said, 'By God, I guess it was. I always liked to smoke, since I was little.' In one sense, I realized that was the beginning of the healing because I took responsibility."

His biopsy was scheduled for a Monday, but it took a couple of days before they took him to surgery. "They basically had a lot of trouble with the biopsy," he recalled. "The tumor was growing outside the lung, although it kind of had its toe in the lung. As they described it to me, it was about the size and shape of a yam." After much discussion in the operating room between the anesthesiologist and the surgeon, he found himself "on the table, the lights are overhead, and these guys are arguing. Finally the surgeon shoves this tube down my throat, right into my lungs in lightning-quick time. And then yanks it out, and a big glob of stuff comes out. At about this time the anesthesiologist leans over, talked to me quietly in the ear, and said, 'Would you like to go under about now? I think it's time.' I said, 'You bet!' So 10 seconds later, I'm out. The next thing I remember is waking up upstairs with tubes coming out everywhere."

When he woke up, his wife was in the room and his two children were with his sister-in-law, whom Frank insisted his wife call to take care of the home front before he went into surgery. Later that night, the surgeon visited him and told him they did a frozen biopsy. Said Frank: "You know, the quickie they do, and it looks like small-cell carcinoma of the lung. And I said, 'What's the outlook on that?' He said, '95 percent fatal.' He doesn't say 5 percent live, he says 95 percent fatal and, of course, that hits you right between the eyes like a sledge hammer." He remembers the day well; it was April Fool's day, and "sure enough, there was a trick pulled on Atlanta. It snowed. I looked out my window at a white world outside." "I was depressed. There was a nurse on my floor; I think she was an angel. I was crying. It wasn't like I needed a handkerchief; I needed a towel. She would come in whenever she could and spent quite a while with me that night holding my hand. It was a really beautiful and healing thing she did. I still remember and I still appreciate.

"It wasn't so much I was afraid of dying. I was thinking of my daughters, one was 4 and a half, the other less than a year old. I was sad for them. I thought, 'They didn't sign on for a dead dad; they signed on for life.'"

The next day, Frank asked his doctor, "Where they get these numbers, 95 percent fatal? The people in this ward, do they all have cancer?" When the doctor nodded and said, "Just about all," Frank said, "These people can't even walk. Are they in your statistics?" When the doctor said that they were, Frank responded, "Well, shit, my odds just really improved."

"I used to ride a motorcycle, and I remember one piece of advice from an old-time motorcycle rider: When you're in a jam, don't hit the brakes. You're just going to die. Find an opening and open the throttle as far as you can and try to shoot through the opening. That's what I was doing; I was looking for an opening. My hand was on the throttle.

"That afternoon I was lying in my bed, and this is where it gets a little mystical. My daughter was in a Montessori school, and every afternoon they had a love circle where each kid would send love thoughts to someone. After my biopsy, all 15 3-, 4- and 5-year-olds decided to collectively send their love to me. And I swear to God I felt it; it came right in the window. Then I started to feel a little better."

The pathology department had sent the biopsy specimen to Emory Medical School for reevaluation to "the guy who had taught just about every oncologist in Atlanta." The new diagnosis was not small cell carcinoma but a large cell carcinoma. "I said, 'What did that mean? What's the survival rate on this one?' And my doctor said, 'Well, 85 to 90 percent die.' I said, 'I just doubled my chances! This is great!' God, what a time in your life and I'm reliving it as we talk. Anyway, with the new diagnosis I felt a little better still. I began to think there might be a chance, and I began to be aggressive about it."

He began radiation treatments immediately. "It was 20 sessions of hell. It burned my shoulders black. They said I would never talk again because the tumor had atrophied my nerves. It was incredibly debilitating. I was good for the session in the morning and maybe a half-hour afterwards. I had to lie down 28 hours a day. After a while, I could hardly eat. It would take me 2 hours to get down a small plate of spaghetti because my esophagus was so badly burned. But I stayed at it."

Sometime during the first week or so, he was alone inside the lead-lined room with this giant machine, and he had an epiphany: "I don't know exactly how to describe this, it wasn't the sky opened, it wasn't the voice of God because there was no voice, but it was a voice, a silent voice came to me inside and said 'You're not going to die. You're not through. You've got work to do.' I'm still trying to figure out what exactly that work is, but I'm doing whatever comes across my path.

"I made friends with all the nurses, the radiology technicians, everybody. I actually had fun most of the time. There were two other women who came for treatment at the same time as me. We made friends, told our stories, supported each other. You could look around and actually see who was going to die. Their heads were down; they accepted what people said."

One night, on the local news, there was an oncology convention in town at the time and Frank heard about visualization. A reporter asked a doctor what she thought about visualization for cancer. "She said, 'That's just false hope; these people die, and they're going to die, and they die thinking they are inadequate because they couldn't cure themselves.' I wanted to jump through the tube and strangle her."

After radiation treatment, every week, Monday through Friday, as a reward, Frank would stop at the shopping center, buy a pack of cigarettes, take out one and throw the rest away, and sit in a "little Italian cafe, get myself something sweet to eat, have an espresso, smoke a cigarette, and read the *New York Times,* before the nausea and weakness started." And he got stronger. He started golfing. "At first, I could go three holes before I lost it. Then I got four. Then I got five, and seven, and I remember the first time I did nine holes."

One day he was reading *Why Me?,* a book about Garrett Porter's recovery from his brain tumor. "I was home alone with my younger daughter; she was about a year old at the time. She woke up from her nap, and I brought her into bed with me, put her on my chest, and started to meditate. She went back to sleep. And for the first time I felt, I don't know what you call it, where you don't exactly leave your body but you sort of do. You're out in space, connecting with everything that lives. Every other human being, every flower, every plant, and I became everything just for those few minutes. I think maybe my baby was a catalyst. I'll never forget it."

It wasn't easy for Frank to keep his belief in himself. His wife told the children he was going to die, his wife told herself he was going to die. "I remember my older daughter came in, and she was in tears. I said, 'What's the matter?' She said, 'Dad, I always thought you were going to be with me forever.' I said, 'I will be. If I live or die, I'll be with you forever, but I'm going to live.' We spent a good deal of time with her grief. And my wife, every time I started crying, she would cry. She thought I was going to die. It's very interesting the way people approach it. Viewing you as already dead. When I was trying to cure myself, I realized my family was interfering. Their grief was interfering with my healing. I encouraged my wife to take a vacation and take the kids, and while they were gone, I had the house to myself and I could focus. I remember I used to listen to a lot of rock and roll; it gets you going and practicing using my voice. And one day, I remember out of my mouth came "AHHHH-HHH. The first clear sound I'd made in months."

At his first CAT scan, maybe a week into the radiation treatments, there was already shrinkage. "I didn't view this incredible radiation as burning the hell out of my body and killing everything in sight; I would lay back and say, 'This is a golden, healing light.' And I would let that healing light flow through my body. I played with all colors of light and finally hit on a pale purple light, which I still use. And by the end of 20 treatments, whether it was the radiation, the prayer from friends, from the lady who cleaned my house and her whole congregation, from my gardener, from all the children at my little girl's school, my attitude, the imagery, the tumor disappeared."

With this news, Frank went out and bought his dream car, "a car that could go 160 miles an hour, the top came down, it was cool, cool, cool. Turbo charge and everything. My wife said it was crazy. If I die, it'll be paid for by the life insurance, and besides, I want to be buried in it if I die, just leave the top open, and when they shovel the dirt on top of me, the most surprised person at the funeral will be me! So I got this car, loaded it up with fishing rods, golf clubs, a change of clothes, cowboy boots, and took off first for a meeting in Washington, saying 'I'll be back. I don't know when.' I had to get away from people who knew I had cancer. I drove up to New York; it was Father's Day weekend. I showed up at a party for my dad. My mom was shocked. I took my dad for a spin in my new car then pointed my car at the George Washington Bridge and never stopped. I didn't even have the license plates yet. I drove and finally wound up in Colorado. Climbed the Rockies at 100 miles per hour with *Graceland* blaring as loud as it could on the speakers and me screaming at the top of my lungs, singing to *Graceland*. I was gone 3 weeks. Finally, I decided I'd better get home. I remember watching this amazing storm. It's like one you see maybe once in 5 years. Off to my left is this big mesa, like a lightning rod. Constant thunder, constant lightning, and I started to try and outrun the storm, next to me is a guy in a big Cadillac with Texas plates, and together we're racing each other and the storm through New Mexico and Texas. The little towns along the way a blur. What an extraordinary night that was!"

Back home, reality struck. He had no cancer and no disability. He had to go back to work. "Sure enough, it was like committing suicide and about 10 or 11 months later, I noticed I was having trouble as I was driving to work. The car seemed to go off to the right. And my wife was saying the side of my face looked odd.

'Brain tumors,' said the doctor. 'Is that bad?' I asked. 'The worst news you can have. I know you're a special case, and you beat the last one through whatever means, whether it's medical or something else, but you can't beat this one. Don't go for extended treatments or experimental therapies. Nobody survives. Get your affairs in order. You've got a couple of months.'

"I went back to the radiologist and said, 'Let's do it again.' I went through it, and I beat it. I went through months of incredible radiation to my head. I knew I couldn't go back to my old job. I had read an article in the *New York Times* that said anger is good for the first year, but after that you need to find peace. You need to find joy. So I sold the house and packed the family up and bought a farm in Pennsylvania. Throughout the first summer, I was getting hoarser and hoarser. I had promised my wife a vacation. I decided whatever it was I would deal with it later, and we left for Bermuda." Frank went back to Atlanta to have a biopsy, and they found a tumor on the vocal cords. They couldn't give him any more radiation. He had had his lifetime limit. The doctors decided to implant radium pellets in the tumor. After surgery, Marty recalled, "I'm all bandaged up and the surgeon comes in and I asked how it went. He said, 'We're done.' I said, 'You got the pellets in?' 'No.' I went ballistic. I said, 'What the hell is going on?' 'We couldn't find it. We couldn't find any cancer.' So now I'm the owner of $1472 worth of radioactive pellets, which I can't sell to anybody. That was in 1989."[13]

Frank died from a recurrence of the cancer on May 8, 2002, at home, at peace, surrounded by those who loved him, 15 years after he was given a few months to live. His experiences with cancer certainly had changed him in many ways, made him more the person he was, and gave him the strength and wisdom to accept his coming death without fear.

"IF THERE IS ADVICE I CAN GIVE...."

Perhaps the most valuable advice for a person with cancer must come from someone who knows the disease from the inside. During a visit at her home in Rotterdam with Geertje Brakel, a woman who was first diagnosed with ovarian cancer over 25 years ago and has experienced both recurrence and recovery, I asked her, given all she had experienced, what she could tell someone with cancer. Several months later, I received a letter in which she wrote:

> If there is an advice that I can give to people and to people with cancer, then it is the following: Let yourself go, let your emotions come out, accept the pain of life, never think that to have pain is no good, look for a person who will listen to you. If you show your hurtness, there will always be a person who sees it and will give you the support you need. You will be surprised who this person is, but begin with yourself, let it all go and be not afraid of the consequences, because they will never be something you cannot bear. Speak out your heart, and when things go wrong with your body, then at

least you will have been yourself for a while, and life feels so much better, so much more honest then. Beware of the people who will not accept this, do not listen to them, but look for the one [person] who will. This can give you all the strength you need for whatever will come.[14]

Commenting on Geertje's extraordinary recovery as the "best-documented case of spontaneous regression that I know of in the world," Dr. Marco deVries said,

> Actually, I think the bottom line of Geertje's history is that for her whole life she really didn't have the courage to live. What she actually did through that confrontation with incurable cancer was she made the choice to live, almost literally. She incarnated (and I hesitate to use that word) in her body. And I have found...because her case brought my attention to this...in questioning other people with cancer, that there are some people who haven't really made the choice to be here, in the world. Often in the past they have been denied, either unconsciously or consciously by parents, by family, by teachers, [told] that they have no right to life, to live. And so the unconscious message is you would rather die because you are not welcome here. And so the lesson I learned is this, and especially it was Geertje who brought my attention to it...that in some cancer patients I've seen, this was the big issue: Do I grant myself the right to be here and to live and to make a dent in this world?[15]

"THERE IS NO SUCH THING AS FALSE HOPE"

The value of faith, hope, and love can only be evaluated in relationship to the whole person—body, mind, and spirit. *Hope* is defined in Webster's dictionary as a "desire accompanied by expectation of, or belief in, fulfillment." The archaic meaning is "trust," and *hopeless* is defined as "having no expectation of good or success, despairing, not susceptible of remedy or cure, incurable, desperate, impossible." There is no question that hope is of immeasurable value to people faced with life-threatening disease.

In October of 1995, a day-long meeting marking the fifteenth anniversary of the Bristol Cancer Help Centre was entitled "The Question of Hope: Does Hope and a Positive State of Mind Affect the Recovery of Cancer Patients?"[16] In the inspiring final address of the day, Penny Brohn, the co-founder of the Centre, diagnosed with breast cancer over 17 years earlier, spoke about hope and false hope:

"I hoped the lump wouldn't be malignant, and it was. I hoped that it wouldn't recur, and it did. I hoped I wouldn't have to have radiotherapy ever, and I did. And then I hoped it wouldn't spread to my bones, and it did. Then I thought, 'Well, please not in my spine,' but I got it in my spine. And then I hoped that the pain wouldn't be absolutely awful, and it was. "So, this is quite an impressive track record of false hopes. But I haven't given up on hoping because I like hoping...the reason there is nothing false about this is that the act of hoping brings with it gains that you didn't look for at the time.... So you get into an optimistic, imaginative, a freer state of mind. Hope gives you an opportunity to expand from the place where you've been locked in by someone else's expectation to a place where you open out into your own.... If you hoped and you got what you wanted, you've succeeded, and if you hoped and you don't get what you wanted, you get something else anyway. It's a win–win situation, so there's no such thing as false hope."[17]

References for this essay are located on the DVD accompanying this book.

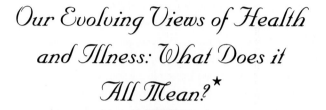

Our Evolving Views of Health and Illness: What Does it All Mean?*

RICHARD B. MILES

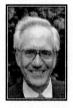

As TODAY'S TECHNOLOGY produces cloned sheep in England and induces septuplets in the United States, it is difficult to realize that less than 150 years ago we had absolutely no idea what even caused disease. Between the end of the U.S. Civil War (1865) and the turn of the twentieth century, massive changes took place in how we perceived our world and our "power" in it. If we explore these changes and the subsequent ideas they have generated, we can see that our beliefs about health and disease are shaped by the larger meaning systems, or worldviews, of the

---

*Adapted from Miles R: Our Evolving Views of Health and Illness: What does it all mean? *Noetic Sciences Connections* 3, February 1998.

175

our evolving views of health and illness: what does it all mean?

culture we share. The emerging noetic view places consciousness and self-awareness as an organizing principle for human experience, including health and disease. This is a crucial dynamic in the integral model. How might all this fit together, and what can it mean?

In a Charles Shultz "Peanuts" cartoon, Lucy, Linus, and Charlie Brown are lying on a hillside gazing at the clouds in a summer sky. Lucy: "Linus, what do you see in the clouds up there?" Linus: "That cloud on the left looks like a map of British Honduras. The cloud in the center reminds me of a bust of the famous artist Thomas Eakins. The cloud on the right shows the stoning of Stephen; you can see St Paul standing there." Lucy: "What do you see in the clouds, Charlie Brown?" Charlie Brown: "I was going to say that I saw a horsie and a duckie, but I've changed my mind."

This insightful cartoon illustrates that when humans look at their world, they impart it with meaning—meaning shaped and bounded by the worldview of the perceiver. We seek what we can grasp and understand within the boundaries of our life experience. The boundaries of our life experience have undergone some profound changes in the last 100 years . . . and our perception of the meaning of health and illness has therefore shifted to grasp these changes.

THE SUPERNATURAL MODEL

In the late nineteenth century, there were essentially three explanations for disease and dysfunction. The Divine Theory proposed that illness resulted as a punishment for sin and misbehavior, a view that is still evident in the AIDS epidemic. The Demonic Theory proposed that people could become possessed by evil forces. The Miasmatic Theory suggested there were hidden entities lingering in the air, the soil, etc. ("noxious exhalations from putrescent organic matter") that emerged when people "had the miasmas"—that is, were feeling poorly.

The common theme of these explanations is a potentially hostile supernatural universe over which humans have little or no control. Fear of disease and death were (and still are) a major organizing element in the dominant worldview. A deep desire to understand and overcome this fear drove human exploration.

THE WARRIOR MODEL

In the late nineteenth century and early twentieth centuries, a fundamental revolution occurred in this worldview. Two major aspects of this revolution are woven together: (1) The explosion of industry and technology, which was "taking over" the world—ships, railroads, steel, mechanized agriculture, manufacturing—all illustrating human capacity to master and manage the forces of nature to create expanding wealth and comfort; (2) The emergence of laboratory science, which revealed the "miasmas" as identifiable bacteria and viruses, not supernatural forces beyond our knowledge.

It is valuable to remember that this second factor came about in the context of the first. Thus, science and technology promised an answer to the fear of death and disease. They were no longer supernatural unknowns over which we were helpless. We might actually learn to master and overcome them in comparable fashion to the amazing feats we were witnessing in other areas of industry. We might actually learn to master the world!

Concurrent with this vision was the widening separation of science and religion and the growing dominance of the "outer rational" view of life and diminution of the "inner subjective" view of meaning. Events, rather than being supernaturally determined, became the result of random probability and bell curve statistics. The universe became indifferent, with no inherent value agenda. Medical information was organized around agents of disease, vectors of attack, and strategies to intervene and stem the disease.

Hence, science and medicine became warriors against disease and death in a quest to overcome nature, and we now participate in the "war on cancer" and the "war on AIDS." The language of medicine is still rife with military analogies.

THE SELF-REGULATING SYSTEMS MODEL

Right at the beginning of the scientific "warrior" model, a profound dialog began between Louis Pasteur, the father of modern bacteriology, and Claude Bernard, the father of modern physiology. In effect, Bernard said, "If a large number of people are exposed to the tubercule bacillus, only a fraction of them become ill, and only a fraction of those who become ill will die. I think it at least as important to study the factors in the lives of those who did not become ill to determine how that came about as it is to study

177

our evolving views of health and illness: what does it all mean?

how to treat those who fall ill." Bernard saw disease as an indication of dysfunction in a connected, self-regulating, and self-healing life system. However, since the worldview of the time was based in mastery and domination of the natural process rather than understanding of its self-regulating framework, his comments were ignored, although some historians report that Pasteur acknowledged the wisdom of Bernard's view in later life.

A factor to consider is that this new understanding of the origins of disease within the interconnected systems of nature generated massive public health measures in the early twentieth century. Refrigerated foods, cleaner water systems, improved sewage disposal, mosquito abatement, antiseptic control in hospitals, and electric indoor lighting (as compared to gas and kerosene lamps) essentially diminished the impact of the major infectious diseases, such as tuberculosis, diphtheria, smallpox, malaria, by 1923. The effective clinical treatments for these diseases (antibiotics) did not become available until the 1940s. Therefore, the public belief that clinical medicine was the "conqueror" of infectious diseases is not validated by history. The current realization of the growing ineffectiveness of antibiotics as the natural system adapts in response to them is a clear illustration of the self-regulating systems model.

Concurrent with the wane of the infectious diseases in the 1920s was the rapid rise of chronic and degenerative disorders–heart disease, cancer, diabetes, and arthritis. The inadequacy of medicine's attempt to treat these conditions in the adversary (germ theory) model has become increasingly evident. Since these disorders are systemic functions in the whole organism, attempting to stem the disease as a separate "entity" can prove difficult, if not counterproductive.

In addition, the emergence of mind-body medicine and psychoneuroimmunology and the importance of subjective factors in illness and dysfunction illustrate that viewing disease as "an adversarial thing," or as an enemy to be overcome, may not be an appropriate view.

A major plus emerging in the systems model is the realization of our interaction within our natural and manufactured environment, and how our physiological systems respond. In just the past 50 years, we have introduced thousands of new materials into our lives, homes, offices, and foods, with little awareness of their cumulative effect on our bodies. In the disease-as-enemy/technology-as-victor model, these effects tend to be denied. We are only now beginning to recognize the extent of the systemic effects they may be generating.

In the systems model, rather than seeking causes to be fixed or symptoms to be modified, the investigator seeks patterns that result in dysfunction. Once the patterns are known, they can be changed and the potential consequences avoided. We have a growing awareness of "lifestyle" medicine and the importance of nutrition, exercise, smoking, and substance abuse, because of our increased knowledge about how life systems operate.

EMERGING CONSCIOUSNESS (NOETIC/INTEGRAL) MODEL

What is the role of human consciousness and intentionality in our interactions within the system of natural life? Is the universe a self-organizing, self-revealing intelligent life process seeking expression through human evolution? Joseph Chilton Pearce once questioned whether we can honestly believe that the evolutionary process that generated human intellect intended for us to become its adversary and try to outsmart it. And Einstein was reputed to ask, "Is the Universe friendly?" rather than hostile or indifferent.

If we considered the life system to be self-regulating and self-revealing, how might we perceive disease and dysfunction? What function would they serve in such a system? If the universe is self-revealing, how can we explore the answers to our deepest questions?

Today's practitioners of somatic psychology, "focusing," inner journal work, and other self-exploration techniques say that if we can clarify our inner questions, "the universe will answer them." Perhaps disease and dysfunction have encoded within them in both a metaphoric and literal sense the message available to us about how best to respond. This shifts the emphasis in healing from "doing to" to "being with."

A potential pitfall in this view is the misdirection of "self-blame." People who explore the cause or meaning of disease should not look upon this process as "creating their own disease" but rather as an insight into the inner process of their life. If the "aha" can be gained, new directions can emerge. This is quite different from "fixing" the problem or

179

our evolving views of health and illness: what does it all mean?

placing the blame. Healing becomes a matter of a shift of personal perspective rather than a rescue achieved.

NEW POWER AND RESPONSIBILITY IN OUR LIVES—INTENTIONALITY

Looking at the evolution of these ideas in just this century, we perceive a profound shift in our sense of what disease is and how we can respond to life circumstances. Just a few generations ago, we felt helpless and victimized by supernatural forces when illness appeared. We are now learning the deeper patterns of living systems, and how our hopes, fears, intentions, and desires may be woven into our lives and our bodies. In this new, more inclusive perspective, we have not only our inner awareness but all of the knowledge of history and science from which to choose to heal and improve our lives. This is both a new responsibility for becoming more self-aware and intentional and a possibility of new levels of health, well-being, and human achievement.

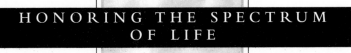

HONORING THE SPECTRUM OF LIFE

The Conflict of Biological and Cultural Imperatives

JOSEPH CHILTON PEARCE

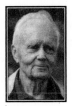

THE ROOTS OF VIOLENCE AND DISEASE

In the early 1950s Harvard University's Medical School did profiles on 200 medical students (all male in that day) to determine, as best they could, the emotional quality of infancy-childhood these students had experienced. Did they have happy or unhappy early memories? Had they felt secure, loved, wanted, accepted, supported by their parents, or had they experienced some degree of psychological abandonment, neglect, lack of love and support, etc? They were grouped under these simple positive-negative categories.

Now, 42 years later, the surviving 160 of these men, in their late 60s and early 70s, were given rigorous physical examinations to determine their overall health. Of those originally reporting a positive early experience, 25% had the "usual" diseases" associated with age: heart trouble, arthritis, and cancer being the big three. Of those reporting a negative infancy-childhood, 89% bore this conventional rostrum of afflictions.[1]

A postscript to the above was provided by the research of Lynda Russek, formerly of Harvard's medical school, and Gary Schwartz, of the medical school at the University of Arizona, Tucson. In the briefest of brief summaries, Schwartz-Russek, using electrocardiogram and brain-wave bio-feedback procedures, ran a further test with a representative number of those surviving medical men, finding that those with positive early experiences, on being interviewed at a close, personal level by an emotionally positive interviewer, showed clear physical-neurological and neuro-cardiological (heart) responses, their heart-brain frequencies going into a matched coherent "entrainment," synchronizing with the heart-brain frequencies of their interviewer, quite beneath their awareness. Such receptivity was not the case with those from a neglected childhood. They had fewer, weaker, and slower-forming signs of entrainment, apparently unresponsive to close positive relations, and implying, possibly, a lifelong state of the isolation and emotional poverty with which they had begun.[2]

Recent research in neurology and neuro-cardiology (the new field of research into the neural components, or "brain," of the heart) clearly show that emotional deprivation in the early formative period results in specific and apparently immutable compromises in neural structure and function, affecting health and all forms of relationship, personal and social, as well as forming subtle barriers that limit intellectual-rational growth, learning, and memory. In this negative case the various neural systems (for thought, feeling, action, relationship, emotional control, etc.) fail to entrain into a single unified response, each function "struggles for dominance" over the other, resulting in functional fragmentation, a conflict within that will express internally as disease and unhappiness or externally as insensitivity toward and/or callous disregard of the welfare of others, including the world, even to the point of violence and harm.[3]

STRANGE-LOOPS

Genetic system and environment are a reciprocal cause-effect loop. Each "gives rise to the other." DNA is experience sensitive, to an indeterminable extent. Without feedback from its environment, a genetic system couldn't build an organism adapted to that environment, and every new creature that appears among us reflects, by default, the environment for which, from which, and by which that development takes place. This is simple adaptability as selected for over the ages. Thus a social environment of anxiety or violence will tend to give rise to a generation genetically built for, and predisposed toward, anxiety and/or violence. By their very presence, such persons produce, or contribute to, a corresponding social environment tinged with and/or giving grounds for expression of their own predispositions. Violence breeds violence; anxiety, anxiety.

Research published in 1998 revealed any mammal's emotional state during conception and gestation of her offspring enters into and determines, to an indeterminable extent, the quality and characteristics of the brain of the infant to which she gives birth. This is critically so with humans. A mother exposed to an external environment of anxiety, violence, or negativity in general, or a mother producing such an environment within herself through her own predispositions and personal history, will give birth to an infant with an enlarged "hindbrain" and smaller "forebrain," terms that will be explained shortly. A mother in a secure, supportive, positive environment, or one that is able to produce and maintain a tranquil inner state regardless of externals, will give birth to an infant with an enlarged forebrain and smaller hindbrain, the opposite of the aforementioned.[4]

The heart is a major endocrine gland in our body, and from the moment of conception forward, it releases specific hormones, (neurotransmitters) designed to keep the mother in a tranquil state, as nature moves to form (or selects for) an infant predisposed toward higher forms of intelligences. A negative cultural environment can, however, overwhelm nature's primary concern and defeat such fail-safe measures.

EVOLUTIONARY BRAIN

The brain that unfolds in the fetus and uterine infant follows the same pattern of neural development observed in evolutionary history. The first to form is the ancient and instinctually powerful "reptilian" or "hindbrain." The "hindbrain" is the foundation of all subsequent formations, providing for our lifelong sensory-motor experience, physical awareness of body and its world, and a corresponding defensive "survival" system to maintain and protect, through ancient, non-negotiable instincts, both body and "self-system." The second and next oldest brain to form is the old mammalian or emotional brain, shared with all mammals, which provides us an objective stance from which we can make a qualitative evaluation of our world-experience. This is an evaluation founded on the simple response of pleasure-pain, feeling safe or threatened, loved and nurtured, or not. These responses are determined, in turn, solely by the infant's experience with the mother, both before and after birth. Learning and memory, immunities, all forms of relationship and emotional capacities center in this old mammalian complex, which clearly imprints to the mother's emotional state as her infant forms. The final neural structure forming in utero is the neocortical or new brain, which provides us the capacity for thought, language, primary reasoning, and so on. That which neuroscience labels the "forebrain" is the old mammalian and neocortical structures combined. The "hindbrain," as pointed out, is that defensive "reptilian" sensory-motor system.[5]

TRANSCENDENT BRAIN

Even a cursory examination of the history of these evolutionary neural structures shows that each evolved to overcome the limitations and constraints impinging on the former systems on which each new brain is based. "Overcoming limitation and constraint" is the dictionary definition of *transcendence*, so we can consider each evolutionary addition to our brain a means of transcending the limitations of the former, and acknowledge that our biological system is itself a transcendent procedure. The unfolding development of the infant-child will follow precisely this same transcendent progression evolution followed, to the extent the biological imperative of appropriate environment and nurturing is met.

A fourth and even more advanced and "transcendent" brain comes onto the scene immediately after birth, but consideration of this late bloomer must hold for the moment.

HINDBRAIN-FOREBRAIN

In summary, up to this point: the mother's emotional state during pregnancy may influence the quality, nature, character, capacity, and even size of her infant's neural system. A state of emotional security and love produces an infant with an enlarged "forebrain" and reduced-sized "hindbrain" as nature assumes the environment safe enough to invest her more advanced intelligences in this new life. A mother experiencing anxiety, insecurity, emotional isolation, or uncaring during pregnancy may give birth to an infant with an enlarged hindbrain and sharply reduced forebrain, since nature finds, in effect, that she can't, in this case, move for her higher evolutionary capacities but must shift her energy back into a successful defense system. Species survival takes precedence in all evolutionary progressions.

Now the very same selective process is involved after birth. The mother's emotional state in responding to her newborn's needs enters as the principal ingredient of the ongoing growth and development of these systems after birth as well.[6]

LATE ADDITION

The issue now is, following birth, that even more advanced or transcendent fourth brain, the prefrontal cortex alluded to above, unfolds for its growth and development. Added only recently in evolutionary history (only some 40,000 to 50,000 years ago, in sharp contrast to the hundreds of millions of years behind the primary reptilian brain), designed to be the largest of all the brains and crucial to civilized life, the prefrontals can only develop after birth and then only to the extent the foundational "triune system" has formed successfully and, as critically, to the extent the newborn is unconditionally nurtured by the mother in the ensuing weeks and months. For this fourth brain is even more critically dependent on and subject to appropriate environmental signals than any of its predecessors, far more susceptible to disruption in its growth and establishment, and equally more difficult to develop.[7] The higher in evolutionary intelligence we move, the more fragile the neural systems involved, though the more powerful they will be on successful maturation.

Just as it took 9 months in utero to develop the basic triune brain, it takes the 9 months following birth to grow and establish this fourth brain. And, just as the actual form and character of the uterine brain is determined by its sole environment, the mother's emotional state, so is the mother's emotional state the major environment and principal factor in the development of the infant's prefrontal cortex.[8] Note that the prefrontals are considered the "governor" of the fourfold brain, designed to modulate or moderate the actions of the other three and entrain them into singular intent or attention, as well as being the medium for translating all the higher human virtues, those that provide for, or give us, the highest dimensions of civilized life: creativity, love, empathy, social-ecological responsiveness, and so on.

TRANQUILIZERS

Earlier we observed that during pregnancy the mother's heart produced or brought about a flood of tranquilizing hormones to offset possible traumas or reactions causing anxiety or fear, as nature tries to ensure her new life's access to higher intelligences. In the same way, the heart provides, or attempts to provide, appropriate emotional responses in the mother for the ongoing postnatal nurturing and emotional support needed for the unfolding of this critical prefrontal cortex.

Indeed, devices for recording brain waves and heart frequencies clearly show that the head-and-heart frequencies of both infant and mother tend to go into entrainment, or coherent synchrony of wave forms, when in direct close interactions such as nursing. If prolonged separation occurs, both infant and mother systems become incoherent, indicating internal stress and release of cortisol and other "flight-fight" alert hormones, along with general survival-defensive reactions. Bring mother and infant back together, and each heart "lifts the other" out of chaos into order—entrainment between the two is reestablished.[9]

Just as the infant's heart has imprinted to and formed according to stimuli from the mother's heart during pregnancy, the ongoing interaction of the mother-infant systems after birth maintains a stabilizing influence each has on the other, and a rich cascade of intricately related sensory feedback loops, far too involved to go into here, opening at the moment of birth if and only if the infant is kept within the mother's immediate heart-field, give rise to that mutually interactive relationship between infant and mother referred to as *bonding*. Through myriad interlocking instinctual responses developed over eons, the infant literally awakens and activates in the mother a compelling desire to nurture her infant in turn. The bonded mother is literally driven with a compulsive and overwhelming passion for such nurturing, and a whole complex of instinctive knowledge of precisely how to nurture and provide all that is needed for the welfare and ongoing development of that new life. This is a joyful union that can sustain both mother and child through extremes of external pressures.[10]

This bonding feedback loop between the two continues unbroken for the first 18 months or so after birth, and on a more relaxed level into the third year and beyond. Nature spent millions of evolutionary years developing precisely this non-negotiable nurturing-protective drive, ensuring a mother who will never abandon her infant nor, as is often the case today, succumb to any of the camouflaged cultural forms of abandonment, as found in day care, foster care, television, playpens, and so on. As we will see, however, this vast and ancient biological imperative has been overridden—indeed all but abolished—by a collective cultural imperative based on fear, distrust of nature, and defensive procedures to predict and control and so protect us from nature, all but destroying her agenda and leaving our children adrift.

SECURITY CHECK

All mammals, when preparing for birth, seek out the safest, most hidden, preferably dark place available, for they are at that point most vulnerable. And at the slightest sign of intervention of any sort, even the cracking of a twig, that mammalian brain controlling birth signals the body to slow or suspend birth proceedings until the coast is clear. We are mammals; our mammalian brain is in charge of birthing, with millions of years of genetically encoded instructions for successful delivery. Interfering with birth in any way, for any reason, disrupts this "cascade" of interacting responses and, in typical domino-fashion, seriously impairs all future infant-mother relations and the ongoing development arising from and dependent on it.

In our day, virtually all births are dramatically, traumatically, indeed violently interfered with, and have been to varying degrees for untold millennia in Western cultures. From the dire pronouncements against women found in the patriarchal-religious myths of Genesis, woman was branded as the primal source of human error and sentenced by the gods to suffer pain and anguish in childbirth as punishment for her sins. Not only was this dark and evil notion slowly embedded into the collective psyche, it became a self-fulfilling prophecy, a morphic-field effect shaping the nature of birth experience. Societies never exposed to these demonic influences know a joyful, generally erotic, and always safer birthing experience than the grisly history of mortality wrought on Western women. Just this darkly negative influence, growing over the centuries, was what exploded exponentially in the twentieth century and engulfed virtually the whole planet.[11]

WITCH HUNTS—OLD AND NEW

Some six centuries ago the church began to systematically eliminate all autochthonic expressions of a nature-based, earth-mother archetype, a spiritual expression of intuitive knowing and capacity which bestowed on women the power to be the mother of our species. Ecclesiastics set about to systematically destroy the wisdom-women, midwives, and crones, their legends and stories carrying on the ancient biological agenda set by nature. English historians estimate some nine million women were murdered by the church over a three century period (dismissed in our history books as rather amusing witch hunts), and males began to fill the vacuum left, slowly taking over all reproductive decisions and childbirth procedures, stripping the power of the mother and her capacity to mother, leaving her dependent on male counterfeits. These maneuvers arose from and sustained the collective cultural imperatives based on fear, sin, retribution, judgment, and punishment, by which social control has been and is still enforced in the West, until today there are few traces of midwifery or natural birthing left. The grossly abnormal has, in fact, become the norm, as with most negative cultural drifts.[12]

No "golden age" is meant to be implied from the above. But somehow our species managed to "muddle-through" terrifying periods of natural and social crises so long as birthing was untrammeled and firmly in the hands of the mother, simply because at least the foundations of nature's biological imperative were established, regardless of what then happened through later cultural impingements and imprinting. And on that thread of sanity established by mother-child bonding, we held at least a fairly viable course. Our populace today seems largely unaware of the vastness of breakdown in species-survival brought to a head in the twentieth century, this past 100 years during which we destroyed 100 million of our own selves. In the second half of the twentieth century, not only did suicide become the third highest cause of death in American children (the number of suicide attempts being far greater than successes), but between 1990 and the year 2000, more American children were killed by the guns of other American children than American soldiers were killed in the Vietnam War. 50,000 children killed each other in that climactic decade, with not one voice raised about causation, not one memorial to those slain victims proposed, nor any move at all to stop the carnage other than self-righteous mutterings about gun control.[13] The American populace simply screens the child crisis from mind, lest our high standard of comfort be disturbed. As Paul MacLean said, there is no historical precedent for a society driving its own children to suicide, a radical innovation in our planet's life and a clear indication of a species on the way out.

The slow erosion of the power of the mother, long under way, increased dramatically some 600 years ago, with males slowly taking over all reproductive issues, particularly birthing, and reached its zenith in the middle of the twentieth century, wherein medicine men with their technologies and hospitals took over birthing in toto and made midwifery and home birth illegal. The fact that home birth, wherever it could be found, was still safer than hospital birth, has been carefully veiled by the medical myth that controls media and minds.[14]

BROKEN BOND

The radical interferences introduced by medical-hospital birthing eliminated all traces of bonding and deliberately eliminated breast feeding in 97% of all infants throughout the century. (Israeli doctors published evidence that any society eliminating breast feeding shows an immediate, one-for-one corresponding increase in breast cancer, studies not published in the U.S.) The recent arbitrary, contrived, and ludicrously ironic legal mandates that hospitals must re-introduce breast-feeding have had feeble results at best, since the bonding instincts involved in that nurturing have been obliterated by the whole technological complex before the issue of mandated breast-feeding could be attempted.

Before this final hospital take-over in mid-century, no suicide in children under 14 years had ever been reported, while within 25 years after the technological takeover, suicide had moved down to age 3, as the social fabric of family, community, education began to come apart at the seams.

Wherein we turned into a nation passionately intent on therapy and healing—opening the door to a new wave of cultural opportunists feeding on the social body's acculturated fear, anxiety, and impotency—while we continued the basic atrocities against mothers and infants unabated.

Few subjects have been more intensely researched than the damage brought about by medical-hospital childbirth, and seldom have we witnessed such a skillful backlash to counter such knowledge and maintain control through fear and deception. Childbirth accounts for some 66% of all hospital revenue, and obstetricians are the second-highest paid of all surgeons, topped only by heart surgeons. After 30 years of attempts to at least communicate this issue to the public, I find the collective cultural imperative too interwoven into the fabric of life, blocking our ability to hear and respond to the situation we face. Throughout, however, a handful of powerful women with remarkable courage and strength have intuitively perceived nature's imperative, or heard about and acted on it. And they have consistently given birth to astonishingly superior children, a fact that is not advertised by these wise women, who intuitively protect their children against the deadly cultural compulsion for conformity and behavioral control. May their number increase, for they may be the seed of a new humanity springing forth, as this present one self-destructs.

NOTES

1.   Song LZ, Schwartz GE, Russek LG: Heart-focused attention and heart-brain synchronization: energetic and physiological mechanisms, *Alt Ther Health Med* 4(5):44-52, 54-60, 62, September 1998.

2.   Russek LG, Schwartz GE: Interpersonal heart-brain registration and the perception of parental love: a 42-year follow-up of the Harvard Mastery of Stress Study, *Subtle Energies* 5(3):195, 1994. Russek L, Schwartz GE: Energy cardiology: a dynamical energy systems approach for integrating conventional and alternative medicine. *Advances: The Journal of Mind-Body Health* 12(4), Fall 1996.

3.   Montessori M: *The secret of childhood*, 1978, Orient-Longman. *The absorbent mind*, 1992, Kalakshetra. Prescott J: Body pleasures and the origin of violence, *The Futurist*

April, 1975. Montague A: *Touching: the human significance of the skin,* New York, 1971, Columbia University Press. Caplan M: *Untouched: the need for genuine affection in an impersonal world,* Prescott, Ariz, 1998, Hohm Press.

4. Bioculturalism, the reciprocal effect of culture on our biology and biology on culture, is explored by Colavito MM: *The myth of Oedipus and the mind-mind split,* London, 1993, Edwin Mellen Press; White LA: Science of culture: a study of man and civilization, Noonday Press; numerous publications by cellular biologist Bruce Lipton since 1970; and several other sources.

5. Cantin M, Genest J: The heart as an endocrine gland, *Sci Am* 9(4):319-327, 1986; MacLean P: *A triune concept of the brain and behavior,* edited by Campbell D and Boag TJ, 1973, Toronto, University of Toronto Press (The Clarence M. Hincks Memorial Lecture Series).

6. See the general work of Allen Schore, Medical School, University of California, Los Angeles, as noted below.

7. Schore AN: *Affect regulation and the origins of the self: the neurobiology of emotional development,* Hillsdale, N.J., 1994, Lawrence Erlbaum Associates.

8. Schore AN: The experience-dependent maturation of a regulatory system in the orbital prefrontal cortex and the origin of developmental psychpathology, *Dev Psychopathol* 89:55-87.

9. From early studies, such as Salk L: Effects of normal heartbeat sound on behavior of newborn babies: implications for mental health, *World Mental Health* 12:4, 1960; on to Childre L, Martin H: *The HeartMath solution,* San Francisco, 1999, Harper; and numerous publications by HeartMath on heart-brain entrainment.

10. As examples of numerous studies, see Klaus M: Human maternal behavior at the first contact with her young, *Pediatrics* 46(2):187-192, 1970; Maternal attachment: importance of the first post-partum days, *N Engl J Med,* 286(9):460-463, 1972; Kennell J, Trause MA, Klaus MH: Evidence for a sensitive period in the human mother, Parent-Infant Interaction *CIBA Foundation Symposium 33,* 1975; Whittlestone WG: The physiology of early attachment in mammals: implications for human obstetric care, *Med J Aust,* 1:50-53, January 14, 1978.

11. From early reports such as those by Ainsworth M: Deprivation of maternal care: a reassessment of its effect *Public Health Papers,* No. l 14: 97-165f; Geneva: World Health Organization, etc; on to the work of Geber M, Pearce JC: *Magical child,* 1977, E.P. Dutton; *From magical child to magical teen,* Rochester, Vermont, 2003, ITI Park Street Press; *Evolution's end,* San Francisco, 1999, Harper; Leidloff J: The c, 1976, Addison-Wesley Press.

13. See the now-classic work by Arms S: *Immaculate deception: A new look at women and childbirth in America,* Boston, 1975, Houghton-Mifflin; or Hunt J: *Natural child,* Sweet B, Sweet W: *Living joyfully with children*; Mendizza M: *Magical parent—magical child.* The list is long.

14. As with child suicide, only the most blatantly lurid and sensational violent killings by and of young people make the news, and figures on both types of death are difficult to dig out of statistics since they are buried under various categories. As of 1995, an estimated 130,000 schoolchildren carried guns to school each day, each day a total of 30 children were struck by bullets from those guns (as well as from wounds inflicted by other weapons), and each day some six of those wounded died. Consider that, as of

the year 2000, suicide was the third-highest cause of death in U.S. children between 5 and 17, which doesn't take into account that far more suicides are attempted than succeed and that more females attempt suicide than males, yet more males accomplish the act. Virtually all suicides in early childhood are recorded as accidental deaths, since, according to a 1989 HEW report, the nation as a whole can't grasp the fact that suicide now reaches down to age 3.

15. The U.S. spends more per capita on medical care than any other nation, and 97% of all infants are (by law) hospital deliveries, yet, according to the 1995 U.S. Bureau of Statistics, the United States stood twenty-third out of 29 industrialized nations in infant-mother birth mortality. At that time, Holland, with 94% of all births midwife-home delivered (for generations), had the lowest birth mortality of any nation. Recently the U.S. Center for Disease Control stated that home birth was as safe as hospital birth, which was quite an admission for a direct branch of the medical establishment. Home birth is far safer, but mortality is only one of the issues. Far more critical is the breakup of bonding that hospitals automatically induce, not just through a series of direct interventions but through the atmosphere of crisis and alarm that fills the scene, as birth is treated as a disease and emergency. Technological birth brings a series of traumas to infants, many of which are lifelong, as explored in many publications, including the forthcoming book, *The Fabric of Autism,* by Judith Bluestone.

References for this essay are located on the DVD accompanying this book.

Aging with Awareness

RON VALLE
MARY MOHS

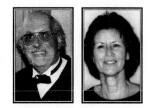

W HEN WE RESIST AGING, we resist life itself, since aging is inherent in living. Suffering results when we push away what is real. Many of us fear growing older; we resist reflecting on our later years, what we will look like, how we will feel, and, hence, we suffer. Healing is the easing of this fear and its resultant suffering. We heal by opening to the changes in life and allowing what is real to naturally evolve. In this chapter, we will explore the anatomy of this process and how wisdom emerges as we bring awareness to the full breadth of our lives.

AGING, GRIEVING, AND THE FEAR OF DEATH

Aging through our later years can be a remarkable time for increasing self-understanding and deepening one's spiritual awareness. To see this opportunity, however, requires a special sensitivity to these possibilities and an atmosphere of mutual support and encouragement. Rather than guiding us in this direction, our society has, regrettably, glorified the benefits of our youthful years while minimizing and degrading the elderly and the value of the aging process. Focusing on youth while pushing away the constant change involved in aging reflects our culture's denial of the ever-changing process that life is, as well as, ultimately, of death itself. Until we accept all of life, we cannot truly live. In light of this, it is essential to recognize the sacredness of every human being, regardless of age, as well as the unfolding wisdom inherent in the aging process itself.

We know in our hearts that living, dying, and grieving are inseparable, each dependent on the other two for its meaning and purpose. In fact, although they are often treated as opposites, life and death are two aspects of a greater, single process, with aging and grieving as the connecting glue. Grieving is the painful response we have to the loss of someone or something we have become attached to, a response we experience quite often to one degree or another, given that change and loss are in the very fabric of life itself. As Levine[1] has pointed out, the degree of grief that we will experience whenever change occurs in our lives is directly related to how much we resist this change here and now in the present moment.

When we begin to live mindful of aging and dying, however, grief is honored as a natural response to loss, and death becomes a mirror in which life is understood and prioritized in a new way. Life, death, and grief are everywhere, whether it be the birth of a new idea, heartbreak at the death of a child, or a leaf falling from a tree. In this way, we begin to accept and celebrate the constant flow of life's transitions rather than fear the next turn in the road. Thus, to the extent that we can let go into the mystery of life, we find true peace and love in the aging process.

Ram Dass[2] and Bianchi[3] both see aging as a means of deepening our spiritual awareness and believe that looking within ourselves is central in this process. Ram Dass, reflecting on his own personal process of growing older and struggling to accept difficult changes in his own life, describes the emotional and spiritual benefits that come with embracing aging, changing, and dying. By shifting our perspective on the nature of pain and loss, new ways of being with grief emerge. Ram Dass expands on this process:

> When we cease to resist our grief, we learn that, painful though it may be, grief is an integral part of elder wisdom, a force that humbles and deepens our hearts, connects us to the grief of the world, and enables us to be of help.

Grief need not paralyze the heart or become a garment for the ego....We must be able to step outside our egos, as Soul. Otherwise we are likely to be swept away by one or the other of grief's common fallouts, either closing our hearts in fear of the magnitude of our own [and others'] feelings and shrinking our lives to a "safe" zone that leaves us feeling half-alive; or becoming professional mourners, caught in the past with its loss and regret, unable to let go or to enjoy the present.[2]

Consistent with Ram Dass' emphasis, Bianchi emphasizes that a spirituality of middle age and elderhood calls for a turning inward, for a deeper contemplative and meditative life.[3] Such an approach stands against the tide of our culture, which expects the middle-aged and even the elderly to compete externally with much of the ardor of youth.

Within our culture, conventional ways of being with suffering and the dying process continue to reflect, on an institutional level, the deepest individual fear: the fear of death. Rather than being recognized as the natural companion of life, death is seen as an outside threat to that life, something to be controlled with our latest drugs and surgical techniques. Or, when the dying process cannot be avoided or significantly delayed, it is often hidden away in nursing homes or the back rooms of special hospital floors.

This same fear of death, left unexamined and unfelt, spills over into our lives. Our need to control others and the environment is our attempt to cope with this fear. Our unwillingness to grow old is one of its manifestations. Restrained by self-imposed limits, we keep ourselves from living in a creative, loving, and meaningful way. We are afraid to live because we don't want to die. We resist change because we don't want to grieve. Rather than celebrating the rich variety and beauty of human expression as it naturally emerges as one grows older and approaches the end of one's life, our emotional and passionate responses are often greeted with disapproval and mistrust. As we progress through our senior years, we are increasingly patronized and treated like children. Gentle acceptance and appreciation are simply not the norm.

UNDERSTANDING ONE'S RESPONSES TO LOSS

A simple awareness of how most individuals typically respond to significant or impending losses in their lives can be very helpful, even healing, in being with a present or soon-to-be realized loss in one's own life. Whether you have just heard of a dear friend's death, realized the natural decline of your health with age, or have just been told by your doctor that you have a terminal illness and have only a month to live, your reactions might very well be intense and very painful. Understanding the natural process of grieving can lessen the fear that often comes when we are lost in overwhelming grief. The following three stages or types of response reflect the process most of us go through when experiencing real or impending loss[4-6]:

1. *Shock can last from weeks to months.* This often includes:
   - Feeling stunned
   - Physical, emotional, and intellectual numbness
   - Denial (e.g., "No! It can't be true!")
   - Feeling confused and crazy
   - Everything in life taking on an unreal quality
   - Loss of self-identity

2. *Reaction and disorganization.* This often includes:
   - Anger and protest (e.g., "The doctors don't know what they're talking about!")
   - Loss of appetite; overeating
   - Self-criticism and guilt
   - Preoccupation with thoughts regarding the loss
   - Absent-mindedness
   - Yearning and searching (for the lost loved one)
   - Avoiding (painful reminders)
   - Having a sense of the loved one's presence
   - Nausea, weakness, shortness of breath, sleep disturbance
   - Increased use of alcohol and other drugs
   - Bargaining ("If I can live until my daughter's wedding, I will die peacefully.")
   - Depression, withdrawal, apathy, and loneliness
   - Aimlessness; restlessness
   - Frequent crying and sighing
   - Anxiety and inactivity

3. *Acceptance and "letting go."* This often includes:
   - Talking about the loss without intense emotion
   - Reorganization—less preoccupation with the loss

- Being more open to new ideas and behavior
- Trusting more in the process of life
- Finding meaning in life and death
- Realizing the grace in grieving
- More interest in serving others
- Seeing relationships as more important than material possessions
- A deepening of spiritual awareness
- Seeing grieving as a personally transforming experience

Although written words themselves cannot truly touch the deep pain of grief, knowing that there is a recognized process that most grieving individuals go through can serve as a ground for one's thoughts, feelings, and sanity itself when the intense waves of grief appear.

OPENING TO THE VALUE OF AGING

During the last phase of life, we have more time to reflect on the nature of life and death. This is a time when we have a special opportunity to open to our inner process and bring greater clarity, meaning, and peace into our lives. In our earlier years, we focused mainly on doing—getting married, buying a house, raising a family, and building our career—and there wasn't much time for simply being or reflecting. In our later years, we are preparing to leave this world. Loss is everywhere. Our friends are dying or moving, our homes and possessions are being sold or given away, we no longer have our careers, our family is often too busy to spend time with us, and our health is deteriorating. We become rigid and resistant to pain to the extent that we hold onto what we are losing. As we let go and open more fully to life, there is a greater realization of what the present moment has to offer. Our deepest wisdom and understanding thereby emerge.

Christine Longaker,[7] hospice director, author, and world lecturer, describes four dimensions or characteristics she has come to recognize in persons who are facing the end of their lives:

1. The elderly look for meaning in their lives. This search for meaning includes exploring past experiences, recognizing the times they felt love for themselves and others, and finding understanding and forgiveness for that which they regret.

2. They reflect on past relationships and wish they could resolve those relationships that are remembered as discordant. Communicating more effectively with their families can be of help in this process. It is, therefore, important to explore where each person feels unfinished with his or her past, since opening to past experiences often helps to resolve these conflicts, relaxing the mind and freeing one's energy.

3. They also want to understand the physical and emotional pain that they are experiencing and to find some relief. Such relief often comes by finding a purpose for this suffering. One purpose that many spiritual traditions recognize is that the experience of suffering provides an opportunity to offer this suffering for the benefit of others. Seeing one's pain in this transpersonal way[8] transforms the solely personal meaning of the pain. This selfless intention leaves its mark in the collective awareness shared by all human beings, thereby reducing the fear and pain of countless individuals throughout the world. Consider Sogyal Rinpoche's words[9]:

Recently one of my students came to me and said: "My friend is in pain, and dying of leukemia. He is already frighteningly bitter; I'm terrified that he'll drown in bitterness. He keeps asking me: 'What can I do with all this useless, horrible suffering?'" My heart went out to her and her friend. Perhaps nothing is as painful as believing that there is no use to the pain you are going through. I told my student that there was a way that her friend could transform his death even now, and even in the great pain he was enduring: to dedicate, with all his heart, the suffering of his dying, and his death itself, to the benefit and ultimate happiness of others. I told her to tell him: "Imagine all the others in the world who are in a pain like yours. Fill your heart with compassion for them. And pray to whomever you believe in and ask that your suffering should help alleviate theirs. Again and again, dedicate your pain to the alleviation of their pain. And you will quickly discover in yourself a new source of strength, a compassion you'll hardly be able now to imagine, and a certainty, beyond any shadow of a doubt, that your suffering is not only not being wasted, but has now a marvelous meaning."

4. Finally, they reflect on death, what it is like and how to prepare for it. Exploring their feelings and beliefs about death can help them discover the depths of their spirituality and can bring a sense of greater peace and joy. Connecting with a respected spiritual leader or teacher and praying or meditating in a way that feels right to them can also be helpful.

Gradually, as one goes within and opens to all four of these dimensions, one becomes more authentic (i.e., true to oneself) and less reactive to life. In this way, we slowly become more accepting of the changes that accompany aging.

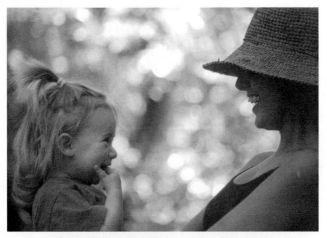

A, "Woman and Child Laughing." (Courtesy David "Dudi" Shmueli.)

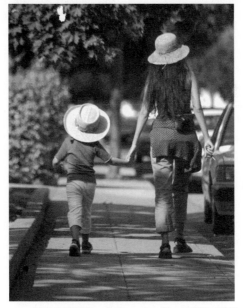

B, "Woman and Child Walking." (Courtesy David "Dudi" Shmueli.)

GROWING OLDER GRACEFULLY

What does the cliché "growing old gracefully" really mean? My (Mary's) mother used to say that one needs to grow old gracefully in order to truly live and feel the joy of life. This requires a true transformation in how we view life as well as, perhaps most important, how we hold on to what is pleasant and familiar. Our youthful identity and vitality are, for example, especially difficult to surrender. The aging process can be an opportunity for such a transformation. In order for this transformation to occur, one must be willing to be present with what is happening in the moment, including opening to one's own inner process. This involves letting go of expectations and past beliefs or experiences that may mask or block what is true in the moment. This letting go allows a deep and natural joy, a joy that lies beyond pleasure and pain, to emerge.

As we become older, we have a tendency to resist change and to close out the world around us. In order to open to life, we need to open our minds and hearts. Whenever we get caught in the grip of our own or others' criticism, or when we ruminate about that which we cannot change, we can consciously and compassionately become more spacious by watching the mind and observing its negative patterns. Rather than trying to analyze why we are feeling frightened, angry, jealous, or lonely, we can observe these feelings, as we sense them in our bodies, with compassion and allow them to simply be.

Working with one's self in this way can be a true spiritual practice. By softening and opening to the painful feelings that we've always run away from in the past, we eventually see what is behind them. We thereby open to the mystery, to the sacred dimensions of life.

CONCLUSION

The approach offered in this chapter is truly integral in that it shares a perspective offered by many of the world's great spiritual traditions—namely, that all apparently separate phenomena and processes in life emanate from the same underlying transcendent reality or source. For example, consider the words of Swami Rama[10] of the Himalayan Yoga Tradition:

Life's purpose is to know the distinction between what is outside and fleeting, and what is inside and eternal, and to discover through practice and experience the infinite value of one to the other. Once this experience is realized, life takes on a joyful meaning and the fear of death evaporates.

Aging while retaining this level of awareness is a challenge in our culture. It is understandable that many of us feel trapped in an aging body while the world around us constantly celebrates the pleasures of youth. Aging with awareness requires being present in each moment and being willing to open to life and all of its complexities. The process of playing one's part in life and then letting go of the effects of one's actions is emphasized in many of the world's scriptures (e.g., the Bible and the Bhagavad Gita). Given that we have become attached to persons and things of the world, letting go is a process that involves grieving the losses in our lives. By opening to this process, we develop gratitude, patience, compassion, confidence, fearlessness, authenticity, harmony, joy, inspiration, and peace of mind.

The value of aging involves the journey within. Meditation, contemplation, prayer, journaling, reading inspirational works, dream-work, poetry, and keeping silence are all means that one can use to enter and explore one's inner space. Ram Dass[2] tells us, "Without acknowledging the soul level or cultivating a soul consciousness, we are like passengers trapped on a sinking ship." If we can see the aging process as an unfolding opportunity to gain deeper wisdom by discriminating external phenomena from internal reality and by opening to the fullness of life, rather than resisting the pain and contracting into our ego-selves, much of our needless suffering will be eased.

References for this essay are located on the DVD accompanying this book.

*Timeless Mind, Ageless Body**

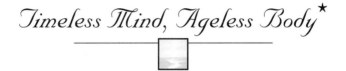

DEEPAK CHOPRA

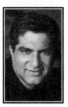

I'D LIKE TO INTRODUCE THE notion of timeless mind and ageless body. I have found we hold many myths about human potential, especially about the aging process. People believe, for example, that aging is fatal. But people don't die of old age—they die of diseases that accompany old age, most of which are preventable.

According to the ancient Indian philosophy of *ayurveda*, one of the reasons people grow old, age, and die is that they see other people growing old, aging, and dying. What we see we become because we have this superstition that seeing is believing. I'd like to persuade you that seeing is not believing, that it is just a superstition, a superstition of materialism.

By the end of this article, at least some of you, I hope, will agree with me that if you can see it and touch it, it's probably an illusion, and it doesn't exist. What we see is the step-child of something that's abstract,

---

*Adapted from Chopra D: Timeless Mind, Ageless Body. *Noetic Sciences Review,* 28:16, Winter 1993. Originally adapted from a keynote talk by Deepak Chopra at the Institute of Noetic Sciences Heart of Healing Conference.

ineffable, unbounded, has no beginning or ending in time—and that "something" is what you and I really are.

The superstition of materialism comes about because we trust our senses. And yet even with common sense we know that, if anything, sensory experience is the least reliable test of reality. After all, my senses tell me that the Earth is flat. Nobody believes that anymore. My senses tell me that the ground I'm standing on is stationary, and yet I know it's spinning at dizzying speeds.

But the superstition of materialism is pervasive. We've been stuck with it for the last 300 years. We each think of ourselves as an encapsulated ego, enmeshed in a bag of flesh and bone, confined to a prison of space, time, and causation, squeezed into the volume of a body and the span of a lifetime. We think of the human body basically as a physical machine that has learned how to think. Consciousness becomes the by-product of matter.

Until recently, all of Western scientific research has been based on this model of the human body. Science has held that if you can understand the mechanisms of disease on the level of matter, then you should be able to get rid of disease. If you can understand, for example, how bacteria multiply and if you interfere using the appropriate antibiotic, then you shouldn't have infections any more. Or if you can understand how cancer cells replicate and you interfere using the appropriate chemotherapy, you should be able to get rid of cancer cells—not realizing that the mechanisms for disease are not the same as origins of disease.

Understanding the mechanisms of disease can be important in eliminating illness, but it really does nothing to alter the overall morbidity or mortality in our population. We simply end up replacing old epidemics with new ones.

Origins of disease have to do with how we live our lives. They have to do with basic life processes such as breathing, eating, digestion, metabolism, elimination, and, most important, the movement of consciousness, which expresses itself as these life processes.

Moreover, origins of disease have very little to do with origins of health, which is a completely different experience. I would venture to say that origins of health have to do with understanding one's own spiritual nature—the essence of life itself. And yet if you ask people what life is, even though they are living it, they are unable to give you any exact description. I asked a friend of mine recently to define life, and he said, "It's a sexually transmitted, incurable disease."

Even in the very act of treating illness, we sow the seeds for illness in the future. I've heard that an estimated 100,000 people die every year in the United States from antibiotic-resistant infections alone, acquired in hospitals. The number-one drug addiction in the world is not to a street drug but to medicine legally prescribed by physicians. It is estimated that in this country 80 percent of the population swallow a medically pre-scribed chemical every 24 hours. Despite the fact that more people are doing research on cancer than have cancer, the incidence of that disease has increased in the last 3 decades.

Something is obviously wrong with our current model of the human body. The reality is that your physical body is not a frozen anatomical structure but literally a river of intelligence and information and energy that's constantly renewing itself every second of your existence. Just as you can't step into the same river twice because new water is always flowing in, the real you cannot step into the same flesh and bones twice. Every second of your existence, you are renewing your body more easily, more effortlessly, and more spontaneously than you can even change your clothes. In fact, the physical body you are using to read this article is not the same as the one you sat down with a short while ago.

Various scientists have calculated that in less than 1 year, you replace about 98 percent of all the atoms in your body, making a new liver every 6 weeks; a new skeleton (which seems so hard and solid and permanent) every 3 months; a new stomach lining every 5 days; a new skin once a month. Even the brain cells you think with, as carbon and hydrogen and oxygen, weren't there 1 year ago, and the actual raw material of the DNA, which holds memories of millions of years of evolutionary time, comes and goes every 6 weeks.

If you think you are your material body, you certainly have a dilemma—which one are you talking about? When I gave my talk in Washington, I used my 1993 model. The previous time I was there, I took with me the same suitcase, some of the same clothes, some of the same lecture notes, but not the same body. The physical body I took with me is merely recycled earth, water, and air.

I'd like to propose that we are not physical machines that have learned how to think. Perhaps it's the other way around: We are thoughts (and impulses, consciousness, feelings, emotions, desires, and dreams) that have learned how to create physical bodies; that which we call our physical body is perhaps just a place that our memories call home for the time being.

I would also suggest that this concept is not just an interesting, esoteric, philosophical speculation based in Eastern mysticism but that, in fact, we can look at it through the window of current science. Today, if you asked a really good physicist to identify the true nature of the physical body, she would tell you that ultimately it's made up of atoms; the atoms are in turn made up of subatomic particles moving at lightning speed around huge empty spaces. These particles suddenly appear, hang on for a fraction of a fraction of a fraction of a second, and then collide, rebound, disintegrate, and disappear into a void; and these subatomic particles are not material things; they are actually fluctuations of energy and information in a huge void.

As you go beyond the facade of molecules into the subatomic cloud, you end up with a handful of nothing. The question is, What is this handful of nothing—is it just an empty void, or possibly the womb of creation? Could it be that nature goes to exactly the same place to create a galaxy of stars or a cluster of nebulae or a rainforest or a human body as it goes to create a thought? Could it be that our inner space is no different from outer space, and could it be that if we could go to this place we could become creators on our own?

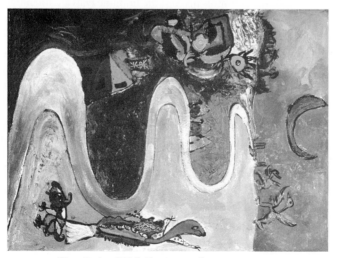

"Jazz Series #12." (Courtesy Eileen G. Hyman.)

Today many scientists recognize that the essential nature of the material world is not material. The essential stuff of the universe is not stuff. What is even more interesting is that it becomes thinking non-stuff; as it thinks, it creates everything from stars to galaxies to human bodies. I would suggest that a thought is nothing but a quantum event in the same unified field from where nature creates everything. A thought is a fluctuation of energy and information in the same void.

I know we experience our thoughts as willfully elite things that are linguistically structured and speak to us in the English language (and mostly with an Indian accent), but before thoughts are spoken, they are just fluctuations in the same quantum fields. Nature is a thinking organism, and our own thinking is just one reflection of nature's thinking. Thoughts transform themselves into molecules, and these molecules, called *neuropeptides* (first discovered in the brain), are literally messengers from inner space. Therefore, to think is to practice brain chemistry and body chemistry because these receptors are not only on the neurons in the brain, they are on all the cells of our body.

If you look at T cells and B cells and lymphocytes, you find they are constantly eavesdropping on your internal dialogue. Somebody inside you is constantly having a conversation with themselves. One thing about this person: He/she/it never shuts up. And the immune cells are listening. Not only are they listening, they are participating in that same conversation, because they make the same peptides the brain makes when it thinks. In fact, there are neurobiologists who say there is no difference between the immune system and the nervous system—the immune system is a circulating nervous system. It thinks, it has emotions, it has memory, and it has the ability to make choices and to anticipate events.

Even more interesting, this is true not only of the immune system but of all the cells in our body. So when you say you have a gut feeling about such and such, you are not speaking metaphorically but quite literally, for the gut makes the same chemicals the brain makes when it thinks. In fact, your gut feelings may be more accurate because gut cells haven't yet learned how to doubt their own thinking.

We are discovering that our body is actually the objective experience of consciousness, just as our mind is the subjective experience of consciousness. But they're both inseparably one. The body is a field of ideas.

When you say, "My heart is heavy with sadness," your heart is literally loaded with fat chemicals. When you say, "I'm bursting with joy," your skin is loaded with endorphins, interleukins, and interferons, which are powerful immunobody regulators and powerful anticancer drugs.

You and I are neither the body nor the mind; we are the creator of both, which is pure consciousness. It's difficult sometimes to express this in words, yet this has been, in fact, the wisdom of almost every spiritual tradition in the world. In ancient Vedic wisdom, for example, there is an aphorism that says, "I am not the mind; I am not the body. I come within myself to create body and mind. I experience myself subjectively as the mind. I experience myself objectively as the body and the physical universe. But I am neither—I am beyond both." The aphorism goes on to say: "I am That, you are That. All this is That. That is all there is."

Understanding that consciousness is the creator of mind and body, I think, is really necessary for us to survive and create a new reality. Not only is the body a field of ideas, but so is the physical universe we inhabit.

The obvious questions to ask are: If it's really true that I create a new body every year and a new skeleton every few months, why do I still have the arthritis? If my blood vessels change every 6 weeks, why are they still blocked? With the cancer cells coming and going with a twitch of an eye, why are they still there?

The answer is that we've become bundles of conditioned reflexes that are constantly being triggered, by people and circumstance, to the same predictable outcomes. We've become victims of the same repetition of unformed memories. Through conditioning, we generate the same impulses of energy and information, the same behavioral practices that result in the same space/time events, the same biochemistry, and, ultimately, the same life experiences. (It is estimated that the average human thinks about 16,000 thoughts a day. This is not surprising, but what is a little disconcerting is that I've heard reports that about 90 percent of the thoughts we've had today are the same ones that we had yesterday.) But it shouldn't have to be like that.

In an interesting experiment at the University of Ohio, scientists put rabbits on extremely high cholesterol diets. To their amazement, they found that one group of rabbits didn't get high cholesterol blood levels or hardening of the arteries. After much investigation, they discovered that the only difference with these rabbits was that the technician who fed them, instead of just throwing the food in to them, would take them out of the cage and cuddle and kiss them. All rabbits were fed the same poisonous food. The addition of the experience of love (I don't usually use that word in speeches—I say "the flow of information") made the crucial difference between life and death from this country's number-one killer.

More recently, *The Journal of Pediatrics* reported on research by scientists at the University of Miami School of Medicine who divided premature infants into two groups; an investigator would reach in and stroke each baby in one group about three times a day for approximately 5 minutes. The babies in this group gained an average of 49 to 50 percent more weight per day, fed on exactly the same formula as the control group. The investigators concluded that tactile kinesthetic stimulation (love) is a positive effective strategy.

A few years ago, the Department of Health, Education, and Welfare in Massachusetts published a study, which has since been replicated in France, in which scientists and statisticians looked once again at the risk factors for heart disease. They found that the number-one predictor of fatal heart attacks, initially described as job dissatisfaction, was more precisely pinned down as lack of meaning or purpose in life.

In fact, the consistent statistic emerging from studies like this is that more people die in our age, in our culture, on one particular day of the week and time of day—Monday morning at nine o'clock. It's a unique accomplishment for which only the human species can take credit.

The point is that our bodies are fields of ideas, and, even more important, our experience of time and space is similarly self-engendered. People think there is such a thing as external time, although no physicist has ever proved within an experiment the existence of the flow of time. We have never experienced the flow of time—all we have experienced is the flow of thoughts or ideas. And our experience of time is dependent on the experience of the flow of ideas. Time is nothing other than the continuity of memory, which uses the self-image as an internal reference point. Time is a conceptual framework in which we measure the experience of sensory change, and that can be a very personal event.

We've all had the experience of timelessness: Perhaps we were in love, praying, listening to music, dancing, reading poetry, walking on the beach, gazing at the stars, or in the silence of meditation, when suddenly we slipped into the timeless. It's when a person says, "The beauty of the mountain was breathtaking—time stood still."

What's that experience of timelessness? Of eternity? It is the experience of unity consciousness, in which we have the knowledge somewhere deep inside us that you and I are not only made up of the same stuff but that we may be the same being in different disguises. The beauty of the mountain was breathtaking because we and the mountain became one. The observer, the process of observation, and that which was being observed became one. The seer and the scenery were the same being. In that moment we escape time-bound awareness and enter timeless awareness, which is the realm of eternity, which is really the reality. We say it was breathtaking because breath comes to a standstill in the moment of transcendence, breath also being the movement of heart. Time separates the observer from the observed.

The next question is, if the body is a field of ideas, who is having these ideas? And where does that person live? At a conference such as the Heart of Healing, we could explore the theory that there is a thinker behind the thoughts, that behind the idea is an idea generator. Every spiritual tradition in the world has said that somewhere deep inside you is some animating force that makes your body alive. It doesn't matter what you call that animating force—the soul or the spirit or the self or consciousness—this is what creates the mind and the body, and this is who you really are.

Scientists brought up in the tradition of materialism will immediately say, "If that's so, show me where it is." In the last century, scientists went to extraordinary lengths to prove the existence of the soul. They would weigh people, for example, just before they died, and then weigh them immediately afterwards to see if something left. They usually didn't find any difference in the weight, but they did reach one reasonably good scientific conclusion: Whatever it is that constitutes the real self, it probably doesn't weigh anything. It has no height and no weight. It is spaceless and timeless. In other words, it is totally dimensionless. Yet it could be who you and I really are.

I believe the reason nobody can find the soul or the spirit inside the brain or the body is because it is not there. We are looking in the wrong place. We are not in the body, the body is in us; we are not in the mind, the mind is in us; we are not in the world, the world is in us. If you are listening to Beethoven on the radio and you take the radio apart hoping to find Beethoven inside, you're not going to find him because he's not there. Similarly, the human body and the human brain are just a set of instruments that take what is universal, unbounded, and infinite and trap it into a local space/time perceptual artifact. To even ask where the spirit is is irrelevant because as soon as you say "where," you have attributed a location in space and time to something that is nonlocal, that is beyond space and time, and is the creator of space and time. It is who you actually are.

Einstein said, "We live in a universe that has no beginning in time, that has no ending in time, that has no outer edges in space."

Spirit is in the silent spaces between our thoughts. If I say I am going to take off my shoe, I'm going to have a glass of water, I'm going to make a phone call—in between one idea and the next, there is a little silent space. That's where I am the orchestrator of the sequence of these thoughts, the infinite choice-maker.

The spirit is a real force. It's as real as gravity, it's as real as time. It's equally as abstract, equally as incomprehensible and mysterious and difficult to grasp conceptually. It's very powerful, and when we touch that spiritual core of awareness, only then can we be healed.

Many of the ancient healing traditions regard cosmic consciousness as the simultaneity of local and nonlocal awareness. Right this moment, your awareness is localized to me, I hope. But the one who is localizing it is nonlocal. If at the time you are reading this you could at the same time just slightly shift your attention to who is reading, you might have it.

It simply means to carry the consciousness of the spirit to the field of matter, to carry the consciousness of eternity to the field of time. And then time, and even your present lifetime, is seen as a flicker of eternity. In that gap of time is the "holographic" imprint of the entire universe.

Deep inside you, even on the level of the cells, is the holographic memory of every experience you had. You and I are different because we have had different experiences. We have walked through different gardens and knelt at different graves and heard different songs and met different people. Every single experience you have or ever have had is recorded in the very cells of your body. Go beyond the superficial memories, and you find memories of gestation and lifetimes, of race, of the species. A friend of mine, an eminent psychologist, said, "I remember the day of my conception." I said, "You do?" He said, "I went to this picnic with my father and came back with my mother."

To go even beyond that, there is the memory of wholeness, the true memory of the experiencer—because you and I are not the experience; we are the experiencer behind the experience. To discover the experiencer behind the experience is to find the timeless factor in every experience. Because of the timeless factor in every experience—experience is timebound, but the experiencer is timeless—if we can find the experiencer in the midst of every experience, then we escape the tyranny of timebound awareness. And we go into the joy of timeless awareness, and then the world becomes magical and different, and healing takes place.

One becomes so defenseless that there's nothing to attack. Spontaneously fear-based behavior is replaced by love-based behavior. Spontaneously one goes beyond time—the barrier of the ego and the continuity of the memory—using the ego as the internal reference point. To the extent you can push through the barrier of the ego and enter the realm of the spirit, you have the experience of immortality.

An Integral Approach to the End of Life

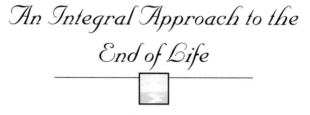

KAREN WYATT

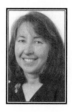

DURING MY MEDICAL career, through my experiences as a hospice medical director, I have spent a great deal of time reflecting upon death as it occurs in our modern society, pondering both the problems and the promises of this final, universal passage. Witnessing a number of deaths and connecting with many who are nearing the end of life, which I consider a privilege of inestimable value, have clarified for me the meaning of my own and mankind's existence. I have come to see a kind of perfection in our human mortality.

It occurs to me now, after experiencing much pain and loss in my own time, that life is a spiritual journey for the purpose of teaching us certain truths and lessons as we travel through this physical realm. Our human bodies are sublime vehicles for gathering information and absorbing the wisdom of the universe: with five senses to experience the diversity of nature manifested through smells, sounds, sights, tastes, and textures; with limbs for mobility and action; with organs for pleasure, performance, and sustenance; with neurological linkages for learning, imagining, and reasoning; and with systems for growth, repair, and healing. What an awesome gift, this physical existence! And yet, it is a transitory gift, at best. Soon enough, the faculties begin to fade and wear as we, ideally, exhaust the learning possibilities provided by this physical body. So, a gradual shift in focus must naturally occur in the end days, from the gifts of the physical world to the truths of the spiritual realm. We practice letting go of the physical body and all its wonders in order to hone our spirits and perfect our souls for the journey that follows this one, whatever that may be. Dying, which is defined by Webster's Dictionary[1] as "drawing to a close," is both a letting-go of what was and a preparation for what will be. The process of dying is meant to be an ending to a story, a final tying together of the threads of a tapestry, to reveal a complete and perfect whole. Dying takes place in the present, where the finale, the finished design, reveals itself moment by moment, until the last breath is taken and the "mortal coil" is shed. The spirit is released to continue a journey into the unfathomable and inexplicable. While the loss of this beautiful physical existence is painful, it is, in my estimation, precisely the impermanence of this life that renders it precious. Knowing that it will come to an end requires us to savor each moment of sweetness and sorrow and waste not one opportunity for learning or love.

Though the dying process is universal and sacred, we live in a society to which death is anathema, an enemy to be avoided at all costs. As nursing homes, hospitals, and mortuaries have allowed us to remove the elderly, ill, and dying from our everyday life, so too is death no longer a part of our everyday consciousness. We have become a society that worships youth, fitness, and health at the expense of the many lessons that could be learned from pain and loss. Bowing down before the altar of beauty, wealth, and power, we fail to notice the spotted wing of the ladybug perched on a blade of grass, or the rosy hue of the last cloud illuminated by the setting sun. Unfortunately, modern medicine plays a role in this massive denial of the true purpose of existence, with promises of new and better drugs and therapies supporting the erroneous belief that no one should ever have to suffer. In a blind attempt to "help," modern medicine has unwittingly served to pave this detour from the true spiritual path of human existence.

What should we, as physicians, as healers of the physical body, contribute to this learning and growing process known as life, for the patients who seek us? How do we interact with our patients in a way that is beneficial to their individual journey, given that true success in the healing process is not really measurable in a laboratory or recordable by radiography? How might we continue to utilize the masterful body of knowledge passed down to us by our forebears and yet integrate it with an understanding of the spiritual realm, which is so desperately needed in our society? The answers to these questions have become clear to me as I have pondered the lessons learned from dying patients. Consider the two stories that follow:

One of the first deaths I witnessed occurred during my internal medicine rotation as a first-year family practice resident. In fact, the patient died beneath my hands in the critical care unit as we carried out a failed resuscitation attempt. I never knew the man's name or the details of his cardiac disease. I was the resident on call that night, and "running codes" was one of my assigned duties. He was referred to as "314-A," since, in the urgent chaos of a "Code Blue" following cardiac arrest, location is a more pertinent designation than a given name. I will never forget the sense of panic I felt, being responsible for my first "code," or the shouting voices, the white noise from the cardiac monitor, the crush of too many bodies jammed into a tiny space, the rhythmic "whoosh" of the Ambu bag, the repetitive counting from one to five as I pushed my hands against his chest, the command to clear, the thud of the defibrillator, the immediate seizing of the body, the resumption of sinus rhythm on the monitor. But I particularly will never erase from my mind the expression on the face of the man in 314-A. Though he was supposedly unconscious, his eyes were wide with fear and his mouth twisted into a grimace. That aura of terror never left him. The nurse called his family to report his condition: comatose and not likely to survive another arrest. Would they like to come in and say their goodbyes? The family expressed two wishes that night: Do everything possible to save him, and don't call again until it's over. We, the members of the code team, felt sick at heart. Our orders were clear. We had no power to change this situation. We were all Mr. 314-A had left to him in this world at that moment, but we could not change his destiny. He arrested four more times that night. On the fifth resuscitation attempt, his heart did not respond to the defibrillator jolt. At last, we were able to allow this man some peace, though his body had long since given up the spirit responsible for its animation. I cringe even now to think of the nature of his closing thoughts, his last sensations, and his final moment of life, surrounded by well-meaning strangers, who nonetheless inflicted a certain torture in the carrying out of their jobs.

Many years later, in fortunate contrast, I was able to share in the dying of Anna, a 93-year-old nurse with unstable angina and congestive heart failure. She had been admitted to our hospice service 9 months before her death by a physician who had taken the time to ask her how she envisioned her last days of life. Because Anna requested that no aggressive measures be taken, that only palliative care be given, and, particularly, that she be allowed to die in her own home, her physician, truly a compassionate healer, turned over her care to our hospice staff. Anna lived alone in an assisted-living facility, and though her family was very supportive and visited frequently, the days often grew long for her. When our team entered her life, weekly visits from our nurses quickly became a highlight for Anna as she delighted in sharing stories of her own days as a nurse, reminiscing and advising her young peers on the art of medicine. Her physical condition stabilized with such positive personal attention and caring relationships, a phenomenon that is frequently seen in hospice care. Our staff found it equally healing to spend time with Anna, as she provided homespun warmth and wisdom with each visit. Eventually, her condition did deteriorate, as was expected. But Anna never saw an emergency room, a critical care unit, a cardiac monitor, or a defibrillator during her last days of life. As she requested, she remained at home, sleeping upright in her favorite recliner, with various family members by her side providing care and administering her medication. I visited her apartment just hours before her death and found Anna in her chair, holding her 3-month-old great-granddaughter in her arms. She grabbed my hand and pulled me close to her. "It's my time, Doctor," she whispered. "I know," I responded, through tears that represented sadness for the loss that was approaching but also awe at the beauty of the scene of her parting. Anna died that evening, with grace and dignity, surrounded by the love that was a reflection of the way she had lived her life. I would think of 314-A that night as I hung up the phone from the nurse's notification call. In our zeal to carry out the orders to "do everything" for him, we deprived him of the one thing every human being must surely deserve at least once before death: to feel loved. I knew that night, as I whispered my last farewell for Anna to the heavens, there would never be another 314-A in my career. I could never again disavow the spiritual aspect of another human being while attending to the physical needs at hand. I was becoming, through hospice work and a certain amount of personal suffering, an integral physician, without even realizing what that term meant.

It is not surprising that this transformation occurred while I was working with dying patients, for medical care in the hospice setting is interdisciplinary or integral in its very approach, offered by a team of providers. Consisting of an MD, a nurse, a home health aide, a chaplain, a social worker, and a volunteer, the hospice team meets the four quadrant needs of Ken Wilber's model of integral medicine.[2] Each of the team members contributes to one of the physical, emotional, spiritual, social, and cultural requirements of the patient. In addition, our hospice had, on occasion, brought in other support people to assist in specific needs of certain patients, including a rabbi, a music therapist, a psychologist, a Native American shaman, and a Buddhist monk. Because the interdisciplinary hospice team meets weekly to discuss patient care, each team member has an opportunity to both teach and learn from the other participants. Such sharing of knowledge and insights is a powerful tool of growth and transformation for everyone involved. Each member of this team, including myself, became increasingly integral in his or her own particular aspect of hospice work because of the influence of the others. And our ability to be a powerful and positive influence in the lives of our patients and their families grew as well.

I believe that the hospice model of medical care evolved into an integral approach because of the needs of the patients themselves. The dying, for the most part, have been stripped of all pretense and that certain brash

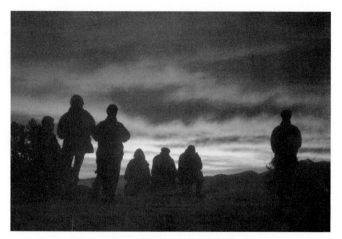

"Sunset Group." (Courtesy Michael Eller.)

arrogance afforded by an intact physical body. Their concerns necessarily involve spirituality in the last-ditch effort to find meaning and purpose in life. While physical pain is an issue for many dying patients, in my experience, spiritual/emotional pain from unfinished business is far more compelling. For this reason, hospice workers must address spirituality in order to perform their jobs. This aspect of human life simply cannot be ignored. It is, to me, unfortunate that it is death that must teach us how to live; that we "rage against the dying of the light"[3] because we never recognized that the light was always meant to be temporary; that we fail to practice for the end of our lives by delving into the "little deaths" life serves us in its buffet of loss and pain, mixed with joy and love. Were we to live our lives with an awareness, every moment, of the nearness of death, would we not accept the end of life with more grace and fulfillment? Would we not transform everything about ourselves? It is the ultimate integral practice to bring this awareness and acceptance of death to every aspect of life.

Once, during my years of work in hospice, I had an amazing dream, or perhaps it was a vision, that has always stayed with me. I was led into a circular room that was filled with an incredible, resplendent light, more beautiful than anything I had ever seen. In the center of the room stood an old white-haired man who was translucent and almost seemed to be composed of the light itself. He pointed to the wall of the room, which was covered with a mural, a collage of pictures. As I looked closely, I saw that each picture was a scene from my life—representing both significant and trivial events, times of celebration and suffering, achievement and failure. I observed that each scene had its own shape and that all of the scenes fit together perfectly, as do the pieces of a jigsaw puzzle. Awestruck, I turned to the old man and whispered, "It's all perfect. Everything that has happened has been perfect!" He nodded in agreement. I went on to bemoan, "Oh, if only I had realized this before. I regret all the time I wasted worrying about things and feeling despair. I just didn't..." He placed a finger on my lips to silence me. Again pointing to the collage, he spoke, "Look! Even the worrying was perfect."

This dream became a new standard in my life, a challenge to view everything that happened as perfect. I would have an opportunity to use this new perspective some months later, when I met Wanda, a retired nurse like Anna but with a very different story. After suffering a life-threatening illness, from which she barely recovered, Wanda had been admitted to a nursing home where I worked. She was very angry that her physical condition forced her to give up her home and move into a nursing home, and she acted upon that anger at every opportunity. Wanda refused her medication and physical therapy, screamed at the nurses, and sometimes threw her food tray on the floor. She would not get out of bed, instead lying there all day moaning, "Why me? Why me?" The staff was exhausted and had considered discharging her from the facility when they asked me to see her and prescribe a sedative to keep her quiet. However, because I could no longer justify treating only a patient's behavior, I had to do some research to help me understand Wanda as a whole person, from all aspects of her being. I learned from her chart that she had been comatose while in the hospital and had been expected to die on three separate occasions. But she pulled through each time and survived her illness, only to find herself in this nursing home. When I met her for the first time, she greeted me with her usual bitter litany of "Why me?" Without thinking about it first, I turned her words around and asked, "Why you?" This brought her whining to an immediate halt as she stared at me, shocked by my impudence. I went on to remind her that she nearly died three times while she was in the hospital and yet she had recovered. Why? For what purpose was she there in that nursing home at that particular time? Why was she still alive? I wanted to know how this particular event fit into the collage of Wanda's life. What perfection had been brought about by her illness and admission to this facility? What gap in her life history had been filled perfectly by the shape of this experience? Wanda turned her head away from me and refused to answer, while I silently kicked myself for speaking so impulsively. I decided to abandon the interaction and try again in 2 weeks, when I was scheduled to return. On that next visit to the nursing home, I found a very different Wanda. When I arrived, she was thumping down the hall in a walker, fully dressed, hair neatly combed in place. "I know the answer to your question, Doctor," she called out to me. Later she would tell me that she had experienced a revelation: She was in that nursing home because the other patients needed her. With her background in nursing and patient care, she knew how to respond to people who are ill and suffering. She knew how to offer comfort. Wanda began visiting other patients on a daily basis, particularly those who received little support from their families. She met with each new patient and family upon their arrival, offering encouragement and friendship. She pointed out to the nurses when other patients weren't doing well but were unable to communicate on their own. She became such a valuable asset that the nursing home administrator joked that he should be paying her to be there. Wanda had managed to turn what seemed to be a tragedy in her life into a blessing for others, as she figured out for herself the perfect purpose for her situation. She transcended loss to arrive at a new higher plane of functioning. No drug, surgery, or therapy could have done that for her. She had to get there on her own, in her own perfect fashion. She had to ask herself the right question, and she had to be willing to look deep inside for her answer. Could we wish anything more than this for our patients or for ourselves? Could we be facilitators of this type of transformation for everyone around us, regardless of the state of their health?

If we choose to bring an integral awareness to the practice of medicine, whether we work with the dying or those whose future death remains a mystery, we must find a way to ask ourselves the difficult questions and search the depths for our answers. To truly participate in integral medicine, we must open our own hearts to suffering and loss, to death in all its forms, to the perfection of this spiritual existence we have been asked to live out in physical bodies. We must see the collage of our lives and understand that at some point, every piece, no matter how misshapen, will fit perfectly into that picture. To practice medicine from an integral perspective is certainly no easy task. But it offers an opportunity to transcend the limits of reductionistic thinking and the possibility of true spiritual growth for ourselves. And once the first step is taken toward this larger view, there is no turning back. To become an integral practitioner is to reach, ever and unceasingly, like the tenacious tendrils of a budding seed, toward the transcendent, ineffable light.

References for this essay are located on the DVD accompanying this book.

Consciousness Beyond Death?[*]

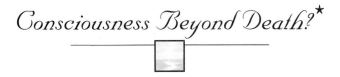

MARILYN SCHLITZ

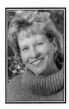

L AST YEAR WAS A CHAL-
lenge for me. Death came for not
one but an even dozen of my friends and colleagues. Since then, I've spent
hours trying to make sense of these losses. I can no longer pick up the
phone and call my friends, or send a hurried e-mail. Death has cut me off
from those who played such important roles in my life. Our communication, once so vital, is now a one-sided discourse. Or is it?

It is easier to avoid or rely solely on faith to answer questions about
survival after bodily death than to seriously consider them as empirical
issues. Yet the mystery of survival can be explored with both critical distance and openness to relevant data—beginning, for instance, with what
the world's religious and spiritual traditions have reported about the possibility of postmortem survival.

---

[*]Adapted from Schlitz M: Consciousness Beyond Death, *Spirituality & Health: The Soul/Body Connection,* July-August, 2003.

Virtually all mystics, of all faiths, maintain that human consciousness continues to exist in a disembodied condition after death. Some Taoist sages have claimed that only a few highly evolved spirits survive, while Hindu and Tibetan Buddhist yogis argue that all living creatures are reincarnated. Considering the diversity of beliefs, it is sensible to remain doubtful about the specifics of most pictures of postmortem existence.

Yet certain claims about the survival of consciousness are founded on the direct experience of people with various beliefs about the afterlife. For example, people in many eras and cultures have enjoyed illuminations or visions in which an eternal or immortal self seemed unequivocally apparent. "Some people imagine that they should see God, as if he stood there and they here," wrote the Christian mystic Meister Eckhart. "This is not so. God and I, we are one in knowledge."[1]

The practices of Stone Age shamans, carried into today's few remaining shamanic cultures, are grounded in a belief that there are multiple levels of reality, and multiple dimensions. By moving between various distinct domains of existence, shamans assert, we can travel to the spirit world, identifying and connecting with our ancestors and the spirits of nature. Shamanism suggests that the line between the living and the dead is arbitrary, less a hard edge than a common boundary.

Various domains of science speak to the question of life after death. Psychologist Gary Schwartz, at the University of Arizona in Tucson, has been testing several well-known mediums under controlled conditions to see whether they can give accurate information about departed loved ones. In one study, a medium was asked to contact a decedent known to a client out of the client's presence, so the medium could not respond to the client's verbal or physical cues. After the reading, the client read several transcripts. One was the medium's report on contacting the client's departed loved one; the others were those of similar readings conducted for other people. If mediums are really in contact with disembodied spirits, then clients should, on average, be able to select their session's transcripts more often than decoy transcripts. In repeated tests with various mediums and clients, Schwartz believes that he has found enough evidence to warrant continuing the work.[2]

Does this mean that we can communicate with the dead? No. But we also don't know that we can't. As studies of mediums are combined with other efforts, such as investigations of reincarnation, out-of-body

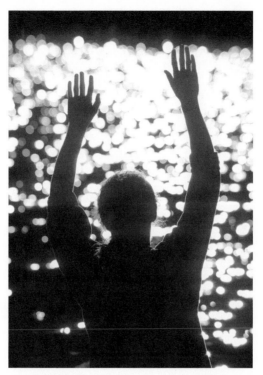

"Noah's Hands." (Courtesy Michael Eller.)

experiences, and near-death experiences, scientists are formulating a new image of death. We are moving from an image of the grim reaper, cutting us off from our loved ones, to what psychiatrist Raymond Moody[3] described as "the being of light." From this perspective, death is seen as a continuum rather than an either/or condition. By reframing death, we may engage in levels of transpersonal growth that provide us with connections to the subtle, causal, and ultimate realms of reality.

This exploration of the possible survival of consciousness, even in the absence of definitive answers, can offer comfort to the bereaved. The burden of grief, the lingering fears and doubts, may be tempered by hope and possibility. Through this process, we may move outside a limited paradigm of separateness and finality and toward a larger sense of self and our connections to the whole.

References for this essay are located on the DVD accompanying this book.

Part Three

HEALING: A MOVE TOWARD WHOLENESS

MARILYN SCHLITZ
TINA AMOROK

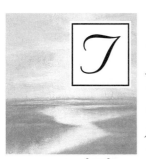

he move toward an inte-gral model of medicine is a move toward whole-ness—embracing the psychological, spiritual, cultural, and environ-mental dimensions of health and ill-ness. Core existential issues about who we are and what we are capable of becoming are deeply embedded in our understanding of health and healing. And how we link inner noetic experiences with collective practice and human biology become key questions.

Today there is a renaissance taking place in the meeting of science on one hand and spirituality and religion on the other. Insights derived from the world's wisdom traditions, combined with advances in scientific understanding, are leading to new and important questions about consciousness and healing. Topics such as love, forgiveness, and gratefulness are no longer abstract plati-tudes—but have now earned an important place in an integral approach to medicine.

PSYCHOLOGY'S MOVEMENT TOWARD WHOLENESS

In our efforts to enlarge our understanding of medicine through the integral lens, we turn now to the fields of psychology and psychiatry to consider the expanded scope of consciousness in health and healing. Integral psychology, according to psychologist Bahman A.K. Shirazi, attempts to cover the body-mind-psyche-spirit spectrum and encompass the unconscious and the conscious dimensions of the psyche. Additionally, it explores the supraconscious dimension traditionally excluded from psychological inquiry. In the author's own words, "Integral psychology seeks to inspire, encourage, and assist humanity in the profound task of healing and evolution toward a future state of existence that is completely attuned to our state of embodied consciousness."

Psychiatrist Stanislav Grof, a pioneer in the study of transpersonal states of consciousness, writes of their significance in a psychology of the future. Grof suggests that in our ordinary state of awareness we are fragmented and identify with only a part of human nature and experience. But in other nonindustrialized cultures, healing always involves expanded states of consciousness. Western psychiatry and psychology have not recognized what Grof refers to as "holotropic states" as potential sources of healing, seeing them rather as pathological phenomena that need to be suppressed through medication. Grof's work teaches us that to achieve an integral and culturally grounded medicine, we need to radically revise our understanding of the nature of consciousness and incorporate non-ordinary domains of consciousness into our appreciation and, when appropriate, our application of what heals.

Building on this expanded view of consciousness, William Braud, a physiological psychologist, summarizes 2 decades of well-controlled experimental research on transpersonal imagery. He argues that imagery functions as a bridge, connecting the conscious, imaginal content or activity of one person with the conscious or unconscious, physiological or psychological activities or experiences of another person. In Braud's words: "Increasing interest and developments in the areas of transpersonal psychology, consciousness studies, the efficacy of prayer, the role of spirituality in health, alternative medical and psychological interventions, and the new positive psychology movement...all promise to cast new light on the nature and power of the imagination and of the imaginal realm."

SPIRITUALITY, RELIGION AND HEALING

In this section we consider more directly the role of spirituality and religion in health and healing. We begin with an essay by Jeff Levin, a social epidemiologist whose pioneering research contributes richly to a theoretical model that restores the spiritual dimension to the prevention of disease and the promotion of well-being. This current turn toward integrating spirit into an integral model of health and healing speaks to a rebirth of long-held wisdom into modern conceptualizations of well-being. Levin writes that findings from this domain of study "suggests something beyond the local mind as part of what it means to be a human being."

Roger Walsh, a psychiatrist and educator, argues that for the first time in human history all of our global problems are human-created; the ills of our time are a manifestation of our individual and collective choices and behavior. Hence, this also indicates that the "state of the world is a reflection of the state of our minds."

We need, he argues, to address and redress the psychological and spiritual roots of our contemporary crisis through reflection on the essential spiritual precepts and perennial practices.

From a different vantage point but with a similar message, we turn to renowned cardiologist, Dean Ornish. Ornish argues that heart bypass surgery—so much a part of American medicine today—has become a metaphor for an incomplete approach to dealing with a life-threatening problem. "It's not enough to deal with the heart as a mechanical device," he writes. "We have to deal with the emotional heart, the psychosocial heart and the spiritual heart. If we can learn to open our hearts in these areas, we may find that the anatomical heart begins to open too, in ways we can measure more easily." This attempt at a redefinition may provide a fundamental shift in understanding where health comes from and how we may grow from the experience of pain and suffering.

Larry Dossey, an internal medicine practitioner, draws from a vast body of evidence indicating that prayer and religious devotion are directly correlated with positive health outcomes. As the evidence on intercessory prayer and distant intentionality reaches the scientific mainstream and lay public, there have been a variety of responses within conventional medicine "ranging from elation to confusion to horror." According to Dossey, even though this debate is fraught with difficulties, it represents a major opportunity for genuine dialogue between science and spirituality and for a "respiritualization of medicine."

ESSENTIAL CAPACITIES

Honoring the development of essential capacities is often neglected when we think about medicine. But there is increasing evidence that the cultivation of love, forgiveness, and gratefulness may be valuable for the healing of ourselves and our relationships with others. Jeff Levin returns and discusses the complexities of engaging in research on such topics as hope, forgiveness, thankfulness, kindness, and love. Levin coined the term "epidemiology of love" as a way of understanding the health correlates of altruism. Based on his preliminary research, he hypothesizes that love may not be just a "host factor, similar to other psychosocial constructs, but also a health-promoting agent."

In the next chapter, research and clinical psychologist Frederic Luskin examines the healing power of forgiveness. As director of the Stanford Forgiveness Projects, Luskin continues to demonstrate through his work that forgiveness has emotional and physical benefits. He writes, "The $64,000 question is, if forgiveness is so good for us, why do so few of us choose to forgive when people hurt us? What I see over and over again from my research and teaching is people have the capacity to make peace with their past.... They learn to forgive and heal in both body and mind."

In a related vein, Brother David Steindl-Rast explores the dynamics of practicing gratefulness. He asks us, "How we can we be grateful in troubled times?" His answer: "The only task in troubled times is to find what opportunity this very trouble offers us to act with gratefulness. To *be* means to be grateful." The Franciscan monk and spiritual teacher discusses the interplay of gratefulness in health and in illness, and the possibility of experiencing a healing crisis as a gift. Like many other authors in this anthology, he suggests that all of life is embedded in the divine mystery. Our deep engagement in this mystery may help to shed light on the foundations of a truly integral medicine

Finally, renown psychologist, Jon Kabat-Zinn, from the Center for Mindfulness in Medicine, Health Care, and Society at the University of Massachusetts Medical Center, suggests that by developing the "inner technologies" or capacities of meditation (mindfulness), we can transform our consciousness and world view. Such individual and collective transformation through the cultivation of "The Contemplative Mind in Society," Kabat-Zinn believes, is seeding a second Italian/European Renaissance in the United States, if not worldwide. Such a Renaissance, Kabat-Zinn writes, will assist us in meeting the challenges of our "technological advances without losing all sense of value and meaning in our individual and collective lives."

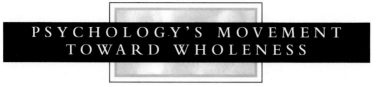

PSYCHOLOGY'S MOVEMENT
TOWARD WHOLENESS

Integral Psychology: Psychology of the Whole Human Being

BAHMAN A.K. SHIRAZI

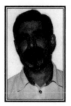

INTRODUCTION

Integral psychology is a psychological system concerned with exploring and understanding the totality of the human phenomenon. It is a framework that not only addresses the behavioral, affective, and cognitive domains of the human experience within a singular system but is concerned with the relationship among the above-mentioned domains in the context of human spiritual development. It is a system that, at its breadth, covers the entire body-mind-psyche-spirit spectrum, while, at its depth dimension, encompasses the previously explored unconscious and the conscious dimensions of the psyche, as well as the supraconscious dimension traditionally excluded from psychological inquiry. It seeks to inspire, encourage, and assist humanity in the profound task of healing and evolution toward a future state of existence that is completely attuned to our state of embodied consciousness.

As Western psychology is historically rooted in Western philosophy, so is integral psychology grounded in, and dependent upon, integral philosophy. At the philosophical level, integral psychology is devoted to addressing the essential issues of human spiritual, natural, social, and psychological alienation through a profound method of reconciliation of the ontological and the existential dimensions of being in the process of integral self-realization.

Integral psychology is inspired and informed by the great teachings of ancient wisdom traditions of the world, as well as the panorama of Western schools of psychological thought and practice. It takes into account the importance of self-knowledge, the multidimensional nature of consciousness and human personality, as well as the multicultural world we live in.

One might expect that with thousands of years of living knowledge traditions, including hundreds of years of academic progress, such a psychological system would be well-developed and advanced by now. Yet it is not an exaggeration to state that up until the present time no singular psychological system, Eastern, Western, or otherwise, has been privileged to benefit from a vision of humanity so comprehensive as to be able to respond to the questions and challenges encountered in such a psychology.

The philosophical outlook required for such a complete vision of psychology is unlikely to be born out of the musings or discoveries of a single human being, or even a single thought system. As the human race proceeds on the path of evolution, new horizons of consciousness, new realities, and new challenges arise. An integral approach to psychology, therefore, needs to have an inherent capability to absorb and benefit from the historical contributions, respond to contemporary issues, provide a vision for the foreseeable future, and anticipate the upcoming challenges of each epoch of human evolution.

Fortunately, the dawn of the twenty-first century carries the promise of a new horizon of human experience and knowledge that, more than ever before, is capable of bringing together various strands of knowledge and other conditions necessary for an appropriate epistemology needed for a comprehensive vision of psychology. Some of the factors involved include the contributions of modern Western psychology, psychological dimensions of several Eastern spiritual traditions, modern consciousness research, the wisdom traditions of nature-based peoples, and the rich cultural exchange between various parts of the world.

WHAT IS INTEGRAL PSYCHOLOGY?

Integral psychology is arguably the latest, and if defined carefully, the last wave of development in the current history of psychology. Although it may not be simply possible to have a system of psychology that would be able to unveil all the mysteries of the human phenomenon at once, it is only common sense that psychology should cover all the known dimensions of the human phenomenon within a singular framework. This psychological framework for understanding the total human being is called integral psychology.

Paul Herman,[1] an early pioneer in the field of integral psychology, described integral psychology as "... an emergent East-West study of the human psyche. It draws upon the findings of both Western depth psychology, and ancient Eastern teachings and yogas, to express a whole, unfragmented view of human functions to resolve human conflicts and open the way toward activating high levels of potential." According to Herman, "integral psychology concerns itself with all phases of human existence, in its multidimensional fullness, which includes physical, emotional, instinctual, mental, moral, social, and spiritual aspects." "Integral psychology seeks to be practical and applicable to the problems of daily life, yet at the same time to lead forward those individuals who are ready to transpersonal dimensions of being where experiences of deep integration, meaningfulness, and fulfillment are possible."

Integral psychology accepts the relative validity of other psychological systems, yet extends the general psychological scope of human development to encompass the full range of the psychospiritual continuum of human existence. Thus, it is concerned with the study of the human psyche in its potential fullness. Accordingly, integral psychology is inspired by and founded upon four general postulates essential to an integral worldview: *nonduality, multidimensionality, holism,* and *evolution.*

The principle of nonduality understands the human being as a continuum of body-mind-spirit; thus it avoids the traditional mind-body (spirit-matter) dichotomy. In an integral framework, human beings can be best understood in terms of a spectrum of qualities, rather than as a set of discrete constituents. Although the three domains of body, mind, and spirit are essentially unified, they manifest as a multidimensional array of distinct qualities and characteristics.

In integral psychology the human psyche is a multidimensional whole, with consciousness comprising its essential structure. However, it must be stressed that although there is an essential wholeness to the psychic structure of body-mind-spirit, this wholeness exists only as a potential. While integral psychology recognizes the urge toward wholeness as the primary motive in the human being, its goal is to actualize this potential wholeness through a process of harmonious self-realization.

Finally, integral psychology recognizes the importance of the evolutionary perspective of life on earth. Sri Aurobindo's[2] insights into the process of life revealed that the human individual is a transitional being, not a final product of creation or evolution. Understood in this light, the goal of spiritual development is not to arrive at a static, final state; rather, human spiritual growth is a dynamic process without any preconceived limits. Thus, an integrally self-realized being is an active key participant involved in perpetual cooperation with the divine in the process of collective transformation of consciousness and manifestation of the divine life on earth.

This requires a radically new understanding of the role of the physical body, embodiment of spirit, the ego-self, and the mind-body relationships, both at individual and collective levels. Sri Aurobindo asked the simple question, why we are embodied beings, in a profound way. He recognized the urgency of including (rather than suppressing) the feminine aspects of the psyche into the overall process of psychospiritual transformation. He was critical of the self-world negating, escapist orientations in many forms of mysticism where the ultimate goal of spiritual practice (at least from a superficial level of understanding) is to avoid being reborn in the physical plane and into the physical body, to ultimately avoid the pain and suffering and dissonance caused by lack of integration of body, mind, and spirit due to ignorance and delusion.

Instead, he affirmed the goal of spiritual practice to be harmonization of the different parts of being through integral yoga and continual cooperation with the Divine in the process of evolution of consciousness on Earth, and the manifestation of the highest of human potential to the point of manifestation of the highest levels of consciousness in the physical body. Integral psychology is, therefore, centrally concerned with the process of embodiment of spirit. Ego is defined as the embodiment principle, and its transformation is key in the overall psychological development of the individual.

DIMENSIONS OF INTEGRAL PSYCHOLOGY

Different approaches to integral psychology may be distinguished on the basis of philosophical underpinnings and epistemological and methodological orientations. So far, three different main approaches to integral psychology have been attempted by Indra Sen[2] (1986), Ken Wilber[3,4] (1997, 2000), and Haridas Chaudhuri.[5] In this chapter I will make an attempt to expound and expand on the integral psychology of Chaudhuri, as his work in this area was never fully published due to his passing away in the midst of this work.

Haridas Chaudhuri's approach to integral psychology may be characterized as an attempt to build a psychological system, from the ground up, using an integrative methodology that brings together some of the most powerful contributions of several systems of psychology, both Eastern and Western. Chaudhuri's integral psychology consists of a *triadic principle* as well as the *principal tenets* of integral psychology, which will be discussed in further detail subsequently. Haridas Chaudhuri's system is inspired by, but does not confine itself to, the scope and terminology of Sri Aurobindo's integral yoga. As an independent and creative thinker, Chaudhuri was little interested in merely reiterating the insights and terminology of Sri Aurobindo. Rather, he began to develop a system that employed an integrative methodology using insights from various schools of Eastern and Western psychology.

Chaudhuri[5] maintains that "integral psychology is based upon experiences and insights affirming the multidimensional richness and indivisible wholeness of human personality. It is founded upon the concept of man's total self as integral unity of uniqueness, relatedness, and transcendence—as the indivisible unity of the existential and the transcendental." Chaudhuri's attempt at integral psychology may be summarized in terms of his proposed tenets for an integral psychology as well as the triadic principle of *uniqueness, relatedness,* and *transcendence.* The following section will briefly introduce and elaborate on this system.

CHAUDHURI'S PRINCIPAL TENETS OF INTEGRAL PSYCHOLOGY

Chaudhuri's approach to integral psychology is not concerned with extrapolation of psychological insights from Sri Aurobindo's overall teachings. Instead, it directly applies an integrative methodology to the existing domain of psychological knowledge in order to construct a system of psychology that is phenomenologically oriented in its methodological outlook, and that holds psychospiritual development as its central objective.

In his effort to explore the basic concepts of integral psychology with a minimum of metaphysical assumptions, Chaudhuri[5] proposed a number of "principal tenets" that form the basis for his approach to integral psychology. Unfortunately, his work in this area remained unfinished. The following is a list of selected principal tenets:

The Wholeness of Personality

The human being is an onto–psycho–somatic continuum, or a spirit–mind–body unity that in the ultimate analysis is an indivisible whole. The reader should be reminded here that the spirit–mind–body spectrum may be experienced and expressed in much more detail. A more detailed version may be represented by the Spirit-Psyche-Mind-Emotions-Body continuum. This may be further understood in terms of further gradations of the mind (such as described by Sri Aurobindo or other systems as summarized in the works of Ken Wilber based on traditional Hindu teachings or other systems of spiritual practice), further gradations of the emotional bodies (such as "lower or higher vital," as described by Sri Aurobindo and others), and gradations of the physical body (such as subtle and gross physical bodies).

The number of bands within the onto-psycho-somatic spectrum depends on the personal experiences and expressions of these experiences, as reported by various mystics, and varies from one system to another. What is important is that all the various bands within the spectrum comprise a single, unified, and nondiscrete multidimensional reality. Changes, disturbances, and developments in any part of the spectrum are bound to affect other bandwidths, and unification of mind-body-spirit requires the inclusion of the entire spectrum.

Different Levels of Consciousness

Consciousness is the basic structure of the psyche according to integral psychology. Thus the various states below waking consciousness, as well as higher meditative states, are worthy of investigation as valid dimensions of human experience.

Importance of All Phases and Areas of Experience

Not only is it important to make direct empirical observations of human experience, it is imperative that all areas of human experience be included in the process of inquiry. Not only wakeful, conscious experiences but also dreams, nondream sleep stages, altered states of consciousness, and creative imagination are important areas of research in integral psychology. Beside ordinary states of consciousness, pathological, paranormal, and peak experiences must be considered.

Need For Personal Integration

A full experience of wholeness presupposes the full integration of the diversified components and aspects of human personality. To this end it is essential to appreciate the role of understanding the self, because it is only by following the inner light of one's own self that the human psyche can be comprehended in its fullness.

The Concept of Integral Self-Realization

Integral psychology holds that integral self-realization is the profoundest potential for the human being. This achievement requires a thorough integration and harmonization of the personal, the interpersonal/social, and the transcendental, and of the existential, and the ontological dimensions of existence.

The Doctrine of Transformation

Integral psychology alerts us to the problem of spiritual by-passing, the attempt to reach the higher realms of consciousness while suppressing, rather than confronting and transforming, the instincts and other unconscious components of the psyche and the associated emotions and mental states.

In integral psychology the doctrine of transformation replaces the kind of transcendence that results from withdrawal from, or negation of, the world. The lower spheres of consciousness (instincts, drives, etc.) are not escaped from or suppressed but are transformed into desirable qualities. Psychological transformation is achieved through a process of purification and psycho-ethical discipline.

The Doctrine of Ontomotivation

"In the course of self-development, ego drives are ultimately transcended and action becomes a spontaneous outpouring of the creative joy of union with Being as the ultimate ground of one's own existence."[5] Chaudhuri extended the notion of ego drives associated with egocentric consciousness and their transformation into higher "Being values," as suggested by Maslow's notion of self-actualization, by pointing out to further and complete transformation of ego/self in the process of integral self-realization.

The Methodology of Integral Experientialism

Integral psychology is comprehensive in its survey of human experience. Critical, experiential investigation and evaluation are encouraged in studying a vast range of states of consciousness and modes and phases of experience. External observations as well as introspective approaches are equally valued in this methodology.

THE TRIADIC PRINCIPLE OF INTEGRAL PSYCHOLOGY

While the preceding foundational principles are useful in understanding the overall parameters, scope, and vision of Chaudhuri's integral psychology, his triadic principle of uniqueness, relatedness, and transcendence provides another set of guidelines for understanding the overall process of psychospiritual development and transformation. *Uniqueness, relatedness, and transcendence correspond to the three domains of personal, interpersonal, and transpersonal psychological inquiry.* According to Chaudhuri,[6]

Broadly speaking, there are three inseparable aspects of human personality: uniqueness, or individuality; universality, or relatedness; and transcendence. In different schools of philosophy, we find that there has been a tendency to over-emphasize one aspect or another. It has not occurred to many people that all these are very essential and interrelated aspects of our being.

The uniqueness principle may be best understood in terms of two ancient yogic principles: *Svabhava* and *Svadharma*. Svabhava refers to the fact that each individual human being is the result of a unique set of qualities and characteristics that are not replicable in their exact configuration. Indeed, no two objects or events are exactly the same in nature. Just as no two leaves of a tree or no two snowflakes are the same despite similarities, no two human beings can ever be identical in the exact configuration of genetic and physiological makeup, temperament, personality traits, cultural and historical conditions, context of personal experience, and potential for spiritual development. In this author's view, the more one understands this profoundly meaningful reality, the harder it becomes to use psychological categories and typologies—including pathological categories.

Svadharma implies that there is a unique path of development, growth, and unfoldment for each individual that must be understood in terms of that person's unique svabhava. Unlike some forms of perennial psychology, integral psychology, then, is extremely sensitive to issues of individuality and the path of individual psychological growth and psychospiritual embodiment and evolution. It is important to note here that most traditional spiritual disciplines, especially those of the East, have overlooked the individual dimensions of personal growth. Individuality has often been associated with egocentrism or selfishness, the antithesis of selflessness, which is a basic tenet of spiritual practice.

In this author's analysis, misunderstanding of the uniqueness principle results in various forms of narcissistic traits and, in many cases, narcissistic personality disorders. Narcissistic individuals are likely to believe in their own uniqueness (specialness) but would not grant others such a privilege. Narcissism is indeed a strong impediment to any kind of real psychological and spiritual growth.

As important as individuality may be, it is not possible to understand the human being only in terms of individuality alone. Relatedness, or the interpersonal dimension, is of equal importance in the triadic formulation. Obviously, human beings are contextualized within numerous holistically organized systems such as the families, cultures, societies, nations, and ultimately the earth and the entire cosmos. Integral psychology holds the assumption that individuals are microcosmic expressions of the greater macrocosm with infinite potential for spiritual realization. Just as an individual needs to maintain harmonious intrapsychic dynamics, she or he needs also to maintain balance and harmony with others and with nature. In this writer's understanding of integral psychology, unhealthy and lopsided growth in the interpersonal realm is likely to lead to enmeshment, co-dependency, and borderline personality disorders.

In integral psychology the human being is understood in terms of both the historical (temporal) and the transcendental, formless/timeless (nontemporal) dimensions. Hitherto Western psychology has been concerned with the historical dimension of the human being, which includes (a) the genetic/biological characteristics or the physical and vital aspects; (b) the emotional aspects; and (c) the mental aspects of human existence. In short, psychology until the present has been concerned with what may be referred to as the body-mind configuration, or personality.

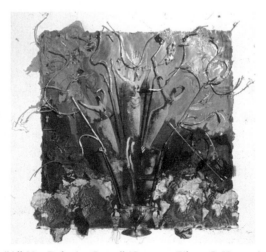

"All Her Paths Are Peace." (Courtesy Eileen G. Hyman.)

However, the transcendental (nontemporal) dimension is of equal importance in integral psychology, which recognizes the importance of the urge toward transcendence and wholeness. Historically the notion of transcendence has been the cornerstone of Eastern psychologies and Western mysticism. Being so, the terminology often characteristic of these systems has been categorically unacceptable to formal Western psychology. On the other hand, traditional mysticism has had little or no concern with the conventional psychological growth and development of the human being. Integral psychology recognizes and emphasizes both of these areas without neglecting either of them.

According to Chaudhuri,[6] "the essential significance of transcendence is that man in his inmost being is a child of immortality, an imperishable spark of the infinite.... As a mode of manifestation of being, his ultimate goal is union with that ground of existence, transcending all other limitations." The notion of transcendence, however, could be misleading if taken in an ultimate or absolute sense. In an article titled "Psychology: Humanistic and Transpersonal," Chaudhuri[7] critiqued one of the early assumptions of transpersonal psychology—the notion of ultimate states—and the notion that transpersonal psychology was concerned with recognition and realization of ultimate states. Chaudhuri did not believe in characterization of mystical experiences in terms of ultimate states. Such characterization, he believed, creates the "dichotomy of the ultimate and the preparatory, the transcendental and the phenomenal... the dichotomy of the lower self and the higher self, the flesh and the spirit, relative knowledge and absolute knowledge, conditioned existence and unconditioned perfection."[7] This problem arises when the principle of transcendence is treated in isolation from the principles of uniqueness and relatedness.

Chaudhuri's integral psychology had anticipated the dilemma of spiritual by-passing, later introduced in the literature of transpersonal psychology. This tendency, especially common among individuals with schizoid personality traits, is characterized by a wish to transcend the physical and affective dimensions through suppression or denial of the body and emotions in order to attain transcendental states of consciousness. It is true that mystical experiences attained in this fashion may have their proper place in the process of psychospiritual development.

But when taken to an extreme, asceticism and denial of the physical-vital energies problematically become the goal of spiritual practice.

It is by now well-established that before attempting to reach higher transcendental states, one must first properly deal with issues of psychological growth and development as well as pathological tendencies and development of a relatively healthy ego and personality. Transcendence, in integral psychology, is replaced by the notion of psychospiritual transformation.

THE PROCESS OF PERSONAL INTEGRATION

The concept of integral self-realization is a key concept in integral psychology, which employs a number of key understandings unique to integral psychology. In order to explore the process of integral self-realization, it is important to briefly discuss the notions of ego and self in integral psychology. The present author[8] has previously developed a model for self that distinguishes three distinct spheres of self-consciousness. These are *egocentric, psychocentric,* and *cosmocentric* spheres.

The egocentric sphere of consciousness has been the topic of traditional psychological study in the West. Three domains—behavioral, affective, and cognitive—compose the basic dimensions of study in this sphere. Western psychology is particularly adept in this area, with a vast number of theories and applications, many of which are at odds with one another. Much of personality theory is concerned with day-to-day waking consciousness as well as what is termed the *unconscious mind*. Recent developments such as transpersonal theories have also included the study of the higher unconscious mind. Transpersonal psychology has extended the boundaries of traditional Western systems by including that which is beyond the immediate ego-based experiences of the self.

In this author's opinion, on the one hand, Western schools of psychology have not yet defined the concept of ego in a way that explicitly includes the somatic/embodied dimension. On the other hand, transpersonal psychologists (excepting Assagioli) have not adequately dealt with what lies beyond the ego by failing to clearly distinguish between the psychocentric and cosmocentric spheres of consciousness.

Ancient Indian teachings referred to the spectrum of consciousness in terms of five main sheaths (*Koshas*). These are, from the outermost to the innermost, the physical, the vital/emotional, the mental, the higher mental/intuitive, and the soul/higher self (*Atman*). Atman is a transcendent principle that lies in the non–spatio-temporal dimension. Individual personality manifests as a result of the projection of Atman onto the spatio-temporal planes of existence. According to integral psychology, projection of the higher self onto the plane of personality results in various personality types (such as Jung's sensate, feeling, thinking, and intuitive), usually with one being dominant. Predominance of the physical results in the sensate personality type, whereas the dominance of the vital results in the feeling type. Dominance of the mental results in the thinking type, and of the intuitive, in the intuitive type. Therefore, the natural state of personality is an imbalanced one. Integral psychology promotes the idea of a balanced and healthy ego development and affirms the role of strong ego-development in the initial stages of psychospiritual growth. But the ego must first be understood as the principle of embodiment. This is quite different from the common definitions of the term ego either as a principle of separation or as defined technically within various schools of Western psychology.

In integral psychology psychocentric consciousness is represented through Sri Aurobindo's "Psychic Being." It is quite important to understand the role of psychocentric consciousness in the overall process of integral self-realization. Many traditional forms of spiritual practice have either overlooked or totally bypassed this area in favor of direct union with the cosmocentric ground of existence—a non–spatio-temporal principle known as God or Brahman, among numerous other terms. Often the body and gross emotions are viewed as a hindrance to spiritual practice. Various forms of self-denial have been attempted in exchange for transcendental or cosmic consciousness.

Integral yoga compensates for this problem by involving the Psychic Being (the subliminal self that is neither totally transcendent nor physically embodied) in the process of self-realization, which facilitates the development of a healthy ego (embodiment principle) and balanced personality. Through the dynamic process of integral self-realization a gradual shift from ego-based to psychocentric consciousness takes place. Initially ego-based personality obscures the subliminal Psychic Being. This condition is due primarily to the fragmented nature of ego-based personality, which creates a dualistic division between the I and not-I, or subject and object of experience. With experiences of self-opening that result from integral yogic and meditative insights, the locus of consciousness occasionally shifts away from the ego and becomes centered in the psychic being. This transition is not possible without meditative and contemplative effort and is not necessarily a developmental consequence of healthy ego-development.

From the psychocentric sphere of consciousness, the ego is not necessarily hidden or absent. In fact, from this point of view a deeper observation of the ego-structure becomes possible. Repeated insights into the ego-structure may bring about transformations of the ego that result in the development of a unified and healthy ego, which is the organizing principle of embodiment.

Continued psychospiritual development makes it possible for the ego to integrate further unconscious contents of the mind. As the ego becomes fully conscious, the locus of consciousness moves to the next sphere and becomes permanently centered in the psychic being. This entire process requires the application of the will and continued effort. It is highly contingent upon the psychoethical development of the individual.

Further development toward integral consciousness may require what Sri Aurobindo called the process of involution (Grace), or descent of higher forms of energy/consciousness. This means that the self becomes receptive to the experience of Being, the cosmic ground of all existence. This is also a gradual process. Once the locus of consciousness becomes focused in the Self, occasional absorption in cosmic consciousness may occur. Eventually this experience becomes possible at will. Unlike traditional linear conceptualizations, this is not a final point in spiritual development. A human being may continue to exist and operate as a unique individual but without an ego/drive-based will. Rather, this individual is ontomotivated.

In short, three levels of integration are involved in the process of integral self-realization: (1) integration of personality; (2) integration of the psychic being into conscious personality; and (3) integration of the existential and cosmic (ontological) dimensions of being. Sri Aurobindo termed the first transition *Psychic Transformation,* and the second transition

Spiritual Transformation. These two transformations are not linearly or developmentally connected and happen differently in different individuals. The third transformation is what Sri Aurobindo called the *Supramental Transformation,* in which every part of the being becomes supramentalized in the Divine consciousness, resulting in the complete transformation of the physical body down to the cellular level. This would result in a complete transformation of mind, life, and body.

The process of psychic transformation (the transformation of ego and egocentric consciousness) is mainly possible by first awakening and engaging the Psychic Being (also known as the Spiritual Heart) because it may be extremely difficult, if not impossible, to begin with the egocentric consciousness due to ego defense mechanisms and the inherent resistance of this sphere of consciousness to spiritual change and transformation. Psychic (Heart) consciousness is capable of seeing through the character structure and defense mechanisms with self-love and compassion, and in due time will help reconcile deeply rooted conflicts between the conscious and unconscious, instinctual and psychic forces, healing the emotional residues caused by the perceived chasm between material and spiritual energies.

In conclusion, today more than ever before there is an urgent need for psychic transformation on both the individual and the collective levels. Integral psychology has the potential to provide a framework for understanding embodied consciousness and its healing and transformation toward a more just and compassionate existence and creative and joyful fulfillment of the purpose of life on Earth.

References for this essay are located on the DVD accompanying this book.

Psychology of the Future: Lessons from Modern Consciousness Research*

STANISLAV GROF

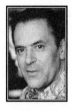

THE OBJECTIVE OF THIS paper is to summarize my experiences and observations concerning the nature of the human psyche in health and disease that I have collected during more than 45 years of research of nonordinary states of consciousness. I will focus specifically on the findings that represent a serious theoretical challenge for academic psychology and psychiatry and suggest the revisions that would be necessary to understand them.

HOLOTROPIC STATES OF CONSCIOUSNESS

Consciousness can be profoundly changed by a variety of pathological processes—by cerebral traumas, by intoxications with poisonous chemi-

---

*Selected and adapted from Stanislav Grof's books and articles.

cals, by infections, or by degenerative and circulatory processes in the brain. Such conditions can certainly result in profound mental changes that would be included in the category of non-ordinary states of consciousness. However, they cause "trivial deliria" or "organic psychoses," states that are very important clinically but are not relevant to our discussion. People suffering from deliriant states are typically disoriented: They do not know who and where they are and what date it is. They typically show a disturbance of intellectual functions and have subsequent amnesia regarding the experiences that they have had.

I would therefore like to narrow our discussion to a large and important subgroup of non-ordinary states of consciousness for which contemporary psychiatry does not have a specific term. Because I feel strongly that they deserve to be distinguished from the rest and placed into a special category, I have coined for them the name *holotropic*.[1] This composite word literally means "oriented toward wholeness" or "moving in the direction of wholeness" (from the Greek *holos*, meaning "whole," and *trepein*, meaning "moving toward or in the direction of something"). It suggests that in our everyday state of consciousness we are fragmented and identify with only a small fraction of who we really are.

Holotropic states are characterized by a specific transformation of consciousness associated with dramatic perceptual changes in all sensory areas, intense and often unusual emotions, and profound alterations in thought processes. They are usually accompanied by a variety of intense psychosomatic manifestations and unconventional forms of behavior. Consciousness is changed qualitatively in a very profound and fundamental way, but it is not grossly impaired as in the delirant conditions. We are experiencing invasion of other dimensions of existence that can be very intense and even overwhelming. However, at the same time, we typically remain fully oriented and do not completely lose touch with everyday reality. We experience simultaneously two very different realities, with "each foot in a different world."

Extraordinary changes in sensory perception represent a very important and characteristic aspect of holotropic states. Our visual perception of the external world is usually drastically transformed, and when we close our eyes, we can be flooded with images drawn from our personal history and from the collective unconscious. We can also have visions portraying various aspects of nature, the cosmos, or the mythological realms. This can be accompanied by a wide range of experiences engaging other senses—various sounds, physical sensations, smells, and tastes.

The emotions associated with holotropic states cover a very broad spectrum that extends far beyond the limits of our everyday experience. They range from feelings of ecstatic rapture, heavenly bliss, and "peace that passeth all understanding" to episodes of abysmal terror, murderous anger, utter despair, consuming guilt, and other forms of unimaginable emotional suffering that match the descriptions of the tortures of hell in the great religions of the world.

A particularly interesting aspect of holotropic states is their effect on thought processes. The intellect is not impaired, but it functions in a way that is significantly different from its everyday mode of operation. While we might not be able to rely on our judgment in ordinary practical matters, we can be literally flooded with remarkable information on a variety of subjects. We can reach profound psychological insights concerning our personal history, unconscious dynamics, emotional difficulties, and interpersonal problems. We can also experience extraordinary revelations concerning various aspects of nature and the cosmos that transcend our educational and intellectual background. The content of holotropic states is often spiritual or mystical. We can experience sequences of psychological death and rebirth and a broad spectrum of transpersonal phenomena, such as feelings of oneness with other people, nature, the universe, and God. We might uncover what seem to be memories from other incarnations, encounter powerful archetypal beings, communicate with discarnate beings, and visit numerous mythological landscapes. Holotropic experiences of this kind are the main source of cosmologies, mythologies, philosophies, and religious systems describing the spiritual nature of the cosmos and existence. They are the key for understanding the ritual and spiritual life of humanity, from shamanism and sacred ceremonies of aboriginal tribes to the great religions of the world.

Holotropic States of Consciousness and Human History

Ancient and aboriginal cultures have spent much time and energy developing powerful mind-altering techniques that can induce holotropic states. They combine in different ways: chanting, breathing, drumming, rhythmic dancing, fasting, social and sensory isolation, extreme physical pain, and other elements. These cultures used them in shamanic procedures, healing ceremonies, and rites of passage—powerful rituals enacted at the time of important biological and social transitions, such as circumcision, puberty, marriage, or birth of a child. Many cultures have used psychedelic plants for these purposes. The most famous examples of these are different varieties of hemp, the Mexican cactus peyote, *Psilocybe* mushrooms, the African shrub *eboga*, and the Amazonian jungle liana *Banisteriopsis caapi*, the source of *yagé* or *ayahuasca*.

Additional important triggers of holotropic experiences are various forms of systematic spiritual practice involving meditation, concentration, breathing, and movement exercises, which are used in different systems of yoga, Vipassana or Zen Buddhism, Tibetan Vajrayana, Taoism, Christian mysticism, Sufism, or Cabalah. Other techniques were used in the ancient mysteries of death and rebirth, such as the Egyptian temple initiations of Isis and Osiris and the Greek Bacchanalia, rites of Attis and Adonis, and the Eleusinian mysteries. The specifics of the procedures involved in these secret rites have remained for the most part unknown, although it is likely that psychedelic preparations played an important part.[2]

Among the modern means of inducing holotropic states of consciousness are psychedelic substances isolated from plants or synthesized in the laboratory and powerful experiential forms of psychotherapy, such as hypnosis, neo-Reichian approaches, primal therapy, and rebirthing. There also exist very effective laboratory techniques for altering consciousness, including sensory or sleep deprivation and biofeedback. My wife Christina and I have developed holotropic breathwork, a method that can facilitate profound holotropic states by very simple means—conscious breathing, evocative music, and focused bodywork.

It is important to emphasize that episodes of varying duration can also occur spontaneously, without any specific identifiable cause, and often against the will of the people involved. Since modern psychiatry does not differentiate between mystical or spiritual states and mental diseases, people experiencing these states are often labeled psychotic, hospitalized, and administered routine suppressive psychopharmacological treatment. Christina and I refer to these states as *spiritual emergencies* or *psychospiritual crises*. We believe that, when properly supported and treated, they can result in emotional and psychosomatic healing, positive personality transformation, and consciousness evolution.[3,4]

Although I have been deeply interested in all the categories of holotropic states mentioned above, I have done most of my work in the area of psychedelic therapy, holotropic breathwork, and spiritual emergency. This paper is based predominantly on my observations from these three areas in which I have the most personal experience. However, the general conclusions I will be drawing apply to all the situations involving holotropic states.

Holotropic States in the History of Psychiatry

It is worth mentioning that the history of depth psychology and psychotherapy is deeply connected with the study of holotropic states— Franz Mesmer's experiments with "animal magnetism," hypnotic sessions with hysterical patients conducted in Paris by Jean Martin Charcot, and the research in hypnosis carried out in Nancy by Hippolyte Bernheim and Ambroise Auguste Liébault. Sigmund Freud's early work was inspired by his work with a client (Miss Anna O.), who experienced spontaneous episodes of non-ordinary states of consciousness. Before radically changing his strategies, Freud initially used hypnosis to gain access to his patients' unconscious.

In retrospect, shifting emphasis from direct experience to free association, from actual trauma to Oedipal fantasies, and from conscious reliving and emotional abreaction of unconscious material to transference dynamics was unfortunate, and this approach limited and misdirected Western psychotherapy for the next 50 years.[5] While verbal therapy can be very useful in providing interpersonal learning and rectifying interaction and communication in human relationships (e.g., couple and family therapy), it is ineffective in dealing with emotional and bioenergetic blockages and macrotraumas, such as the trauma of birth.

As a consequence of this development, psychotherapy in the first half of this century was practically synonymous with talking—face-to-face interviews, free associations on the couch, and the behaviorist deconditioning. At the same time, holotropic states, initially seen as an effective therapeutic tool, became associated with pathology rather than healing. This situation started to change in the 1950s, with the advent of psychedelic therapy and new developments in psychology. A group of American psychologists headed by Abraham Maslow, dissatisfied with behaviorism and Freudian psychoanalysis, launched a revolutionary movement—humanistic psychology. Within a very short time, this movement became very popular and provided the context for a broad spectrum of new therapies.

While traditional psychotherapies used primarily verbal means and intellectual analysis, these new, so-called experiential therapies emphasized direct experience and expression of emotions and used various forms of bodywork as an integral part of the process. Probably the most famous representative of these new approaches is Fritz Perls' Gestalt therapy.[6] However, most experiential therapies still rely to a great degree on verbal communication and require that the client stay in the ordinary state of consciousness.

The therapeutic use of holotropic states is the most recent development in Western psychotherapy. Paradoxically, it is also the oldest form of healing and can be traced back to the dawn of human history. Therapies using holotropic states actually represent a rediscovery and modern reinterpretation of the elements and principles that have been documented by historians and anthropologists studying the sacred mysteries of death and rebirth, rites of passage, and ancient and aboriginal forms of spiritual healing, particularly various shamanic procedures. Shamanism is the most ancient religion and healing art of humanity, the roots of which reach far back into the Paleolithic era.

The fact that so many different cultures throughout human history have found shamanic techniques useful and relevant suggests that they address the "primal mind"—a basic and primordial aspect of the human psyche that transcends race, culture, and time. All cultures, with the exception of the Western industrial civilization, have held holotropic states in great esteem and spent much time and effort to develop various ways of inducing them. These cultures used such states to connect with their deities, other dimensions of reality, and the forces of nature for healing, for cultivation of extrasensory perception, and for artistic inspiration. For pre-industrial cultures, healing always involves non-ordinary states of consciousness—either for the client, the healer, or both of them at the same time. In many instances, a large group or even an entire tribe enters a non-ordinary state of consciousness together, as do, for example, the !Kung bushmen in the African Kalahari Desert.

Western psychiatry and psychology do not see holotropic states (with the exception of dreams that are not recurrent or frightening) as potential sources of healing or of valuable information about the human psyche but basically as pathological phenomena. Traditional psychiatry tends to use indiscriminately pathological labels and suppressive medication whenever these states occur spontaneously. Michael Harner,[7] an anthropologist of good academic standing who underwent a shamanic initiation during his field work in the Amazonian jungle and who also practices shamanism, suggests that Western psychiatry is seriously biased in at least two significant ways.

It is *ethnocentric,* which means that it considers its own view of the human psyche and of reality to be the only correct one and superior to all others. It is also *cognicentric* (a more accurate word might be "pragmacentric"), meaning that it takes into consideration only experiences and observations in the ordinary state of consciousness. Psychiatry's disinterest in holotropic states and disregard for them has resulted in a culturally insensitive approach and a tendency to pathologize all activities that cannot be understood in its own narrow context. This includes the ritual and spiritual life of ancient and pre-industrial cultures and the entire spiritual history of humanity.

IMPLICATIONS OF MODERN CONSCIOUSNESS RESEARCH FOR PSYCHIATRY

Traditional academic psychiatry and psychology use a model that is limited to biology, postnatal biography, and the Freudian individual unconscious. This model has to be vastly expanded and a new cartography of the psyche has to be created to describe all the phenomena occurring in holotropic states. The new understanding has to include additional realms of the psyche, transbiographical and trans-personal in nature, as potential sources of emotional problems. Indeed, many of the experiences and observations that occur during this work are so extraordinary that they cannot be understood in the context of the Newtonian-Cartesian materialistic paradigm and undermine the most basic metaphysical assumptions of the entire edifice of Western science.

In an effort to account for the experiences and observations from holotropic states, I have suggested a cartography or model of the psyche that contains, in addition to the usual *biographical level*, two transbiographical realms: *the perinatal domain*, related to the trauma of biological birth, and *the transpersonal domain*, which accounts for such phenomena as experiential identification with other people or with animals, visions of archetypal and mythological beings and realms, ancestral, racial, and karmic experiences, and identification with the Universal Mind or the Void.

Postnatal Biography and the Individual Unconscious

There are a few important differences between exploring postnatal biography through verbal psychotherapy and through approaches using holotropic states. First, one does not just remember emotionally significant events or reconstruct them indirectly from dreams, slips of tongue, or from transference distortions; rather, one experiences the original emotions, physical sensations, and even sensory perceptions in full age regression.

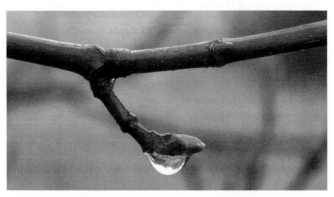

"Water Drop." (Courtesy Michael Eller.)

This means that during the reliving of an important trauma from infancy or childhood, one actually has the body image, naive perception of the world, sensations, and emotions corresponding to the age he or she was at that time. Besides confronting the usual psychotraumas known from handbooks of psychology, people often have to relive and integrate traumas that were primarily of a physical nature. As it surfaces, people realize that these physical traumas have actually played a significant role in the psychogenesis of their emotional and psychosomatic problems. The reliving of such traumatic memories and their integration can then have very far-reaching therapeutic consequences. This contrasts sharply with the attitudes of academic psychiatry and psychology, which do not recognize the direct psychotraumatic impact of physical traumas.

Emotionally relevant memories are stored in the unconscious in the form of complex dynamic constellations, not as a mosaic of isolated imprints. I have coined for them the name *COEX systems,* which is short for the phrase "systems of condensed experience." A COEX system consists of emotionally charged memories from different periods of our life that resemble each other in the quality of emotion or physical sensation that they share. Each COEX has a basic theme that permeates all its layers and represents their common denominator. The individual layers then contain variations on this basic theme that occurred at different periods of the person's life. Particularly important are COEX systems that contain memories of encounters with situations endangering life, health, and integrity of the body.

When I first described the COEX systems in the early stages of my LSD research, I thought they governed the dynamics of the biographical level of the unconscious. As my experience with non-ordinary states became richer and more extensive, I realized that the roots of the COEX systems reach much deeper. Each of the COEX constellations seems to be superimposed over and anchored in a particular aspect of the trauma of birth.

As we will see later in the discussion of the perinatal level of the unconscious, the experience of birth is so complex and rich in emotions and physical sensations that it contains in a prototypical form the elementary themes of all conceivable COEX systems. In addition, a typical COEX reaches even further and has its deepest roots in various forms of transpersonal phenomena, such as past life experiences, Jungian archetypes, conscious identification with various animals, and others. At present, I see the COEX systems as general organizing principles of the human psyche.

The similarities and differences between the concept of COEX systems and Jung's concept of complexes have been discussed elsewhere.[8]

Before we continue our discussion of the new extended cartography of the human psyche, it seems appropriate to emphasize in this context a very important and amazing characteristic of holotropic states that played an important role in charting the experiential territories, one that also is invaluable for the process of psychotherapy. Holotropic states tend to engage something like an "inner radar," bringing into consciousness automatically the contents from the unconscious that have the strongest emotional charge and are most psychodynamically relevant at the time. This represents a great advantage in comparison with verbal psychotherapy, where the client presents a broad array of information of various kinds and the therapist has to decide what is important, what is irrelevant, where the client is blocking, etc. The holotropic states save the therapist such difficult decisions and eliminate much of the subjectivity and professional idiosyncrasy of the verbal approaches.

The Perinatal Domain of the Psyche

The domain of the psyche that lies immediately beyond the recollective-biographical realm seems to have close connections with the beginning of life and its end, with birth and death. Many people identify the experiences that originate on this level as the reliving of their biological birth trauma. The use of the term *perinatal* in connection with consciousness reflects my own findings and is entirely new.[8]

As the name indicates, an important core of perinatal experiences is the reliving of various aspects of the biological birth process. As I mentioned before, these experiences represent a very strange mixture and combination of two critical aspects of human life—birth and death. They involve a sense of a severe, life-threatening confinement and a desperate and determined struggle to free oneself and survive. They often involve photographic details and occur even in people who have no intellectual knowledge about their birth. The replay of the original birth situation can be very convincing. We can, for example, discover through direct experience that we had a breech birth, that a forceps was used during our delivery, or that we were born with the umbilical cord twisted around our neck. We can feel the anxiety, biological fury, physical pain, and suffocation associated with this terrifying event and even accurately recognize the type of anesthesia used when we were born.

However, the spectrum of perinatal experiences is not limited to the elements that can be derived from the biological processes involved in childbirth. The perinatal domain of the psyche also represents an important gateway to the collective unconscious in the Jungian sense. Identification with the infant facing the ordeal of the passage through the birth canal seems to provide access to experiences involving people from other times and cultures, various animals, and even mythological figures. It is as if by connecting with the fetus struggling to be born, one reaches an intimate, almost mystical connection with other sentient beings who are in a similar difficult predicament.

Perinatal phenomena occur in four distinct experiential patterns characterized by specific emotions, physical feelings, and symbolic images. Each of them is closely related to one of the four consecutive periods of biological delivery. At each of these stages, the baby undergoes a specific and typical set of experiences. In turn, these experiences form distinct matrices or psychospiritual blueprints that later manifest in non-ordinary states of consciousness and that we find echoing in individual and social psychopathology, religion, art, philosophy, politics, and other areas of our life. We can talk about these four dynamic constellations of the deep unconscious that are associated with the trauma of birth as *Basic Perinatal Matrices (BPMs)*. Each perinatal matrix has its specific biological, psychological, archetypal, and spiritual aspects. In addition to having specific content of their own, BPMs also function as organizing principles for experiential elements from other levels of the unconscious—namely for biographical material and for some transpersonal phenomena. Individual matrices thus have fixed connections with certain categories of postnatal experiences arranged in COEX systems. (For more detail on Basic Perinatal Matrices and COEX systems, see my book, *Realms of the Human Unconscious,* 1975.)

The Transpersonal Domain of the Psyche

The second major domain that has to be added to mainstream psychiatry's cartography of the human psyche when we work with holotropic states is now known under the name *transpersonal,* meaning literally "beyond the personal" or "transcending the personal." The experiences that originate on this level involve transcendence of the usual boundaries of the individual (his or her body and ego) and of the limitations of three-dimensional space and linear time that restrict our perception of the world in the ordinary state of consciousness.

In the ordinary, or "normal," state of consciousness, we experience ourselves as Newtonian objects existing within the boundaries of our skin. The American writer and philosopher Alan Watts referred to this experience of oneself as identifying with the "skin-encapsulated ego." Our perception of the environment is restricted by the physiological limitations of our sensory organs and by physical characteristics of the environment.

Transpersonal experiences can be divided into three large categories. The first of these involves primarily transcendence of the usual spatial barriers, or the limitations of the "skin-encapsulated ego." Here belong experiences of merging with another person into a state that can be called "dual unity," assuming the identity of another person, identifying with the consciousness of an entire group of people (e.g., all mothers of the world, the entire population of India, or all the inmates of concentration camps), or even experiencing an extension of consciousness that seems to encompass all of humanity. Experiences of this kind have been repeatedly described in the spiritual literature of the world.

In a similar way, one can transcend the limits of the specifically human experience and identify with the consciousness of various animals, plants, or even a form of consciousness that seems to be associated with inorganic objects and processes. In the extremes, it is possible to experience consciousness of the entire biosphere, of our planet, or the entire material universe. Incredible and absurd as it might seem to a Westerner committed to Cartesian-Newtonian science, these experiences suggest that everything we can experience in the everyday state of consciousness as an object has in the non-ordinary states of consciousness a corresponding subjective representation. It is as if everything in the universe has its objective and subjective aspect, the way it is described in the great spiritual philosophies of the East (e.g., in Hinduism all that exists is seen as a manifestation of Brahma, or in Taoism as a transformation of the Tao).

The second category of transpersonal experiences is characterized primarily by overcoming of temporal rather than spatial boundaries, by transcendence of linear time. We have already talked about the possibility of vivid reliving of important memories from infancy and of the trauma of birth. This historical regression can continue further and involve authentic fetal and embryonal memories from different periods of intrauterine life. It is not even unusual to experience, on the level of cellular consciousness, full identification with the sperm and the ovum at the time of conception. But the historical regression does not stop here, and it is possible to have experiences from the lives of one's human or animal ancestors, or even those that seem to be coming from the racial and collective unconscious as described by C.G. Jung.[9] Quite frequently, the experiences that seem to be happening in other cultures and historical periods are associated with a sense of personal remembering; people then talk about reliving of memories from past lives, from previous incarnations.

In the transpersonal experiences described so far, the content reflects various phenomena existing in space-time. They involve elements of the everyday familiar reality—other people, animals, plants, materials, and events from the past. What is surprising here is not the content of these experiences but the fact that we can witness or fully identify with something that is not ordinarily accessible to our experience. We know that there are pregnant whales in the world, but we should not be able to have an authentic experience of being one. The fact that there once was the French Revolution is readily acceptable, but we should not be able to have a vivid experience of being there and lying wounded on the barricades of Paris. We know that there are many things happening in the world in places where we are not present, but it is usually considered impossible to experience something that is happening in remote locations (without the mediation of the television and a satellite). We may also be surprised to find consciousness associated with lower animals, plants, and with inorganic nature.

However, the third category of transpersonal experiences is even stranger; here consciousness seems to extend into realms and dimensions that the Western industrial culture does not consider to be "real." Here belong numerous visions of archetypal beings and mythological landscapes, encounters or even identification with deities and demons of various cultures, and communication with discarnate beings, spirit guides, suprahuman entities, extraterrestrials, and inhabitants of parallel universes. Additional examples in this category are visions and intuitive understanding of universal symbols, such as the cross, the Nile cross or ankh, the swastika, the pentacle, the six-pointed star, and the yin-yang sign.

In its farther reaches, individual consciousness can identify with cosmic consciousness or the Universal Mind known under many different names—Brahman, Buddha, the Cosmic Christ, Keter, Allah, the Tao, the Great Spirit, and many others. The ultimate of all experiences appears to be identification with the Supracosmic and Metacosmic Void, the mysterious and primordial emptiness and nothingness that is conscious of itself and is the ultimate cradle of all existence. It has no concrete content, yet it contains all there is in a germinal and potential form.

Transpersonal experiences have many strange characteristics that shatter the most fundamental metaphysical assumptions of the Newtonian-Cartesian paradigm and of the materialistic worldview. Researchers who have studied and/or personally experienced these fascinating phenomena realize that the attempts of mainstream science to dismiss them as irrelevant products of human fantasy and imagination or as hallucinations—erratic products of pathological processes in the brain—are naive and inadequate. Any unbiased study of the transpersonal domain of the psyche has to come to the conclusion that the observations represent a critical challenge not only for psychiatry and psychology but for the entire philosophy of Western science.

These observations indicate that we can obtain information about the universe in two radically different ways: Besides the conventional possibility of learning through sensory perception and analysis and synthesis of the data, we can also find out about various aspects of the world by direct identification with them in a non-ordinary state of consciousness. The reports of subjects who have experienced episodes of embryonal existence, the moment of conception, and elements of cellular, tissue, and organ consciousness abound in medically accurate insights into the anatomical, physiological, and biochemical aspects of the processes involved. Similarly, ancestral, racial, and collective memories and past incarnation experiences frequently provide very specific details about architecture, costumes, weapons, art forms, social structure, and religious and ritual practices of the culture and historical period involved, or even concrete historical events.

The philosophical challenge associated with the already-described observations, as formidable as it is all by itself, is further augmented by the fact that the transpersonal experiences correctly reflecting the material world often appear on the same continuum as and intimately interwoven with others that contain elements that the Western industrial world does not consider to be real. Here belong, for example, experiences involving deities and demons from various cultures, mythological realms such as heavens and paradises, and legendary or fairy-tale sequences.

For example, one can have an experience of Shiva's heaven, of the paradise of the Aztec rain god Tlaloc, of the Sumerian underworld, or of one of the Buddhist hot hells. It is also possible to communicate with Jesus, have a shattering encounter with the Hindu goddess Kali, or identify with the dancing Shiva. Even these episodes can impart accurate new information about religious symbolism and mythical motifs that were previously unknown to the person involved. Observations of this kind confirm C.G. Jung's[9] idea that in addition to the Freudian individual unconscious we can also gain access to the collective unconscious, which contains the cultural heritage of all humanity.

It is not an easy task to convey in a few sentences conclusions from daily observations in the course of over 35 years' of research of non-ordinary states of consciousness and make this statement believable. It is not realistic to expect that a few sentences would be able to override the deeply culturally ingrained worldview in those of the readers who are not familiar with the transpersonal dimension and who cannot relate what I say to their personal experience. Although I myself had many experiences of non-ordinary states of consciousness and the opportunity to observe closely a number of other people, it took me years to fully absorb the impact of this cognitive shock.

Because of space considerations, I cannot present detailed case histories that could help to illustrate the nature of transpersonal experiences and the insights that they make available. I have to refer those readers who would like to explore this area further to my book, *The Adventure of Self-Discovery*,[10] where I discuss in detail the various types of transpersonal experiences and give many illustrative examples of situations where they provided unusual new information about different aspects of the universe.

The same book also describes the method of holotropic breathwork, which opens the access to the perinatal and transpersonal realms for anybody who is interested in personal verification of the above observations. Comparable information about psychedelic sessions can be found in my book *LSD Psychotherapy*, which has recently been published in a new edition.[11]

The Nature and Architecture of Emotional and Psychosomatic Disorders

Traditional psychiatry uses the medical model and the disease concept not only for disorders of a clearly organic nature but also for emotional and psychosomatic disorders for which no biological cause has been found. Psychiatrists use quite loosely the term "mental" or "emotional disease" and try to assign various disorders to specific diagnostic categories comparable to those of general medicine. Generally, the time of the onset of symptoms is seen as the beginning of the "disease," and the intensity of the symptoms is used as the measure of the seriousness of the pathological process. Alleviation of the symptoms is considered "clinical improvement," and their intensification is seen as "worsening of the clinical condition."

The observations from the study of holotropic states suggest that thinking in terms of disease, diagnosis, and allopathic therapy is not appropriate for most psychiatric problems that are not clearly organic in nature, including some of the conditions currently labeled as psychoses. To exist in a material form, to have experienced the embryological development, birth, infancy, and childhood has left traumatic imprints in all of us, although we certainly differ as to their intensity, extensiveness, and also availability of this traumatic material for conscious experience. Every person is carrying a variety of more-or-less latent emotional and bioenergetic blockages, which interfere with full physiological and psychological functioning.

The manifestation of emotional and psychosomatic symptoms is the beginning of a healing process through which the organism is trying to free itself from traumatic imprints and simplify its functioning. The only way this can happen is by emergence of the traumatic material into consciousness and its full experience and emotional and motor expression. If the trauma that is being processed is of major proportions, such as a difficult birth that lasted many hours and seriously threatened biological survival, the emotions and behavioral expressions can be extremely dramatic. Under these circumstances, it might seem more plausible that it is a result of some exotic pathology than to recognize that it is a potentially beneficial development. However, when properly understood and supported, this process can be conducive to healing, spiritual opening, personality transformation, and consciousness evolution.

The emergence of symptoms thus represents not only a problem but also a therapeutic opportunity; this insight is the basis of most experiential psychotherapies. Symptoms manifest in the area where the defense system is at its weakest, making it possible for the healing process to begin. According to my experience, this is true not only in relation to neuroses and psychosomatic disorders but also in relation to certain conditions traditionally considered psychotic (psychospiritual crises or "spiritual emergencies").

Therapeutic Mechanisms and the Process of Healing

The work with holotropic states has thus discovered that emotional and psychosomatic problems are much more complex than is usually assumed and that their roots reach incomparably deeper into the psyche. However, it also revealed the existence of deeper and more effective therapeutic mechanisms. Traditional psychotherapy treatments of psychogenic disorders recognize only therapeutic mechanisms related to various manipulations of biographical material, for example: lifting of psychological repression and remembering or reconstructing events from infancy and childhood; emotional and intellectual insights into one's life history; or transference neurosis and analysis of transference.

The new observations show that these approaches fail to recognize and appreciate the amazing healing potential of the deeper dynamics of the psyche. Thus, for example, the reliving of birth and the experience of ego death and spiritual rebirth can have a far-reaching therapeutic impact on a broad spectrum of psychological disorders. Similar beneficial results are often associated with various forms of transpersonal phenomena, such as past life experiences and identification with various animals or archetypal figures and energies. Of particular importance in this sense are ecstatic feelings of cosmic unity, which—if properly integrated—provide a healing mechanism of extraordinary power.

When confronted with the challenging observations from modern consciousness research, we have only two choices. The first one is to reject the new observations simply because they are incompatible with the traditional scientific belief system. This involves an arrogant assumption that we already know what the universe is like and can tell with certainty what is possible and what is not possible. With this kind of approach, there cannot be any surprises, but there is also very little real progress. In this context, anyone who brings critically challenging data is accused of being a bad scientist, a fraud, or a mentally deranged person.

This is an approach that characterizes pseudoscience or scientistic fundamentalism and has very little to do with genuine science. There exist many historical examples of such an approach: people who refused to look into Galileo Galilei's telescope because they "knew" there could not be craters on the moon; those who fought against the atomic theory of chemistry and defended the concept of the nonexistent substance flogiston; those who called Einstein a psychotic when he proposed his special theory of relativity; and many others.

The second reaction to challenging new observations is characteristic of true science. It is excitement about and intense interest in such anomalies, combined with healthy critical skepticism. Major scientific progress has always occurred when the leading paradigm seriously fails to account for significant findings and is subsequently seriously questioned. In the history of science, paradigms come, dominate the field for some time, and then are replaced by new ones. If, instead of rejecting and ridiculing the new observations, we would consider them an exciting opportunity and conduct our own study to test them, we might very likely find that the reports were accurate.

It is hard to imagine that Western academic science will continue indefinitely to censor all the extraordinary evidence that has in the past been accumulated in the study of various forms of holotropic states, as well as to ignore the influx of new data. Sooner or later, it will have to face this challenge and accept all the far-reaching theoretical and practical consequences. When that happens, we will realize that the nature of human beings is very different from what is being taught at Western universities and what the industrial civilization believes it to be. It will also become clear to us that materialistic science has an incomplete and inadequate image of reality and that its ideas about the nature of consciousness and the relationship between consciousness and matter (particularly the brain) have to be radically revised. It is my firm belief that we are rapidly approaching a point when transpersonal psychology and the work with non-ordinary states of consciousness will become integral parts of a new scientific paradigm of the future.

References for this essay are located on the DVD accompanying this book.

Transpersonal Images: Implications for Health*

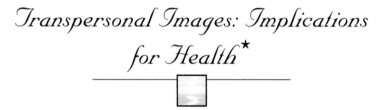

WILLIAM BRAUD

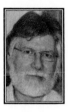

> *The imagination of man can act not only on his own body, but even on others and very distant bodies. It can fascinate and modify them; make them ill, or restore them to health.*
>
> IBN SÎNÂ[1]

TRANSPERSONAL IMAGERY

Jeanne Achterberg, in discussing the role of imagery in healing, distinguished between two types of imagery. *Preverbal imagery* acts upon one's own physical being to alter cellular, biochemical, and physiological activity. *Transpersonal imagery* "embodies the assumption that information can

---

*This chapter is an abridged version of Braud WG: Transpersonal images: implications for health. In Sheikh AA, Editor: *Healing images: the role of imagination in health,* Amityville, N.Y., 2003, Baywood Publishing Company, pp 444-466.

be transmitted from the consciousness of one person to the physical substrate of others...."[2]

In its most straightforward sense, transpersonal imagery is imagery that can exist or act *across* persons—i.e., from one person to another. Here, imagery functions as a bridge, connecting the conscious, imaginal content or activity of one person with the conscious or unconscious, physiological or psychological activities or experiences of another person.

There is another meaning of *trans*—as *beyond*—that is of great importance in the relatively young disciplines of transpersonal psychology and transpersonal studies. These fields of study explore experiences and processes that extend beyond the conventionally understood stages of personal development, beyond what is ordinarily understood as the individual ego or personality, beyond one's ordinary conditions of consciousness, and beyond the usual modes of knowing, being, and doing. Transpersonal experiences are those "in which the sense of identity or self extends beyond (trans) the individual or personal to encompass wider aspects of humankind, life, psyche, or cosmos."[3] This emphasis does not exclude or invalidate the personal; rather, it places the personal in a larger context, and it recognizes that the transpersonal or the transcendent can be expressed *through* the personal—in still another meaning of trans. The emphasis on a beyond or a something more—which can be contrasted with a reductionistic, "nothing-but" mindset—is congruent with William James'[4] view that one can become conscious of and in touch with a "More" with which one is "conterminous and continuous" and that such forms of awareness are at the heart of what we today call spiritual experiences.

THE REALITY OF THE IMAGINAL

In transpersonal experiences, there can be an expansion of one's identity to include much more of the world, and there can be a greater appreciation of one's interconnectedness with all of nature. Some of these apprehensions may be represented in one's imagination and imagery. Are such awarenesses and images momentary illusions or merely ways of speaking, or is there some sense in which they partake of "reality"?

Certainly, perceptions and images can be illusory and have no correspondence with conventional reality. There is a tendency, especially among Western, Eurocentric thinkers, to attribute a status of unreality to all aspects of the imagination. The usual connotations of words such as *imaginary* or *fantasy* reveal such a mindset. However, there always has been a parallel stream of thought in which the transpersonal and the imaginal are considered *real*—although this reality may be of a different character than that of the physical entities with which we are familiar. A sampling of systems of thought in which a special reality is attributed to the imaginal realm includes shamanic worldviews[5-7]; the Tantric Buddhism of Tibet[5]; descriptions of the spiritual and creative imagination in Ibn al-'Arabî and Suhrawardî, within mystical Islam[5,8]; the Western hermetic and magical traditions[9,10]; various mystical traditions[5]; and the views of Romantic poets such as Blake, Wordsworth, Coleridge, Keats, and Shelley.[11,12] More recent are the works of Carl Jung, James Hillman's archetypal psychology, Henry Corbin's writings on the imaginal faculty, Jess Hollenback's treatments of the empowered imagination, and Stanislav Grof's research on the transpersonal realm.[13-19]

Key considerations regarding different forms of imagery and their nature and "powers" have been provided by Henry Corbin,[8,14] in his elaboration of Ibn al-'Arabî's description of *himmah*—a kind of transfigured or empowered imaginal process or creative imagination, through which it becomes possible to directly perceive subtle or spiritual realities and to endow products of one's imagination and intention with a form of external reality, capable of being perceived by others—and by Jess Hollenback's[5] treatments of *enthymesis,* or empowered imagination, with properties identical to those of *himmah*. In these systems of thought, ordinary imagination may remain "local" in what it may know and accomplish. However, a special form of concentrated, empowered, transformed, or dynamized imagination can know and act veridically and "nonlocally."

The imaginal is emphasized and is active in both the Era II and Era III categories of Larry Dossey's schema for medical paradigms.[20-22] The validity (as an accurate means of knowing) and efficacy (in producing objectively measurable changes) of preverbal imagery have been demonstrated repeatedly in Era II contexts—through immunological, physiological, and behavioral studies. Here we will explore indications of the reality, validity, and efficacy of transpersonal imagery in nonlocal, or what Dossey calls "Era III," contexts. The imagery to be discussed is called "transpersonal" because it acts upon a person other than the person who is its "source."

USE OF IMAGERY IN NONLOCAL INTERVENTIONS: EMPIRICAL INVESTIGATIONS

The use of imagery in the nonlocal production of health-related outcomes, or of physiological or psychological changes with health-related potentials, has been documented not only in everyday life but also in carefully designed and executed laboratory studies. In this chapter, I will summarize the methods and findings of a research program in which my colleagues and I have been involved since 1977. This program involves laboratory experiments exploring what is now commonly known as "direct mental interactions with living systems (DMILS)." We have published seven reports and reviews of these experiments[23-29]; interested readers are referred to these reports for specific details and additional information.

In these experiments, one person, sometimes called the "sender" for expository convenience, uses imagery and intention to exert a direct mental influence upon the objectively measured physiological activity of another person isolated at a distance, nominally called the "receiver." Precautions are taken to prevent sensory cueing, inference, expectation, and placebo-like confounds from influencing the receiver in any systematic way. Changes in the receiver's physiology are monitored and recorded by electronic equipment, and blind or computer-scoring methods used to prevent recording errors or motivated scoring errors. The resulting data are then analyzed to determine whether the sender's intention causes physiological changes in the receiver.

In many of our studies, electrodermal activity (EDA) was used as the dependent variable, primarily for its ease of measurement, its sensitive reflection of sympathetic nervous system changes, and its relationship to emotional and psychological changes that are relevant to physical and psychological health and well-being.

EDA is recorded continuously throughout a session, and short-term fluctuations in EDA serve as the specific physiological measure of interest. The receiver is asked to remain seated in a comfortable chair for about 30 minutes, in a dimly illuminated room; to not to become overly excited or relaxed; and to be open to the possibility of distant mental influences from the remote sender.

Meanwhile, the sender is presented with instructions—either by the experimenter or in more recent studies automatically by a computer—to try either to influence or to not influence the receiver. A random process determines the type of condition and the timing of each influence period. During non-influence periods, the sender rests and thinks about matters that are not related to the experiment. During influence periods, the sender's aim is to either activate or calm the remote receiver using mental imagery and intention.

So far we have conducted 15 such experiments involving 323 separate sessions contributed by 271 different receivers, 62 senders, and 4 experimenters. Cumulatively these studies have provided repeatable, statistically significant evidence for the existence of nonlocal, direct mental influences (overall p = 0.000023; mean effect size r = 0.29).[27] As compared with baseline measures, receivers' EDA increased during periods in which remotely situated senders used activating imagery, and it decreased during periods in which calming, relaxing imagery was used. After our first cumulative article published in 1989, four replication studies, involving a total of 75 experimental sessions, were attempted elsewhere. In 1997, we updated our work to include these replications and determined the grand p-value to be 0.0000007 and a mean effect size of r = 0.25.[29]

Besides the studies focusing on EDA measures, we also conducted experiments measuring subtle muscular movements, muscular tremor, blood pressure, the spatial orientation of fish, the locomotor activity of small mammals, and the rate of hemolysis of human red blood cells in vitro. Positive results were obtained for all of these new living systems with one exception—muscular tremor. In 1991, we published a grand meta-analysis of all of our DMILS studies conducted up to that point. The research program included 37 experiments, 655 sessions, 449 different receivers, 153 different senders, and 12 different experimenters. The overall results yielded a combined p value of 2.58×10^{-14} and a mean effect size of r = +.33.[28]

Influences "Across Time"

In the studies described above, process-oriented and goal-oriented imagery acted nonlocally with respect to space—a person's direct mental influence was monitored in a distant living system. We have also conducted sessions in which the to-be-influenced living system was distant in *time*. The procedures and analysis methods for these temporally nonlocal experiments are similar to those of the concurrent influence studies, with the important difference that the activity of the living "target" system was monitored and recorded *before* the influence attempts were made. Thus, any systematic results in such experiments involved time-displaced influences. Although such outcomes might seem to be impossible given conventional apprehensions of time and causality, there is nonetheless both theoretical and empirical support for such outcomes. Discussion of these issues is beyond the scope of this chapter, so the reader is referred to an article that describes these studies in detail.[30,31] For present purposes, I will simply say that there exists both anecdotal and laboratory evidence supporting the possibility of apparently "backward-acting," time-displaced, direct mental influences of living systems. Our imaginal processes appear to be capable of exerting objectively measurable influences not only upon present, distant biological and physical systems but also upon the past and future activities of these systems.

ROLE OF IMAGERY IN NONLOCAL KNOWING: EMPIRICAL INVESTIGATIONS

The studies briefly summarized in the preceding pages explored processes that could be considered models of nonlocal imaginal *interventions* that may occur in everyday life. In addition to these, there have been numerous laboratory studies of processes equivalent to nonlocal imaginal *diagnosis*. In these studies, imagery can serve as a vehicle for veridical perception or knowledge of physical, biological, or psychological events that distance and other barriers have placed beyond the reach of the conventional senses. There are extensive empirical studies of remote knowing through imagery.

Our access to information beyond the reach of our conventional senses can be revealed in many ways. This "knowing" can be expressed in clear, information-rich thoughts—as when the name of an illness or condition comes to mind. Equally unambiguous are specific bodily conditions that may be felt that correspond clearly to those of a distant person;

these could be described as empathic or telesomatic indicators.[21,32] Other expressions can take the form of behavioral, perceptual, or memory-related changes that indicate a "knowing" that has not yet reached conscious awareness; these are the psi-mediated instrumental responses (PMIR)—e.g., finding ourselves at the right place at the right time, and thereby avoiding an accident or gaining access to needed information—that have been well-described and studied by Rex Stanford.[33,34] Knowledge of events beyond sensory range can also be indicated by subtle physiological changes, of which we may be unaware; by a diffuse awareness too vague to be articulated; or by a direct experience of "knowing" that also is difficult or impossible to put into words. Perhaps most commonly, our knowledge of distant or otherwise inaccessible events is expressed by imagery that bears some resemblance to the distant event or circumstance.

Methods and Findings

In order to qualify imagery as transpersonal, it is necessary to distinguish images that carry information about distant events from other forms of imagery. Some of the latter include imagery that might arise naturally independent of distant events, images that might be triggered by common, conventional events that influence both the distant event and the person generating the imagery, or images that may correspond to distant events by coincidence. Our experimental designs allow us to make these distinctions through the use of sensory shielding, truly random selection of events, blind evaluation of imagery correspondences with the true target event versus randomly selected non-target "decoys," and statistical analyses that compare obtained results with theoretically or empirically derived baselines.

We have conducted experiments in which spontaneously arising imagery, in suitably prepared individuals, could be shown to correspond to distant, randomly selected target events. These events could be randomly selected pictures or objects, or their representations in the thoughts, images, and sensations of other persons. In some cases, the research participants were in ordinary states of consciousness (e.g., in remote viewing studies); in other cases, participants were studied under more imagery-rich conditions provided by relaxation, autogenic, sensory restriction (e.g., the *ganzfeld* state), hypnotic induction, guided imagery, "waking dream," or nocturnal dream conditions.[35,36] In these and related studies transpersonal imagery has been demonstrated to have a veridical, *noetic* character—allowing accurate access to information temporarily unavailable to the conventional senses.

The focus of such imagery can be "targeted" to physical or psychological conditions of distant persons for purposes of remote or augmented diagnosis. For example, in one test session, a participant was asked to describe the health condition of an absent "target person." The participant described a young girl with blonde hair in ringlets, a metal brace on one of her legs, her heart "blown up, like a big red balloon," and the unusual circumstance of her heart displaced to the "wrong" side of the body. Each of these images corresponded perfectly to the conditions of the target person. Such accurate correspondences of "local" imagery with remote realities have been observed in numerous formal and informal experiments.

MODULATING FACTORS

Although considerable uncertainty and mystery continue to exist with respect to the nature of these transpersonal imagery effects and the conditions that influence them, we are able to make certain generalizations about the factors that seem to facilitate or impede their occurrence. These empirical generalizations are based upon our own research, conducted over a span of 30 years, and upon a huge database of similar research findings reported by others.[37-44]

PHYSICAL FACILITATORS AND INHIBITORS

Transpersonal imagery effects, in both their influential/intervention and noetic/diagnostic forms, are relatively independent of physical influences. Factors such as distance, time, physical barriers, and the physical nature of the events to be known or influenced do not appear to play critical roles in transpersonal imagery outcomes. One factor that does seem to be important is the amount of free variability that is inherent in the system to be influenced. Random or labile physical systems that are relatively free from internal or external constraints or structure seem most amenable to being influenced through transpersonal imagery.

Three additional, possible physical correlates have been suggested. A tantalizing one, in terms of potential medical applications, is that water that has been "treated" through transpersonal imagery or related intention techniques may be physically altered. Such treated water appears to have decreased hydrogen bonding, compared with untreated control water.[45] To the extent that changes in hydrogen bonding characterize either disease conditions or therapeutic agents, this possible mode of action of nonlocal influence may provide a useful entry point for health applications.

Two other physical factors have recently been found to correlate with the likelihood or accuracy of nonlocal knowing—one is a decrease in the activity in the earth's geomagnetic field (roughly equivalent to a reduction in the amount of "noise" in the earth's electromagnetic "atmosphere")[46,47]; a second is the local sidereal time (i.e., time according to the "fixed" stars rather than local clock time) at the site at which a nonlocal knowing experiment is being conducted.[48]

Physiological Facilitators and Inhibitors

Although the nonlocal knowing effects we have been considering probably can occur in any physiological state, they appear to occur most readily or most accurately—or, at least, are most readily *noticed* or *detected*—under conditions of reduced muscular activity, reduced sympathetic autonomic activation, and a freeing of the brain (of the knower) from heavy information-processing demands.[36,37] There also are indications—but not as definitive as the foregoing—that heightened sympathetic nervous system arousal in the influencer may be associated with the production of some forms of nonlocal influence effects.[49]

Complementary principles may apply to what is to be known or influenced. For example, heightened physiological arousal (which might be associated with increased *need*) in one person may make that person or that person's circumstances more discernible to others via the latter's nonlocal knowing. A person whose internal systems are relatively quiet and free from energetic- or information-handling demands may be more susceptible to nonlocal influence than would overly structured, constrained, or burdened physiological systems.

Psychological Facilitators and Inhibitors

It is in the psychological area that we have learned most about facilitating and inhibiting factors. Many of the psychological facilitators of transpersonal imagery effects are closely related to the virtues of faith, hope, and love, and many of the inhibitors are related to the opposites. Space permits only a brief mentioning of these factors here; more extended treatments are available elsewhere.[37,44,50] Psychological facilitators of transpersonal imagery effects include attitudes of belief, confidence, trust, hope, expectation of a successful outcome, the presence of strong motives and incentives, need, positive dispositions, caring, and a reduction in egocentric motives, strivings, or involvements. Psychological inhibitors include attitudes of disbelief, distrust, doubt, suspicion, absent or negative expectations of success, increased egocentric motivation or too-effortful striving, and the absence of sufficient need, motivation, or purpose for the task at hand.

Additional facilitators include psychological comfort and absence of stress; freedom from distractions; conditions of relaxation and quietude; and the ability to direct attention inwardly and access inner processes, to concentrate attention, to generate vivid imagery, to reduce "left-hemispheric" analytical thought and increase "right-hemispheric" intuitive modes of mentation, engage in intention that is more "passive" and less effortful (akin to wishing rather than willing); freedom from excessive cognitive structure or information-handling demands; the presence of openness; and the absence of defensiveness.[51,52] Psychological inhibitors include the absence or opposites of these facilitators.

Also important to the occurrence of these transpersonal imagery effects is the preparedness, adequateness, and predisposition of the participant. The most effective participant is one who is familiar with the imaginal world, skilled in negotiating this realm, and skilled in the use of creative imagination. Training in active imagination, psychophysiological self-regulation, concentration, meditation, and related psychospiritual practices may be useful preparations for engaging in transpersonal imagery exercises and nonlocal knowing and influence attempts.

IMPLICATIONS AND POTENTIAL APPLICATIONS

The most obvious health-related applications of nonlocal knowing and influence mediated by transpersonal imagery are in the areas of diagnosis and intervention in physical and psychological health disturbances. Just as *preverbal* imagery may serve these functions within a given individual, transpersonal images may provide diagnostic information and serve an intervention function with respect to *other* individuals. These complementary functions may already be present even in local, personal uses of imagery. In learning more about, and possibly influencing, one's own bodily and psychological circumstances, imagery may act *directly*, as well as through conventionally understood mediating channels of neurological and immunological secretions and processes.[53] The direct action of imagery may even be present in the familiar processes of volitional action, memory, perception, and so on.

A similar mix of local and nonlocal effects may be present in any and all diagnostic and healing interventions provided by health practitioners and may, indeed, be an important component of the mysterious art of healing. The nonlocal working of imagery may be a crucial aspect of such common phenomena as accurate intuitions about a patient or client, the efficacy of therapeutic touch and similar techniques, accurate diagnoses by physicians or therapists, physicians' bedside manners, the ways in which voiced (or unvoiced) prognoses fulfill themselves, nonspecific influences of medical or therapeutic interactions, spontaneous remissions, and placebo effects. If this is the case, then we could make greater use of our knowledge of the facilitators and inhibitors of transpersonal imagery to amplify any of the processes just mentioned for the increased benefits of our patients, our clients, and ourselves.

The experiments summarized in this chapter, along with those of other investigators, help us discern nonlocal from local aspects, and they provide indications of what is possible when the nonlocal aspect is acting alone. These experiments have indicated that the active and creative imagination is able to provide accurate knowledge about, and influence, physical, physiological, and psychological circumstances related to health issues. In one study, we found that these remote mental influences were greater for persons who had a greater "need" to be influenced—i.e., for persons with overly active autonomic activity.[26] In other experiments, persons were able to remotely help others focus their attention, helping them calm and focus their wandering thoughts—an outcome that could have well-being implications in the psychological realm. Although these are basic research studies, conducted in the laboratory, they involve actual forms of healing. Other forms of direct, imagery-mediated, remote healing effects or healing analog effects have been well-documented elsewhere.[54,55] So, we have both direct evidence of remote healing, as well as many more instances of influences that indicate this possibility more indirectly and in an "in principle" form. Similar evidence—some direct, some indirect—exists for the reality of the diagnostic modes of these effects.[56]

The important next steps in these areas involve exploring more thoroughly what may be accomplished through transpersonal imagery. It would be unwise to underestimate the power of imaginal, adjunctive techniques. Even small remote mental influences upon the more labile, more susceptible earliest stages or seed moments of illnesses or of health can become amplified and blossom into much larger, later outcomes with definite health relevance. Research in the area of chaos studies has shown that the later, very large-scale activities of certain animate and inanimate systems can be extraordinarily sensitive to very slight changes in initial conditions.[57,58] The imaginal processes treated in this chapter may be capable of exerting comparably large, later effects through their initial, subtle influences in critical stages of the developmental processes of symptoms and syndromes—both physiological and psychological, both harmful and healthful. Specific examples of actual and hypothetical health applications, especially in the context of time-displaced, direct mental influences, have been described elsewhere.[31]

At a more theoretical level, the findings reviewed in this paper have important implications for our understanding of the imagination. In traditions going back to early Greek and Persian thinkers, the imaginal has been considered a special and powerful human faculty with noetic and creative properties of its own.[13,14] In these traditions, the active and creative imagination has been viewed as a bridge between the sensory realm (of the body) and the intellectual realm (of the mind), between the conscious and the unconscious, between mind and matter, and between possibility and actuality. The imagery effects noted in this chapter are consistent with such a view. Increasing interest and developments in the areas of transpersonal psychology, consciousness studies, the efficacy of prayer, the role of spirituality in health, alternative medical and psychological interventions, and the new positive psychology movement within the American Psychological Association[59] all promise to cast new light on the nature and power of the imagination and of the imaginal realm.

References for this essay are located on the DVD accompanying this book.

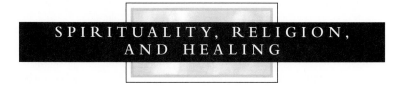

SPIRITUALITY, RELIGION, AND HEALING

Etiology Recapitulates Ontology: Reflections on Restoring the Spiritual Dimension to Models of the Determinants of Health*

JEFF LEVIN

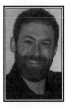

BACKGROUND

This paper's subtitle promises reflections on restoring the spiritual dimension to a theoretical model for the prevention of morbidity and promotion of health and well-being. There was certainly a time in human

*This paper was originally published in *Subtle Energies & Energy Medicine*, Volume 12 No. 1, pages 17-37 (published by the International Society for the Study of Subtle Energies & Energy Medicine, 11005 Ralston Rd. 100D, Arvada, CO 80004) and was based on a presentation at The Heart of Energy Medicine: A Renaissance of Health & Healing, the Tenth Annual ISSSEEM Conference, Boulder, CO, June 19, 2000. The author would like to thank Dr. Lea Steele and Dr. Larry Dossey for comments on earlier versions of this manuscript.

history when spirit was a central, not peripheral, focus in matters of health and illness and healing. With the advent of science, this perspective changed. The realm of spirit was relegated to religion and philosophy, which were other than science. Science is the measurable, the observable, the impersonal, the objective, the rational. It is the opposite of the unmeasurable, the unobservable, the ineffable, the personal, the subjective, and the intuitive. Somewhere along the way, it was determined that health, illness, and healing had more to do with the former than the latter.

In other words, the psychosomatic or mind-body revolution of the past several decades, and more recent explorations of possible body-mind-spirit connections in medicine, are not so much new developments as a renaissance of ideas that have long been a part of human understandings of health and well-being. Practitioners, scientists, and laypeople are increasingly aware of this fact.

The thesis reflected in the title of this chapter, "Etiology Recapitulates Ontology," is a play on the familiar biological dictum "ontogeny recapitulates phylogeny." Prevailing biomedical and clinical theories on the causes of disease (etiology) precisely reflect prevailing beliefs on what it means to be a human being (ontology). If nothing exists but atoms and empty space, to paraphrase Democritus, then the biomedical paradigm is complete. If the mind is real, and not solely an epiphenomenon of our neurochemistry, then psychosomatic medicine is a possibility. And if humans possess a soul or a spiritual nature or life force, and if this becomes widely acknowledged by clinicians and medical scientists, a new spirit-filled medical paradigm may emerge.

SPIRIT AND MEDICINE

The idea that we are on the frontier of a new medical paradigm—a successor to the mind-body perspective—has been advanced by many commentators. This new medicine goes by many names: Dossey's "Era III,"[1] Gerber's "vibrational medicine,"[2] Green's "energy medicine,"[3] Dacher's "spiritual healing system,"[4] and my own "theosomatic medicine."[5] Regardless of what it is called or how exactly it is described, a consensus seems to be building that our health is determined by not just physical, mental, and emotional factors but by something more. Religiousness, spirituality, faith, consciousness, subtle energy, the bioenergy field, non-local mind, our relationship with God or the divine—each of these concepts suggests something "beyond" the local mind as part of what it means to be a human being. Many of these concepts are being increasingly validated through empirical research as relevant to health, healing, and human physiology. Nearly all of these concepts are seen as imaginary and/or irrelevant to health by the mainstream biomedical model.

A body-only view of what it means to be a human being has distinct implications for medicine. The corresponding body-only view of the determinants of health as limited to physical factors—heredity, health history, physiological parameters, etc.—results in (a) reinforcement of a mechanized and reductionistic view of human beings as a collection of parts, (b) promotion of depersonalized care that seeks to fix or manage these parts, (c) emphasis on discrete biological outcomes as markers of the proper or improper functioning of these parts, (d) a concomitant disease-entity orientation that focuses clinical attention on conditions defined by signs and not symptoms, (e) therapeutic metaphors based on warfare (e.g., words and phrases like "attack," "bomb," "war on cancer"), (f) an economic-driven ethics that sanctions decision-making strategies that uphold all of these features, and (g) reliance upon high-tech invasive therapies.

These therapies are precisely routinized, target discrete outcomes, are managed and reimbursed. Alternative clinical approaches are based on holism, whole-person-centered care, psychosocial and behavioral causation of illness, the desubordination of symptoms to signs, non-hierarchical patient-practitioner relations, therapeutic objectives grounded in functioning and general well-being, and hands-on healing.

Because the prevailing scientific worldview excludes spirit, so-called scientific medicine excludes it as well. These same forces support and reinforce the body-as-machine metaphor that informs thinking in modern medicine, lending it public status, authority, and sanction. We can never have a truly "integral medicine" until we have an integral body-mind-spirit model of what it means to be human. Without the latter, we will not be able to acknowledge all of the myriad potential determinants of health.

Many scientists and physicians are reluctant to discuss, or acknowledge, the idea of a human spirit. Perhaps this is because acknowledging the role of spirit would question the hegemony of left-brained reason and logic as means of determining scientific truth and medical reality.

Currently, medical progress is predicated on an ethic that seeks to control and correct nature—including human nature. Proponents seeking to reconfigure medicine around body-mind and body-mind-spirit principles would risk being dismissed by the mainstream as "antiscientific" or "pseudoscientific." Not all scientists, of course, find the consideration of the human spirit a nuisance. According to Einstein, for example, that science should someday come to consider the role and salience of spirituality was inevitable and welcome:

> "Everyone seriously involved in the pursuit of science becomes convinced that a spirit is manifest in the laws of the Universe—a spirit vastly superior to that of man. . . ."[4]

Disbelief in God or spirit, or in models of human life that encompass more than just the body, certainly inhibits acceptance of a broader model of the determinants of health and healing. Skeptics and debunkers, however, invariably deny that their philosophy of life drives their defense of the biomedical paradigm. The onus is placed on proponents of a more holistic model who, it is asserted, have failed to produce any empirical evidence in support of their claims.[7] In order for such a dramatic transformation to occur—a shift to a new medical paradigm—it is always asserted that there first needs to be a scientific basis. This is a fair stipulation. Physicians and scientists require evidence.

RELIGION, HEALTH, AND HEALING: THREE TYPES OF SCIENTIFIC EVIDENCE

According to a now enormous and well-publicized volume of empirical research findings and scholarly reviews, religiousness and spirituality, broadly defined, have been found to be associated with myriad indicators of health status, physical functioning, physiology, morbidity, mortality, and healing or recovery from illness.[8] Research findings in this field come from three general categories of studies.

First, there have been experimental and quasi-experimental trials and experiments of the therapeutic efficacy of prayer and other sorts of absent or distant intentionality. Outcome variables in these studies have included a variety of indicators related to healing of disease or restored functioning. Moreover, studies have been conducted not just in humans but in a variety of biological systems, from domestic and laboratory animals to bacteria, viruses, and fungi. According to Dr. Daniel J. Benor, a leading expert on the scope and content of this literature, nearly 200 such studies have been conducted, about half to two thirds of which show statistically significant impacts on healing.[9]

A second category of religion and health studies consists of basic research on spiritual consciousness and psychophysiology. A steadily growing body of research has investigated the impact of psychological characteristics of religious participation, spiritual experience, and mystical or transcendent states of consciousness on cognitive or affective correlates or markers of psychophysiology. Included are studies of transcendental meditation and the relaxation response,[10] research on the physiological effects of yogic practice,[11] biofeedback investigations of autonomic self-regulation in adepts,[12] and analysis of the association between intrinsic religiousness and absorption.[13]

Finally, hundreds of peer-reviewed journal articles have reported findings from epidemiologic and social science studies investigating the effects of dimensions of religious involvement on population health parameters such as rates of morbidity or mortality or indices of health status or psychological well-being.[8] These include studies of religious affiliation or membership, church or synagogue attendance, public or private prayer or worship, adherence to specific religious beliefs, profession of faith in God, and religious or mystical experiences. This field of study, which has come to be known as the "epidemiology of religion,"[14] has produced empirical findings identifying significant religious differences in rates of health and illness, as well as significant salutary effects of religious indicators on indices of physical and mental health and well-being.[15] Further, these findings seem to persist regardless of the religious affiliation of those being studied, the diseases or health conditions under investigation, or the age, sex, race or ethnicity, or nationality of study respondents or subjects![16]

The interested reader is referred to resources such as the academic *Handbook of Religion and Health*[8] and my own recently published *God, Faith, and Health: Exploring the Spirituality-Healing Connection.*

THE ROLE OF NORMAL SCIENCE

The past decade has witnessed tremendous growth in all three classes of religion and health studies. Especially popular has been research on religious determinants of population health, as well as clinical investigations of spiritual issues. Original empirical investigations funded by the National Institutes of Health (NIH) or by established foundations have proliferated. Many such studies have been conducted by well-known researchers at leading universities and medical centers. Additionally, many excellent theoretical, conceptual, and methodological contributions have appeared in print, more often than not in mainline peer-reviewed social science and medical journals, especially in the field of gerontology. This mainstreaming of religion and health research has occurred so rapidly and so completely, and the field has become so institutionalized, that it appears to have entered a state of what philosopher and historian Dr. Thomas S. Kuhn called "normal science."[17]

By normal science, Kuhn was referring to the "mop-up work"[17] that inevitably occupies the time and effort of most of the scientists employed in research sanctioned by an existing paradigm. Instead of the envelope-pushing, giant intuitive leaps, and inspired stabs in the dark by lone geniuses that characterize shifts in paradigms—breakthroughs to new ways of conceiving some reality—normal science is more about filling in the blanks. This is the kind of work that serves to transform a novel or revolutionary idea into an established institution, and to maintain the institution against assaults by subsequent new ideas. Kuhn lamented the "drastically restricted vision"[17] of scientists operating within the bounds of normal science:

> Closely examined, whether historically or in the contemporary laboratory, that enterprise seems an attempt to force nature into the preformed and relatively inflexible box that the paradigm supplies. No part of the aim of normal science is to call forth new sorts of phenomena; indeed those that will not fit the box are often not seen at all. Nor do scientists normally aim to invent new theories, and they are often intolerant of those invented by others. Instead, normal-scientific research is directed to the articulation of those phenomena and theories that the paradigm already supplies.[17]

As momentum has built in the religion and health field, the attributes of normal science have arrived. These include (a) research funding by several branches of the NIH (e.g., the National Institute on Aging, the National Institute of Mental Health, and the National Center for Complementary and Alternative Medicine) and by important foundations, such as Templeton, Fetzer, and Robert Wood Johnson; (b) the establishment of scholarly journals and of academic centers and institutes at leading medical schools (represented by the Consortium of Academic Health Centers for Integrative Medicine); (c) the convening of study sections, expert panels, and expert working groups at the NIH and elsewhere; (d) the issuance of white papers, consensus reports, and research agendas; (e) the release of Requests for Proposals and Requests for Applications by both the NIH and foundations; (f) the publication, and solicitation of publication, of original research and review articles in leading peer-reviewed journals, including *JAMA*; (g) the proliferation of conferences, symposia, and Continuing Medical Education opportunities, and the endowment of named addresses (e.g., at Columbia University) and chairs (e.g., at Emory University); (h) the successful navigation by the first cohort of researchers through academic appointments and promotions committees and tenure committees; and (i) the attention of the mass media, as evidenced by cover stories in *Time* and *Readers' Digest* and major stories on all of the television networks and on National Public Radio.

Once a state of normal science is reached, the creative spark that lit the original fire may be extinguished. The maintenance and regulation of routine becomes the *raison d'être* of the field. Dr. Richard L. Garrison outlined a process with reference to revolutionary innovations in medical thinking. In his brilliant essay entitled "The Five Generations of American Medical Revolutions," he described how the first generation of proponents of change is characterized by a small cohort of inspired innovators.[18] Subsequent generations synthesize the innovation into an established agenda; found and administer institutions of normal science; rationalize and bureaucratize the original idea, centralizing gatekeeping functions within a cabal; and perpetuate field-defining authority by repressing or withholding sanction of developments that threaten their oligarchy. Granted, the imagery used by

Garrison is stark and may be overstated with respect to the religion and health field.

The phenomena of routinization may be manifest in many ways: Anything beyond incremental change is resisted; true innovation is stifled; groupthink is rewarded; the rethinking of paradigms is discouraged and perhaps seen as crankish; and outcroppings of genius, originality or creativity are plowed under or ignored. The camaraderie of early innovators may be replaced by turf battles and self-promotion. Worse, a kind of worker-bee mentality is sanctioned, in contrast to the envelope-pushing that got the field established in the first place. Scholars occupy themselves with the work described by Kuhn—the unending fill-in-the-blanks sorts of studies.

Although a body-mind-spirit perspective has not attained paradigmatic status within medicine, a paradigm is emerging within the religion and health field.

THE FACTIONING OF RELIGION AND HEALTH

An effect of attaining normal-science mode for the study of religion and health has been the premature and increasing sanction of certain ideas or concepts at the expense of others. As this field has begun to enter the mainstream, and as institutions have sprung up to serve gatekeeping functions, the boundaries of acceptable discourse have predictably narrowed. Particular theoretical and religious perspectives have attained a sort of "approved" status; others have been relegated to the margins, where all of this field once resided.

The clearest example that this field is entering a state of normal science is its rapid fragmentation into three camps or factions, and the marginalization of two of these groups. The first group (call it Faction I) is composed of academic physicians and clinical researchers, primarily but not exclusively conservative Christians. These individuals have been most successful in staking out a position in the mainstream, as seen by research funding, academic acceptance, CME conference appearances, popular writing, and media coverage. Faction II includes those scientists and clinicians working in the complementary and alternative medicine, consciousness studies, and mind-body fields—areas already held to be marginal by mainstream medicine and science. These individuals seem to operate in an alternative universe of conferences, publications, and institutions. Members of Faction III, a relatively small group of social scientists, have actually conducted much of the empirical research in this field over the past 15 to 20 years. These investigators typically work alone, do not exhibit much interest in popular writing or publicity, are not medical scientists, and do not conduct clinical studies, strictly speaking; nearly all have principal research interests outside of religion and health. They are also largely unknown to both the general public and many investigators in the first two factions.

Finally, while members of these factions sometimes do attend the same meetings and on occasion take part in collaborative efforts, overlap among these three groups is minimal.

An unsettling outcome of this fragmentation has been the success of Faction I in defining the field, its own work, and the ideas and work of the other two groups. An example was the recent publication in a leading "debunker" magazine of an essay signed by many of the leading figures in Faction I.[19] This article roundly denounced exploration of parapsychology, of alternative medicine, of "metaphysics," and of types of distant healing, while putting over religion and health research as "distinct and separate"[19] and thus worthy of acceptance by the debunkers. The article was meant to sound conciliatory and reasonable, but Faction I's embarrassment over this more cutting-edge work, and their urgency in distancing themselves from it, was transparent.

A response to this article was penned by Dr. Larry Dossey, a leading light of what has been termed Faction II. His response, published in the journal *Alternative Therapies in Health and Medicine,* was cogent:

Why did these researchers choose parapsychology as a disreputable referent for their own field, and why did they bracket complementary and alternative medicine (CAM) with parapsychology? . . . In effect, the religion-and-health researchers are proclaiming to the scientific community, 'Like you, we oppose this spooky, distant, mental stuff. We're against parapsychology and its bedfellow, CAM.' . . . This move, however, places the religion-and-health researchers in a double-bind. How can they be considered open-minded and scientific while denying the increasing evidence that psi-like, distant healing is real?[20]

Faction I has positioned itself as the proponent of the re-introduction of spirituality into medical practice and medical education, principally on the basis of the growing research evidence outlined earlier. The preponderance of the evidence that they draw on, however, is the data of Faction III: population-based sociological and epidemiologic studies of general communities investigated cross-sectionally or prospectively in order to identify religious correlates or determinants of health and well-being. This body of research is not based on medicine, physicians, patients, illness, the clinical setting, medical therapies, or healing. It does not and cannot provide any evidence for or against principal features of the broader Faction I agenda, such as physicians praying with patients.

The two bodies of findings that can and do provide such supportive evidence, and in spades, are the studies of nonlocal healing and absent prayer and of psychophysiological correlates of consciousness. But these studies are squarely in the tradition of parapsychological and mind-body research, many of the leading investigators follow non-Western or non-mainstream spiritual paths, and study results often report salutary effects of Eastern or esoteric spiritual practices. Thus, to Faction I, this work—probably the best work to cite to advance their agenda—is condemned or ignored.

The marginalization of Faction III is more subtle. As social scientists with other interests besides studying religion and health, their work is not as heavily promoted and is thus easily overlooked. Most of the leading figures in this faction are probably unknown to individuals in Faction II, while their work is drawn on (whether cited or uncited) and often misinterpreted by Faction I. Many investigators in Faction III are perhaps unaware of this or may not be particularly concerned.

CONDUCTING PARADIGM-CHALLENGING RESEARCH

In order to conduct exciting, cutting-edge research—paradigm-challenging research—one does not require normal science. If anything, the rewards of normal science—even the lure of such rewards—may serve primarily to inhibit such research. The kind of mop-up work mentioned by Kuhn is by its very nature constrained by the parameters of a given field—by the boundaries of its dominant paradigm. It is unlikely that researchers operating within normal-science mode can even conduct envelope-pushing research; this would require first "stepping out" of the paradigm. What one does need to conduct such research is actually quite modest. For many types of scientific research, a formal academic appointment or scholarly position may not even be necessary. In fact, it may introduce intractable barriers preventing such research from ever taking place.

AN AGENDA FOR A NEXT GENERATION OF BODY-MIND-SPIRIT RESEARCH

By now, nearly a generation of scientific research has explored the interconnections among religion, spirituality, health, and healing. A cohort of researchers has helped this field to come of age since its earliest emergence in the middle 1980s. Normal science seems to have taken hold. With increased attention from the NIH, prominent foundations, and academic medicine has come increased involvement in the direction, content, and application of research in this field. This field is capable of more than surveys correlating the frequency of church attendance with self-ratings of health in subgroups of telephone-surveyed community-dwellers or hospitalized psychiatric patients. Researchers, constrained by circumstances, are directed by the availability of funding to drive their decisions as to what to research.

Freed from the constraints of normal science, here are some thoughts about a possible next generation of body-mind-spirit research. These include issues germane to each of the three categories of religion and health research summarized earlier. They are the kind of topics that I have heard some of my colleagues express an interest in while remarking sadly that such research is too "out there" to be feasible at the present time.

First, much of the clinical research on prayer has up to now focused on the effects of Christian intercession on patients in Western medical facilities. The efficacy of non-Western intercessors, prayers, or healers is a frontier that ought to be explored in greater depth than it has up to now. Concomitantly, little effort has been made to compare the therapeutic effects of prayers from different religious or metaphysical traditions. It may be that liberal-minded researchers are skittish of tackling such a controversial and potentially embarrassing research question. They may be genuinely uneasy over the possibility of producing information that might offend or challenge the faith of certain believers. On the other hand, some resistance to this type of study may come from religious partisans who are not anxious to discover that the healing effects of prayer are no respecter of creed, culture, religion, or denomination. My experience as a researcher in the religion and health field suggests that the latter explanation is more likely.

Second, psychophysiological research on the correlates and sequelae of certain spiritually induced states of consciousness has produced some of the most exciting yet underpublicized findings in the religion and health field. Basic-science research in general has been particularly lacking, as compared with clinical trials and population-based social and epidemiologic research. One reason may be that the basic sciences of healing (as opposed to pathogenesis) are underdeveloped in Western biomedicine. Contrast this with non-Western systems of medicine, such as *Ayurveda*, traditional Chinese medicine, and various esoteric schools. All sorts of interesting research projects can be envisioned: mapping the human subtle-energy anatomy; identifying physiological pathways by which love, hope, forgiveness, and other examples of "positive psychology" impact on health; and documenting the anatomy, physiology, nosology, etiology, pathophysiology, and therapeutic options available in esoteric healing systems. A certain stigma may be attached to ideas like these, but an investigator with a thick skin would not find that a particular barrier.

Third, population-based epidemiologic and social research on religious involvement has proved to be the bread and butter of religion and health studies. Much of this research, though, has lost its creative edge. Nearly all of this work has focused on the health effects of formal, institutional, or public types of religious participation—denominational affiliation, church or synagogue attendance, public prayer, sanctioned religious beliefs. Much could be gained by extending consideration to more "inner" states of spiritual expression, such as mystical or transcendent experience.[21] (See "The Epidemiology of Love" in *Essential Capacities*.) A proposal has recently been made for development of an "epidemiology of love,"[22] and new empirical evidence supports the health benefits of a loving relationship with God or the divine.[23]

These ideas are admittedly outside of the mainstream—even outside of the mainstream of what now encompasses religion and health research. This field came into being because a cohort of investigators willingly broke through the bounds defined by the existing body-only paradigm and maintained by the biomedical research establishment. Today, within the religion and health field, a paradigm of sorts is taking hold. Efforts should be expanded to study how the spiritual, mental, emotional, and physical domains of life interact to the benefit of human health and well-being. Innovation and creativity in research can proceed outside of the range of normal science; indeed, this may be the only way it can proceed.[24]

References for this essay are located on the DVD accompanying this book.

The Practices of Essential Spirituality*

ROGER WALSH

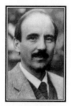

DO YOU REALIZE THIS IS the first time in history that publicly acknowledging that you follow two or more distinct spiritual traditions would not have you burned at the stake, stoned to death, or facing a firing squad?

We tend to forget what an extraordinary time this is, that for the first time in history we have the entirety of the world's spiritual and religious traditions available to us, and we can practice them, at least here, without fear.

We are discovering that underlying this vast array of practices and traditions and theologies and beliefs is a common core of wisdom and practices. Beneath the surface we find a deeper wisdom, not usually recognized but hidden in the depths of each and every one of the great religious traditions, a wisdom known as the perennial philosophy and the perennial psychology, which encompass a set of perennial practices.

---

*Adapted from a plenary talk "The Seven Practices of Essential Spirituality" given by Roger Walsh at the Institute of Noetic Sciences Conference, "Spirit Rising: Taking the Next Step, July 11-16, 2001 and from *Essential Spirituality*, John Wiley & Sons, 2000.

THE PERENNIAL PHILOSOPHY

The perennial philosophy has been known for some time, and at its heart are four statements about the nature of reality: The first is that this physical world we live in and see and touch is not all there is to reality, that underneath it—in fact, at its source—is another world, a sacred world, a world of spirit or consciousness or Mind with a capital "M," or Geist, or Tao.

The second of the four claims is that we as human beings partake of this reality. We are rather like amphibians. We have a part of our life and being in this world we see and touch, but in a deeper part at the core of our being, at the center of our minds, at the center of our awareness, we experience this other sacred realm, and we partake of it, and we are it.

The third claim of the perennial philosophy has to do with epistemology: It states that we are capable of knowing this other realm. If we train and develop the mind sufficiently, if we hone our awareness, develop our attention, refine our perception, then we can come to know this reality directly for ourselves. This is what differentiates the perennial philosophy from dogma. It is not a truth-claim to be believed simply on someone's word. It is an experiment that is offered to us, one that each and every one of us can try.

The fourth claim is an ethic. It states that coming to know this sacred realm and coming to recognize it as ourselves is the highest good and the highest goal of human existence—that it is the means by which we can best serve ourselves and others.

THE PERENNIAL PSYCHOLOGY

Closely married to this perennial wisdom is a perennial psychology, an understanding about the nature of mind. The perennial psychology tells us that our usual state of mind, our usual state of consciousness, is underdeveloped. We are immature. What we have taken for normality is actually a form of collective developmental arrest. The perennial psychology tells us that because of our immature states of mind, we do not perceive accurately; our beliefs are distorted; our understanding is awry; we don't recognize our true nature. In fact, we suffer from a case of mistaken identity!

On a more affirmative note, the perennial psychology says it is possible for us to restart the growth process. It is possible for us to grow up, and to wake up. As the greatest gift of all, the great spiritual traditions offer road maps and means for doing just that. They offer a variety of practices, the so-called perennial practices, designed to help us awaken. And whether they're known as the yogas of Taoism and Hinduism or the Eightfold Path of Buddhism or the contemplations and commandments of the monotheistic traditions, we find a set of practices designed to hone and train the mind.

At first glance these practices may seem disparate and conflictual. But when we look more deeply, when we look at their contemplative core, we find they are road maps for training the mind and inducing the same states of consciousness, the same wisdom, the same love as their various founders discovered.

We find, also, that underlying this vast array of practices is a common set of perennial practices of which there seem to be seven—seven practices that each and every one of the world's great religions says is essential for any of us who would come to awaken to our true potential and recognize our true identity.

These seven are: redirecting motivation, transforming emotions, living ethically, developing attention or concentration, refining awareness, cultivating wisdom, and expressing these in service. I view these seven practices as part of an essential transformative curriculum.

In this talk I focus on those practices particularly relevant to the fostering of a Wisdom Society: emotional transformation (the cultivation of love), ethics, the training or cultivation of wisdom, and the expression of that in service.

THE CULTIVATION OF LOVE

Numerous emotions pour through our minds each day, but among the great traditions, there's unanimity that one emotion is to be valued above others, and that emotion is love.

Love, of course, has been the subject of myth and poetry, the object of study of philosophers and sages, the source of meaning and purpose for countless lives. Millions of people have lived and died for it. *The*

Encyclopedia of Religion has this to say about love: "The idea of love has left a wider and more indelible imprint upon the development of human culture in all its aspects than any other single notion. In fact, many great figures have argued that love is the single most potent force in the universe, a cosmic impulse that creates, maintains, directs, informs, and brings to its proper end every living thing."

But what is love? If you turn on your radio, you have about a 50 percent chance of hitting a "love song." These are wonderful studies in pathos and pathology. They have such great lines as "I can't live without you; I'm thinking about you all the time; I break out in sweats; I can't sleep." These are the symptoms of heroin withdrawal! Our culture has totally conflated love and addiction.

And yet the great religions point to something much more profound, a love that is vaster, more stable, more encompassing, a love that, as Saint Paul said, "Bears all things, believes all things, hopes all things, endures all things." Or as the Buddha said, "As a mother watches over her child, willing to risk her own life to protect her only child, so we too, with a boundless heart, should cherish all living beings, suffusing the whole world with unobstructed loving kindness."

This spiritual love, then, is something far deeper, far more profound than the romantic love that is almost the sole focus of our culture. This of course is Christianity's *agape*, Confucianism's universal love, the *bhakti* of Hinduism, or the *metta* of Buddhism. And it raises a very important question: Can love be cultivated?

Our culture has a very curious answer to this. In our culture, love is something you feel when you're with the right person, someone who looks the right way and who says the right things to you. Then love will probably descend on you like an attack of epilepsy. You'll be taken and swirled around, then left bereft and wondering what the hell happened. But the great religious traditions suggest there's another possibility, that love is an art, a skill, something we can cultivate and develop. And they lay out a very specific road map for how to do so. This map consists of four strategies:

1. Reducing barriers to love, such as fear and greed and anger and jealousy and pride, which are seen to be incompatible with love.

In contemporary psychological terms, we would say they reciprocally inhibit one another. Take anger, for example. We would want to reduce anger, because as we all know, anger has an extraordinary power; it can take us over. Here's a wonderful example: Two psychiatrists were talking, and one said to the other, "You know, I was having dinner with my mother the other day and I made this terrible Freudian slip. I meant to say, 'Mother, would you pass the peas, please?' And instead, I said 'You bitch! You ruined my life!'" So anger will come out. Of course sometimes we can use it skillfully, but it is like playing with fire. When Ram Dass' teacher Neem Karoli Baba was saying one had to let go of anger, Ram Dass asked, "Baba-ji, can't I even use anger for teaching?" Neem Karoli Baba leapt up and came face to face with him and yelled "NO!"

But how do we reduce anger? The great religious traditions give us a variety of practices. They would suggest, for example, reflecting on how it feels when you're angry. Stop, be mindful; be aware of what it feels like; it doesn't feel so good.

Alternatively, reflect on your life and the nature of life itself, and recall that you are mortal and the person you're angry with is mortal. If you're really angry and you wish someone were dead, be patient! They will be. And so will you. And then it won't seem so important.

Another recommended strategy is to reflect on your own mistakes. I am repetitively humbled whenever I'm angry with others if I just take a moment to reflect. Then I realize it wasn't all that long ago that I just did what I'm angry at them for doing. You can practice forgiveness, letting go of anger. Lao Tzu said it wonderfully: "Only pursue an offender to show them the Tao."

2. Cultivating supporting attitudes and emotions such as gratitude and generosity. Stop for a moment to recall how much we have to be grateful for. For example, think of all the people who were involved, all the work they did so we could be together today at this conference. It's inconceivable how many people's work our well-being and coming together is dependent on. Most people are grateful because they're happy: Wise people are happy because they're grateful. It's a recurrent theme across traditions. St. Paul recommended, "Be thankful in all circumstances."

3. Cultivating love directly through prayer, contemplation, or meditation, for example. Here is one very simple meditation. Just close your eyes for a moment . . . and take a couple of breaths to relax . . . . Now bring to mind someone who's pretty angry . . . and notice how you feel . . . and let that go . . . . Now bring to mind someone who's loving and kind . . . notice how you feel . . . and when you're ready, bring your awareness back to the room. Isn't the difference remarkable! By meditating on loving people, one cultivates love itself. What we meditate on, we become.

4. Looking deeply into reality, with the understanding that the deeper we see into reality, the more we recognize that, at its heart, wisdom merges or unites with love. At its deepest, we find beautiful words such as these in the Gospel of John, "God is love, and those who abide in love abide in God, and God abides in them."

ETHICS

Ethics is regarded not as conventional moralism but as a foundational practice for anyone who would really wake up. However, this practice is much misunderstood. As Confucius said, "Rare are those who understand virtue." But the essential message is very simple. It's the golden rule of Christianity, "Do unto others as you want them to do unto you," or the silver rule of Confucianism, "Don't do to others as you don't want them to do to you." But this is done with a very interesting twist, because ethics as the great spiritual traditions define it is not done as sacrifice. Ethics comes from a recognition that an ethical life is a superb means for training the mind and coming to awakening. It's based on a very sophisticated understanding of the way the mind works. It's based on an understanding that unethical behavior, behavior in which we deliberately intend to harm ourselves or others, springs from destructive and painful mind states such as fear, greed, anger, and jealousy and reinforces them. That's the kicker. Unethical behavior drives these factors deeper into our minds; it reinforces them, it conditions them, or, in spiritual terms, it carves karmic traces deeper into our awareness.

On the other hand, ethical acts designed to enhance the well-being of everyone, including ourselves, spring from motives and emotions such as love and joy and generosity and compassion, and strengthen them. So from this perspective, we can begin to understand that ethics is not sacrifice. It is a very sophisticated approach to train the mind and refine our awareness so as to wake up. A study in 1996 found that those people who felt they were trying to live their lives ethically were twice as likely—twice as likely—to report themselves as happy compared with those who weren't. I love it when modern scientific research catches up with perennial wisdom.

CULTIVATION OF WISDOM

A beautiful quote from the Jewish Torah states, "Happy are those who find wisdom. She is more precious than jewels, and nothing you desire can compare with her. Her ways are ways of pleasantness, and all her paths are peace. Get wisdom. Get insight. Do not forget."

What is wisdom? It is a lot more than knowledge. Knowledge acquires information, but wisdom requires understanding. Knowledge informs us, but wisdom transforms us. Knowledge empowers; wisdom enlightens. Knowledge is something we have, but wisdom is something we have to become. I suggest that wisdom is a deep understanding and practical skill with the central—especially the existential and spiritual—issues of life.

How do we cultivate wisdom? The Torah says, "Wisdom will not enter a deceitful soul." Therefore an ethical foundation is essential. The next step is to recognize how much we don't know. As the Buddha said, "The fool who thinks he is wise is a fool indeed." One of my favorite stories comes from Seung Sunim, the Korean Zen master who teaches "Don't-know mind, just keep don't-know mind, don't know." He tells the story of a rabbi in Russia at the turn of the last century who was crossing the village square to go to pray. On his way he ran into the Cossack, who was in a lousy mood and said, "Hi Rabbi, where are you going?" Rabbi said, "Don't know . . ." The Cossack said, "What do you mean you don't know? For 20 years you've crossed this square, you've prayed in the tabernacle; you're trying to tell me you don't know where you're going?" He was so angry he grabbed the rabbi and hauled him off to the village jail. Just as he was throwing him in the cell, the rabbi said, "See, you just don't know!"

The great spiritual traditions suggest wisdom can be found in five places. First, we find wisdom in nature, which winnows away the transient and unimportant. Second, they suggest that one should turn to silence and solitude. Father Thomas Keating, the popularizer of centering prayer, said it wonderfully: "Silence is the language God speaks, and everything else is a bad translation." And Taoism says: "In stillness the mind becomes clear; in clarity it becomes bright, and this brightness is the radiance of the Tao within."

There is a third place to find wisdom: from the wise. I spent 3 years researching this topic, writing the book *Essential Spirituality,* and the thing that surprised me most in those 3 years of surveying the world's spiritual traditions was how tradition after tradition said, "If you want to develop this quality, whether it's love or compassion or wisdom or generosity, hang out with people who have it." This common thread was so repetitive that it really surprised me

The fourth place to look for wisdom—surprise—is in yourself. "Those who know themselves know their Lord," said Mohammad. The fifth place to look is in the nature of life and death, to realize our mortality, and to realize how brief our time here is. To recognize that, as the Taoists say, "Our lives last but a moment." Or as the Jewish Psalms state, "They are soon gone. They come to an end like a sigh, like a dream."

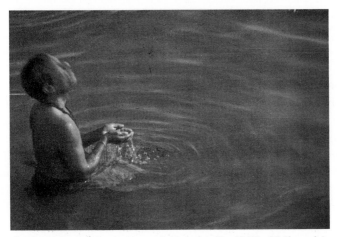

"Indian Man Praying in Ganges." (Courtesy David "Dudi" Shmueli.)

When we do these practices, they culminate, finally, in what's called liberating wisdom, a wisdom that is of a different order. It's not so much a conceptual understanding but a transrational intuition—a direct transrational, transconceptual seeing into the nature of mind, and into the depths of awareness. We can penetrate the very nature of consciousness and thereby into the nature of reality, and discover that our minds are unbounded and one with reality.

We recognize that who and what we are is far more than we first realized. Our true nature is not only intimately linked with but embraced by and even one with the sacred. The words from various traditions are different, but they all echo the same theme. In Christianity: "The kingdom of heaven is within you." In Islam: "Those who know themselves know their Lord." In Confucianism: "Those who know completely their own nature know heaven." Or, "In the depths of the soul, one finds the Divine, the One." In Hinduism: "Atman, the individual consciousness, and Brahman, the universal consciousness, are one." Or in Buddhism: "Look within—you are the Buddha." "Who chants the name of Buddha? Buddha."

This depth of wisdom leads to service, to expressing our understanding and insights in contribution and service to others, which is the final practice, the culmination. All of the great traditions emphasize service as a means to, and an expression of, awakening. We go into ourselves to go more effectively out into the world, and we go out into the world to go deeper into ourselves. This is the so-called cycle of withdrawal and return that the great historian Arnold Toynbee found was the one common characteristic of the lives of those people who he felt had contributed most to the development of civilization and human well-being. Each of these persons had taken time out from society to turn their attention inward, to wrestle with the fundamental questions of existence, to plumb their own nature, and when they finally found some illumination or understanding, then they returned to the world to heal and help. This is Plato's reentry into the cave; it's Zen's final ox-herding picture, entering the marketplace with help-bestowing hands. In Christianity, it's the fruitfulness of the soul that follows after the sacred marriage.

In Buddhism, there's the extraordinary ideal, the Bodhisattva, the person who dedicates his or her life to the welfare and awakening of all.

And our world desperately needs such people, more than ever. We all know that never before have we faced such enormously complex and demanding problems, not only to ourselves but to our planet and all species. We all know the litany of problems: overpopulation, pollution, starvation, ecological decay, resource-depletion.

Yes, there are problems, but we also have extraordinary opportunities. Never in human history have we had such an array of technologies or communication tools or resources. We have the power to leave our planet as a radioactive, polluted, plundered place or to turn it into a heaven on Earth. It's our choice.

OUR CHOICE

The perennial practices are rooted in ancient traditions and at the same time are critical in today's world. For the first time in human history every single one of our global problems is human-created. Every one is a reflection of our individual and collective choices and behavior. Every single global problem is a symptom, a symptom of our collective and individual psychological and spiritual distortions. And this means that the state of the world is a reflection of the state of our minds. If we are to truly heal the world, we need not only to reduce nuclear stockpiles, not only to care for and feed the hungry. We also need to deal with the psychological and spiritual pains and forces within us and between us that created these things in the first place. Otherwise we are only dealing with symptoms. We need, in short, to address and redress the psychological and spiritual roots of our contemporary crisis.

The methods for doing so are found in the perennial practices, the essential curriculum. We do these practices not only for ourselves but for the welfare and awakening of all. We do them in order to become an optimal instrument of service, an optimal instrument of help and healing. And we do our service as karma yoga, as part of our own awakening, so that there is nothing we do that isn't service. Our world is in grave trouble; we all know this. Our world is in grave, grave trouble, but our world also rests in good hands, because, actually, it rests in yours.

Opening Your Heart: Anatomically, Emotionally, and Spiritually*

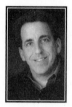

DEAN ORNISH

WHEN I WAS A STUDENT, A renowned spiritual teacher, Swami Satchidananda, often asked me the same question over and over: "Yes, but what is the cause? And what is the cause of that? And what underlies that cause?" His questions were a simple yet powerful means of getting to—well, to the heart of what is really important.

Nowhere is that easier to see than in the area of cardiology. I got interested in underlying causes early on as a medical student during my surgical rotation. We would cut people open to bypass their blocked arteries. The patients' chest pain would go away, and they would think they were cured. Then, more often than not, they would return home, eat the same food, continue smoking, and not meditate or exercise. Often, they would come back, sometimes years or sometimes a few months later, because even their bypasses had clogged. We would

---

*Adapted from a presentation at the Institute of Noetic Sciences' Heart of Healing conference in June 1993.

cut them open again and bypass the bypass, sometimes two or three times.

Bypass surgery became, for me, a metaphor for an incomplete approach to dealing with a life-threatening problem. The heart is more than just a pump. It's not enough to deal with the heart as a mechanical device; we have to deal with the emotional heart, the psychosocial heart, and the spiritual heart. If we can learn to open our hearts in these areas, we may find that the anatomical heart begins to open too, in ways we can measure more easily.

This vision of the "open heart" is at the core of the work that my colleagues and I have been doing for years. It's a vision that attempts to integrate medical knowledge with a deeper, ancient wisdom. Our lifestyle program is not new; it has been around for thousands of years. In modern medical terminology, we could call our program "a multifactorial intervention that includes diet, stress management, smoking cessation, exercise, and group support" or, perhaps more simply, "psychoneurocardiology."

REVERSING HEART DISEASE

Taken together, diet, stress management, and other lifestyle changes may often reverse serious illness. When I was a second-year medical student I became a little obsessed with the idea that maybe heart disease could be reversed. Shirley Brown and I took a year off between our second and third years of medical school. We took 10 heart patients, housed them in a hotel for a month and put them on our program. We used a new test, a thallium scan. The injected thallium was taken up by the heart and served as a tracer to measure improvements in blood flow to the heart. After 30 days, we found the subjects not only felt better but also were better in ways we could measure.

Again in 1980, after finishing medical school and before our internship, we decided to take another year off. We studied 48 heart patients, including a randomized control group for comparison. We tested for how well the heart was pumping blood. After 3 and a half weeks, the patients on our lifestyle program showed an improvement while those in the usual-care control group actually got worse. The differences between these groups were highly statistically significant, and we published the results in the *Journal of the American Medical Association* in January 1983.

In 1990, we published the 1-year results of a more definitive third study: The Lifestyle Heart Trial. The group of patients who received our lifestyle program reduced their blood cholesterol levels by almost 40 percent. We found a 91 percent reduction in chest pain, mostly in the first week—a powerful motivator. These patients showed improved blood flow to their hearts, as measured by cardiac PET scans, and an overall reversal of the build-up of coronary artery blockages, as measured by computer-analyzed X-ray movies called *coronary arteriograms*.

In contrast, the control group, following the conventional lifestyle, including a 30 percent fat diet, showed an increase in chest pain of 165 percent, a decrease of blood flow to the heart, and a worsening in coronary artery blockages. After 4 years, patients in the lifestyle group showed even more reversal, whereas the control group patients became even worse. Instead of getting progressively worse—the so-called natural history of heart disease—our results showed that many people can, in fact, continue to improve over time. Our results are giving many people new hope and new choices.

We found a strong correlation between adherence to the program and outcome. Surprisingly, the more people adapted their lifestyle, the better they got. That was not what I expected. I thought the younger patients with milder disease would be more likely to show reversal, but that was not the case. In fact, the most reversal was in the oldest patient, now 79, and in patients who had the most severe disease but whose adherence was the best. The primary determinant of improvement was not how old they were or how sick they were; it was how much they changed their lifestyle. Changes in arterial blockages were strongly correlated with the degree of changes in lifestyle.

THE DEEPER CAUSES OF HEART DISEASE

These results highlight the wisdom of pursuing causes, as my teacher impressed on me. If we don't deal with the cause, the problem keeps coming back or we find new problems and side effects; but if we do, the results are much more effective. What causes heart disease? Essentially, it's when your heart doesn't get enough blood. What causes that? If the arteries get clogged, if they constrict, if blood clots form, each of these mechanisms can reduce blood flow to your heart. Let's go back another step. What causes these mechanisms to be activated? What you eat, how you respond to stress, your use of nicotine, cocaine, and other stimulants—these all play a role. Let's focus on one factor, emotional stress. What causes that? Go back another step. Stress is not just what you do, it's how you react to what you do. Take two people in the same job: One may thrive, one may have a heart attack. What's the difference? Why do some people react to emotional stress in ways they thrive on while others get sick from it? That's where it gets very interesting.

In doing this work, I have had a chance to spend a lot of time with the same group of patients over a period of many years. We got to know each other very well. They were about as different from each other as you could imagine—in age, race, religion, socio-economics, demographics, sex, sexual preference, disease severity, you name it. At first, it seemed the only thing they had in common was heart disease. But over time we began to realize that many of them had something else in common: an emotional or spiritual heart disease. By that I mean the sense of loneliness, isolation, and alienation that I think is epidemic in our culture.

One hundred years ago people had social networks, they had extended families, they had a church or synagogue that they went to regularly, they had a neighborhood that they grew up in, they knew their neighbors, and they had a job that they worked at for many years. These days, many people don't have such a sense of community and belonging. Even the nuclear family has melted down. The two-parent family, with children from the same two parents, is in the minority now in many parts of this country.

I think we are paying a high price for these changes. Part of that price is chronic stress, rooted in widespread feelings of isolation. Many patients I work with tell me, "I feel isolated and alone. I must be lacking something or I wouldn't feel this way, so if only I had more ... (fill in the blank: more money, more power, more accomplishment, more love), then I would be okay, then people would love and respect me, then I wouldn't feel so lonely and isolated."

Once they set up that view of the world, however, it turns out they're likely to feel more stressed. There's a lot at stake, because it's not just winning and losing—it's *being* a winner or a loser that's on the line. They believe that losers will be shunned and isolated, whereas everybody loves a winner. Winning (at whatever fills the blank) holds out an illusion of intimacy. Later, they find out life doesn't work that way. Until they get what they think they need, they feel stressed. If somebody else wins and they don't, then they feel really bad, confirming their belief that we really live in a dog-eat-dog, hostile world of scarcity. "The more you get the less there is for me." "You only live once, so get it while you can."

Even if they get it, it's satisfying only for a little while. It reinforces their belief that their sense of peace and well-being comes from outside themselves—and that is what's so seductive. But it is soon followed by "Now what?" or "So what? Big deal!" One patient told me he can't even enjoy the view from the mountain he's climbed; he's already looking over at the next peak. "This one didn't quite do it," he says to himself, "maybe the next one will." Another patient said, "The letdown that comes after I get what I thought would bring me happiness and intimacy—but doesn't—is so great that I keep 15 projects going at the same time so I can quickly go on to the next one." And so the never-ending process continues. It's like being on a treadmill.

HOW CAN WE BREAK THE CYCLE OF STRESS?

Most of us are deeply attached to our belief systems and are resistant to change. However, when we are in pain, the status quo becomes less desirable. There is an opportunity for real change. Our lifestyle program is not just about teaching people how to manage stress, or cope with it—it addresses deeper issues.

The ancient swamis and yogis, rabbis and priests, nuns and monks didn't develop mind-body techniques to get cholesterol down, or unclog arteries, or help people lose weight, or perform better at board meetings. Their techniques are tools for transformation and transcendence that can help us quiet the mind and body, and experience an inner sense of peace and joy and well-being.

This experience may provide a fundamental shift in understanding where health comes from, where we think our well-being and our peace of mind and joy come from. I've had patients say "My health is in this bottle of pills." Traditional medicine tends to define health or well-being as something that we get instead of something that we have. Once we realize that well-being is usually something we have until we disturb it, the question then becomes "What am I doing to disturb it?" At that point, we can start paying attention to how we live, how we think, how we behave, how we eat, how we relate. The world itself then becomes our teacher rather than something punishing us.

People who meditate on a regular basis may ultimately find it leads to a direct experience of transcendence. Beyond just quieting their minds, they may experience that although on one level we're all separate, and we can enjoy the differences, on another level we're part of something larger that connects us all—whatever spiritual, religious, or secular context we may experience that in.

We work with people within their own belief systems. We're not trying to change them; we're just trying to expand their understanding of what they already believe. I think that anything that promotes a sense of intimacy is healing. Conversely, anything that promotes a sense of isolation may lead to chronic stress and, ultimately, to illnesses such as heart disease. Even the word "heal" comes from the Indo-European "to make whole." And in Sanskrit, the word "yoga" means "to yoke," to bring together, sometimes translated as "union." These are very old ideas.

When we talk about "the heart of healing," it brings us to the question: "What can we do to try to heal that sense of isolation?" Meditation is one way. Communication skills are another: learning how to talk to people in ways that don't feel like attacks or judgment.

Group support is another way. Our groups started out as places where people could exchange shopping tips, recipes, or types of running shoes—and it evolved into something much deeper. We realized that people need a sense of safety, a place where they can let down their walls and defenses and talk about what's really going on in their lives without fear that anyone is going to judge or reject them. Too often people think, "I feel lonely. But I have to hide parts of myself because if people really knew me they'd like me even less." That way of thinking sets people up for losing either way. If they don't get the love and respect they want, they lose; and even if they succeed in getting it, it's not for who they really are but only for the image they're projecting.

Having a "safe space," therefore, is important; a place that feels safe enough for people to say things like "You know, I may look like I'm really wealthy" (as one patient said), "but I've been bankrupt for years, and even my own wife doesn't know about it." A safe environment that enables truth like that to be expressed without fear of being judged, rejected, or given advice opens the way to real healing and is profoundly transformative. It is transformative in ways that go beyond what we can measure, and ultimately it is such experiences that are often the most motivating and valuable to people.

BIG CHANGES ARE EASIER

Many people are willing to make these changes. I think big changes are often easier than small ones. When you make small changes, such as going on a 30 percent fat diet, you have a sense of deprivation because you're not getting to eat or do everything that you want, but you're not making changes big enough to feel much better. Weight, blood pressure, and cholesterol levels do not decrease very much, and chest pain and heart disease tend to worsen. When people make big changes, however, most find they feel so much better, so quickly, that the choices become much clearer and, for many people, are worth making. People are not afraid to make big choices if they understand the benefit, and if the benefit is immediate.

Efforts to make people change habits out of fear of dying don't work very well. A couple of weeks after someone has had a heart attack, perhaps they might be motivated to change, but then the denial comes back. I never tell people what to do. Telling people what to do makes them just want to cringe. Even more than feeling healthy, people want to feel free and in control of their lives. I offer people a range of choices and discuss the risks, benefits, costs, and side-effects of these choices. I say, "It's your life, you're the one who is going to take the consequences. I'm here to serve you in whatever way I can. Whatever you choose is fine with me." Then we both remain free.

I asked people in our studies, "Why do you eat so much, work too hard, or drink too much, or smoke?" They say, "To you, as a doctor, it looks maladaptive for us to do these things because it increases the risks something bad may happen to us. But to us, it's very adaptive because it helps us get through the day." For many people, just getting through the day is a lot more important than living to be 86 instead of 85. People often use these behaviors as ways to deal with isolation and to ward off emotional pain. A well-known food writer told me once, "Fat coats my neurons and numbs the pain." Some people use the TV control as an anesthetic, surfing through the channels as a way to numb themselves.

The modern epidemic is not just physical heart disease but also emotional and spiritual heart disease: the loneliness, isolation and alienation that we discussed earlier. Change is difficult; the status quo is familiar. When it becomes sufficiently painful, there is an opportunity for transformation. We can use the pain to begin healing in ways that go beyond unclogging our arteries or losing weight. We may use our pain to open our hearts.

If we work at these deeper levels, people are much more likely to choose and maintain lifestyles that are life-enhancing rather than self-destructive. They may say, "Maybe I'll live longer, but that's not the point. Health is only a means to an end, not an end in itself. What matters is the quality of my life." To the extent any of us realize and remember this, I think we're already healthier. It's a different kind of "open heart surgery"—one that's based on altruism, compassion, and love, not just unclogging arteries.

The Return of Prayer*

LARRY DOSSEY

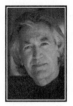

MARGARET MEAD,[1] THE noted anthropologist, once said, "Prayer does not use any artificial energy, it doesn't burn up any fossil fuel, it doesn't pollute." It has another attribute Mead didn't mention, which should be of interest to all healthcare professionals: It apparently works. An impressive body of evidence suggests that prayer and religious devotion are associated with positive health outcomes.[2] As this information has become increasingly known, prayer is returning to medicine after sitting on the sidelines for most of this century. This phenomenon has evoked a variety of responses, ranging from elation to confusion to horror.

"PRAYER ACTUALLY WORKS?"

I bumped into the latter of these responses in 1996 when I was invited to lecture and consult at a large hospital in New York City. The day began with an address to the house staff, in which I discussed the emerging

*From Dossey L: The Return of Prayer. *Altern Ther Health Med* 3(16) 10-17, 113-120, 1997.

scientific evidence for the effectiveness of intercessory prayer. I reviewed several of the salient experiments that had captured the attention of the medical profession, and I summarized some of the studies that were currently in progress. Later in the day I met with the staff of the hospice department in a follow-up meeting. Before our discussion could begin, I was approached by a clergyman who was obviously quite disturbed. He worked full-time in the hospice area and devoted his life to offering spiritual guidance and prayer for dying patients and to providing psychological and spiritual support for the hospice staff. He said, "Look, I need to get something straight. I heard your lecture this morning—and if I understand you correctly, you're claiming that intercessory prayer actually works?"

For a moment I was speechless and did not know how to respond. Although this man's life was immersed in prayer, he obviously harbored deep doubts about whether his prayers had any effect whatever. When confronted with evidence that intercessory prayer might actually be effective, he was astonished and confused. We chatted privately for a few moments, and I affirmed my earlier comments. I admired his honesty; most of us aren't as courageous as he was in expressing our doubts about prayer.

This experience confirmed my belief that even "true believers" often doubt, at some level of the mind, the effectiveness of prayer and that even religious professionals can be shocked to discover that science has something positive to say about prayer. The reasons are no doubt complex but are related to the stormy relations that have existed between science and religion for the past 2 centuries, particularly since the time of Darwin. When battles between these two camps have arisen, religion usually has not fared well. As a result, most religious believers are understandably leery of "what science says" about their faith.

Another reason many religious folk object to the entry of science onto their turf is the stereotypical attitude toward science that most of us have developed during the process of becoming educated and socialized in twentieth-century America. The following message has been driven home to almost all of us in our colleges and universities: "There are two ways to live your life. You can choose to be intellectual, rational, analytical, logical, and scientific; or, on the other hand, you can choose to be intuitive, spiritual, and religious. These two vectors of the psyche are incompatible and cannot be brought together; you cannot have it both ways."

Most of us choose one path or the other and suffer the rest of our life as a result of this artificial, schizophrenic split. The recent developments in prayer research show, however, that these choices are not incompatible. Science and spirituality can come together; we can have it both ways.

WHAT IS PRAYER?

I have discussed with thousands of Americans what they believe prayer is. I have concluded that the most common image of prayer in our culture is something like this: "Prayer is talking aloud or to yourself, to a white, male, cosmic parent figure, who prefers to be addressed in English."

Of course, this is an extremely limited and culturally conditioned view of prayer. It disenfranchises large proportions of the world's population as well as those in our own society who do not share this perspective. For example, many people believe that prayer can go beyond words to involve silence. For some, prayer is more a matter of being than doing—such as Thomas Merton, who once remarked that he prayed by breathing. Moreover, most people who pray worldwide are not white and don't speak English (nor did Jesus or any of the founders of the world's major religions). Also, many people who pray are not fond of the idea of a male god or a personal god of any kind. Consider Buddhism, one of the world's great faiths: Buddhism is not a theistic religion, yet prayer is central to the Buddhist tradition. Buddhists offer their prayers to the universe, not to a personal god. Buddhism therefore violates most of the cultural assumptions we make about the nature of prayer. Shall we inform Buddhists and others who differ from our cultural norm that they aren't really praying?

In the following discussion I want to employ a deliberately broad and ambiguous definition of prayer: "Prayer is communication with the Absolute." This definition is inclusive, not exclusive; it affirms religious tolerance; and it invites people to define for themselves what "communication" is, and who or what "the Absolute" may be. This definition is broad enough to include people of the various faiths who have participated as subjects in prayer research.

What is intercessory prayer? "Intercessory" comes from the Latin *inter*, or "between," and *cedere*, meaning "to go." Intercessory prayer is therefore a go-between—an effort to mediate on behalf of, or plead the case of, someone else. Intercessory prayer is often called "distant" prayer, because the individual being prayed for is often remote from the person who is praying.

SURVEYING THE FIELD

How much of the experimental data supports intercessory prayer? There is a significant difference of opinion. If one performs an electronic database search using "prayer" as a keyword, one will probably retrieve around a half a dozen studies of dubious quality. On the other hand, physician Daniel J. Benor[3] has written a four-volume work, *Healing Research,* which cites nearly 150 studies in this field, many of which are of excellent quality and over half of which show statistically significant results.

Part of the problem in identifying work in this field is the lack of agreement on language. Many researchers shy away from using the word "prayer" in favor of a more neutral term such as "distant intentionality." Even though their experiment may actually involve prayer, they often do not use this term in the titles of their papers. If their subjects pray, the researcher may say instead that the subject "concentrated" or applied "mental effort" to produce the effect being studied, or they may use terms such as "mental healing," "psi healing," or "spiritual healing" to describe their work.

Perhaps we should not be too critical of researchers on this point. Research into the distant effects of consciousness is generally considered to be the domain of parapsychology. This field is sufficiently controversial without adding the furor surrounding the concept of distant, intercessory prayer. But the aversion of experimenters to using "prayer" comes with a price—the difficulty of identifying prayer-and-healing studies, and the underestimation of the number of prayer experiments that exist.

ABOUT PRAYER AND PARAPSYCHOLOGY

Many religious people are exceedingly uncomfortable about "parapsychology," and they deplore the practice of parapsychologists equating prayer with mental intentionality, focused attention, concentration, or even meditation. They often feel that parapsychologists dishonor prayer and are disrespectful of the spiritual traditions in which prayer is embedded. I sympathize with these reservations, but after exploring prayer and parapsychology for several years, I feel that a clean separation between these fields does not exist and is impossible to achieve. In experiments in parapsychology in which individuals attempt to influence living things at a distance, participants often actually pray or enter a sacred, reverential, prayerlike state of mind to accomplish their task. On the other hand, when people pray, they often have paranormal experiences such as telepathy, clairvoyance, precognition, and so on. Anyone doubting this would do well to read philosopher Donald Evans's[4] scholarly work *Spirituality and Human Nature,* or historian Brian Inglis's[5] classic book *Natural and Supernatural: A History of the Paranormal.*

Fortunately, the long-standing antipathy between religion and parapsychology appears to be diminishing. *The Journal of Religion and Psychical Research,* published in the United States, and *The Christian Parapsychologist,* published in Great Britain, are notable examples of bridge-building between these fields (see note 1). The latter publication was begun in 1953 by a group of British clergy and laymen who were "convinced that psychical phenomena [have] great relevance to the Christian faith, both in life and death ... [but that] psychical studies are as likely to lead to harm as to good if pursued outside the realms of the spiritual life ... through the practice of prayer, worship, and service to [our] fellow creatures."

As further evidence of the emerging religion-and-parapsychology dialogue, Michael Stoeber, assistant professor in the Department of Religion and Religious Education at The Catholic University of America, and Hugo Meynell, professor in the Department of Religious Studies at the University of Calgary, have co-edited a critically acclaimed book, *Critical Reflections on the Paranormal,*[6] which examines issues of mutual interest to both parapsychology and religion.

As a single example of how parapsychology (often called "psi") and prayer are difficult, if not impossible, to keep separate, consider a study by Haraldsson and Thorsteinsson,[7] in which subjects attempted mentally to cause increases in the growth rate of yeast cultures. The title of the paper, "Psychokinetic Effects on Yeast: An Exploration Experiment,"[7,8] gives no hint that spiritual healers and prayer were involved. The researchers recruited seven subjects—two spiritual healers who used prayer, one physician who employed spiritual healing and prayer in his practice, and four students with no experience or particular interest in healing. The subjects were asked to "direct their healing effects" to increase the growth of yeast in 120 test tubes. The study was well designed and employed appropriate controls. The results indicated that "mental concentration or intention" indeed affected the growth of the yeast. The bulk of the scoring was done by the two spiritual healers and the physician and yielded a p-value less than 0.00014—meaning that the odds against a chance result were less than 14 in 100,000. By contrast, the students, who had little interest in either prayer or healing, scored at chance levels. The title of this article suggests that it was a study in parapsychology and psychokinesis ("mind over matter"), but a closer look shows that it was clearly an experiment in the effects of prayer. Because of this study's title, however, a survey of the prayer-and-healing literature would probably not identify it. This experiment is a typical example of why the boundaries between prayer and experimental parapsychology are artificial.

THE MOST FAMOUS PRAYER STUDY

The most celebrated twentieth-century prayer study involving humans was published in 1988 by physician Randolph Byrd,[9] a staff cardiologist at UC San Francisco School of Medicine. Byrd randomized 393 patients in the coronary care unit at San Francisco General Hospital to either a group receiving intercessory prayer or a control group. Intercessory prayer was offered by groups outside the hospital; they were not instructed how often to pray, but only to pray as they saw fit. In this double-blind study, in which neither the patients, physicians, nor nurses knew who was receiving prayer, the prayed-for patients did better on several counts. There were fewer deaths in the prayer group (though this factor was not statistically significant); they were less likely to require endotracheal intubation and ventilator support; they required fewer potent drugs, including diuretics and antibiotics; they experienced a lower incidence of pulmonary edema; and they required cardiopulmonary resuscitation less often.

Byrd's study illustrates some of the difficulties in studying the effects of intercessory prayer in humans.[10] In one variation of a controlled study—the testing of a new drug, for example—the control group does not receive the treatment being evaluated. But in prayer studies involving humans who are seriously ill, subjects in the control group may pray for themselves or their loved ones and friends may pray for them: the problem of "extraneous prayer." Even though the degree of outside prayer may equalize between the treatment and control groups, a major problem remains. If both groups are prayed for, the experiment becomes not a test of prayer versus no prayer but a test of the degree or the amount of prayer. "It could be that the efforts of these strangers [who are recruited to pray for the 'prayer treatment' group] will be swamped by the heart-felt prayers of those directly involved with the patients," says professor of physics Russell Stannard[11] of the Open University in England. If so, both groups might benefit equally from prayer, with no significant differences detectable between them. In technical jargon this is called "reduction of the effect size" between the two groups. This can be a vexing methodological problem, because it means that prayer can appear ineffective even when it works. Although this problem can be dealt with through sophisticated research methods, it is a significant obstacle in perhaps all prayer studies involving sick people.

Researchers have considered ways of overcoming the problem of self-prayer by individuals in the control group—for example, using as subjects sick infants or newborns, or unconscious, brain-damaged adults who do not or cannot pray for themselves. But this still does not eliminate the confounding effect of prayer by loved ones and friends.

Critics have therefore charged that controlled studies of prayer are impossible, because extraneous prayer cannot be eliminated from the control group. However, a controlled study does not always require that the control group not be exposed to the variable being tested. An example is the controlled testing of high-dose versus low-dose treatment regimens of a particular drug, in which both the control and treatment groups receive the drug being evaluated. This is analogous to most of the human studies involving intercessory prayer.

In any case, as we have seen, these research difficulties can be completely overcome if nonhumans instead of humans are used as subjects. If bacterial growth rates are being manipulated through prayer, for example, the organisms in the control group presumably do not pray for themselves, nor do their fellow bacteria pray for them. This makes it possible to achieve great precision in nonhuman prayer studies and may account for why the effect sizes of these studies often dwarf those seen in human experiments. Although the design of Byrd's study could have been improved, he deserves immense credit for undertaking the experiment. He established a principle: that distant, intercessory prayer can be studied like a drug in humans in a controlled fashion in a sophisticated medical environment. Byrd's contribution is monumental—not because it was the first prayer study (many others preceded it), or because it was flawless, but because it helped break a taboo against prayer as a subject of medical research.

A LOOK TO THE FUTURE

Although we can always benefit from more experimental data (scientists in every field say this), the major obstacle in taking intercessory prayer seriously is not, I think, a lack of empirical evidence. Our major difficulty is that we seem to be suffering from a failure of the imagination. Unable to see how prayer could work, too many people insist that it cannot work. Unless we learn to see the world in new ways, we shall remain unable to engage the evidence for intercessory prayer that already exists, and we shall be tempted to dismiss future evidence no matter how strong it proves to be. Physician-researcher Jan Ehrenwald,[12] writing in the *Journal of Nervous and Mental Disease*, describes what we're up against:

> It is paradoxical that more than one-half century after the advent of relativistic physics and the formulation of quantum mechanics, current theories of personality are still steeped in the classical Judeo-Christian, Aristotelian, or Cartesian tradition. Our neurophysiological models of the organism, our psychological and psychoanalytic concepts about the 'mind,' are located in Euclidean space and conform to essentially mechanistic, Newtonian, causal-reductive principles.
>
> What are the hallmarks of the classical model? It conceives of personality as a closed, self-contained, homeostatic system operating in a universe extended in pre-relativistic space and time and subject to the ironclad laws of cause and effect. It found its classical pictorial representation in

Leonardo da Vinci's figure of a male of ideal proportions, safely anchored in the double enclosure of the circle and the square, setting him apart from the rest of the world.

Even those who believe in intercessory prayer generally seem wedded to the classical images to which Ehrenwald refers, a stance that seems hopelessly flawed.[13] They generally conceive of prayer as some sort of energetic signal that is sent up and out to the Almighty, who functions as a kind of satellite relay station who passes on the effect to the recipient of the prayer. There is no evidence whatever in studies of prayer and distant intentionality that these images apply. Still, the cherished hope of many seems to be that some sort of "subtle energy" will one day be detected to explain the distant effects of prayer. Although this conceivably could happen, current evidence suggests that the old energy-based, classical concepts will remain unable to explain the workings of intercessory prayer, and new images will be necessary (see note 3).[14-16]

Until adequate scientific explanations of intercessory prayer arrive, we need not suspend our belief in prayer nor deny the evidence for it. Even when future explanations are in place, "God does it!" will remain a perfectly reasonable alternative, because any new theory is certain to raise more questions than it will answer. After all, it is impossible in principle for any scientific theory to disprove the existence and workings of the Absolute.

Another major obstacle to engaging the evidence for intercessory prayer is fear.[17] The instant we acknowledge the data that we can affect living systems positively at a distance through prayer, the possibility is raised that we may be able to harm them as well. This consideration prompts almost everybody to run for cover, including believers in prayer—because, as philosopher Alan Watts once put it, we want to keep God's skirts clean. It is going to be difficult to do so. As we've seen, several studies in distant intentionality using bacteria and fungi strongly suggest that we can not only increase their growth rates but inhibit them as well.[17-19,20] This prospect should not horrify us. Sometimes we need prayer to be injurious—as when we pray for a cancer to be destroyed, for an obstruction in a coronary artery to be obliterated, or for AIDS viruses to be killed (see note 2).

THE RESPIRITUALIZATION OF MEDICINE

The studies in intercessory prayer and distant intentionality represent a major opportunity for a genuine dialogue between science and spirituality. This debate needs desperately to go forward, particularly within medicine. Modern medicine has become one of the most spiritually malnourished professions in our society. Because we have so thoroughly disowned the spiritual component to healing, most healers throughout history would view our profession today as inherently perverse. They would be aghast at how we have squeezed the life juices and the heart out of our calling. Physicians have spiritual needs like anyone else, and we have paid a painful price for ignoring them. It simply does not feel good to practice medicine as if the only thing that matters is the physical; something feels left out and incomplete.

André Malraux, the late French novelist and minister of culture of France, said that the twenty-first century will be spiritual or it will not be at all. I often feel the same way about medicine. It will be respiritualized or it may not be at all—at least not in any form we would desire. Yet there is great hope, and the scientific research into the healing effects of prayer, empathy, and love bodes well for a respiritualization of medicine.

The dangers in the prayer-and-science dialogue are quite real, and so we must navigate these waters carefully. But if we do so—and I am convinced that we can—medicine may once again deserve to be called the healing profession.

NOTES

1. *The Journal of Religion and Psychical Research* is published by The Academy of Religion and Psychical Research, P.O. Box 614, Bloomfield, CT 06002. *The Christian Parapsychologist* is published by The Churches' Fellowship for Psychical and Spiritual Studies, South Road, North Somercotes, North Louth, Lincolnshire LN11 7PT, United Kingdom.

2. Dr. Thomson's arguments concerning prayer are presented at some length in his Point/Counterpoint article on pp 92-96 of *Alt Ther Health Med* 3(16).

3. The reasons "energy" is inadequate to explain nonlocal, distant healing are discussed in my editorial "The Forces of Healing: Reflections on Energy, Consciousness, and the Beef Stroganoff Principle," *Altern Ther Health Med* 3(5):8-14, 1997.

References for this essay are located on the DVD accompanying this book.

A Prolegomenon to an Epidemiology of Love: Theory, Measurement, and Health Outcomes*

JEFF LEVIN

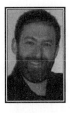

| *"The greatest science in the world, in heaven and on earth, is love."*

MOTHER TERESA[1]

FOR NEARLY 50 YEARS, social and behavioral scientists have investigated the effects of a wide range of social, psychosocial, and behavioral constructs on health. Considerable work has explored the effects of important personal characteristics and interpersonal states, such as life stress, social support, Type A behavior, locus of control, religiosity, self-esteem, and coping.[2-6] However, constructs tapping more fundamental

*Adapted from Levin J: A Prolegomenon to an Epidemiology of Love: Theory, Measurement, and Health Outcomes, *Journal of Social and Clinical Psychology* 19(1):117-136, 2000. The author thanks Lea Steele Levin, Berton H. Kaplan, and Larry Dossey for comments on an earlier draft of this article.

characteristics of the human psyche and its social context have been relatively unexplored. Hope, forgiveness, thankfulness, and kindness have no tradition of epidemiologic research. Nor is there a tradition of research on what may be the most fundamental resource: love.

Poets, philosophers, mystics, theologians, and saints from across religions, cultures, and historical epochs have proclaimed the experience of love—given or received—to be the sine qua non of a life well lived. To the thirteenth-century Sufi master, Jalaluddin Rumi, "through love all that is bitter will be sweet."[7] In the Dhammapada (15:197), the Buddha implores, "O let us live in joy, in love..."[8] For the sixteenth-century Spanish Carmelite nun and mystic St. Teresa of Avila, "love alone gives value to all things."[9]

Among scientific disciplines, psychology has directed systematic though sporadic attention to love. Most of this work has described features or sequelae of the romantic side of love and its associated phenomena (e.g., spousal affection, dating behavior, sexual attraction, devoted attachments, and relationships between two people). This collection of research and writing constitutes the new field that has been termed "the psychology of love."[10]

THE PSYCHOLOGY OF LOVE

Theoretical Perspectives on Love

Since the middle 1970s, the psychological study of love has proceeded in earnest, with a twofold emphasis on defining and delineating the boundaries and formulating theories and models of this construct.[11] It was not always so—an oversight that Allport[12] long ago termed "[a] persistent defect of modern psychology." The publication of the definitive volume, *The Psychology of Love*,[10] signaled the maturation of this topic into a recognized field of study.

Depending upon one's perspective, love has been conceptualized as an affect, an attitude, a behavior, or a judgment or cognitive decision.[13] Love has been described as "a subject whose boundaries recede with each attempt to characterize them."[14] Empirical science and its underlying theories probably cannot be the source of a definitive answer as to what "love" is.

One prominent and influential approach to the psychology of love has been Lee's[15] conceptual model of the six "colors of love," also known as love-styles. These represent variant styles or ways of loving and being loved by another—preferences deeply held, but not so intransiently as traits. This approach has spawned numerous attempts to develop measurement instruments. According to Lee,[16] "Love-styles are not like signs of the zodiac. You are not born with a particular preference, and you can have more than one preference in a lifetime."

In this theory,[16,17] three colors, or styles, of love are primary: *eros*, or romantic/passionate love, including "love at first sight"; *ludus*, or game-playing love, as manifest in the seeking of serial love experiences; and *storge*, or friendship love, exemplified by loving affection and companionship. Three secondary love-styles, formed by compounding combinations of the primary styles, include *mania*, the product of eros and ludus, characterized by being "in love with love itself"; *pragma*, the product of ludus and storge, seen in those who select lovers or partners through a "shopping list" method or through computer dating or in the arranged marriages of yesteryear; and *agape*, the product of eros and storge, known through the familiar Christian ideal of selfless altruistic love guided by duty and "more expressive of will than emotion."[16]

A less influential but perhaps more theoretically grounded approach to a theory of love has been the characterization of love within the context of Bowlby's[18-20] attachment theory. According to this theory, affectional bonding systems develop in infants as evolutionary adaptations that provide security in the face of temporary separations (from the mother); thus, they permit exploration of the local environment. Attachment theory has been applied to the study of various intrapsychic and interpersonal phenomena, including theistic religions,[21] in which, as a result of early-life experiences, a child may develop "cognitive-emotional schemas about interpersonal relationships that later may be associated with a supernatural attachment figure."[22]

Shaver, Hazan, and Bradshaw[23] provide a thorough outline of the shared dynamics of infant-mother attachment, as well as affectional bonds between adult lovers in nearly 20 categories. These categories include intense desire for the love object's interest and reciprocation; feelings of confidence, security, and safety and happiness and positive affect in the reciprocant; anxiety and preoccupation in the nonreciprocant; wanting to spend time with the love object, distress at separation, and ecstasy at reunion; desire for shared experiences and prolonged eye contact; powerful empathy; high dependence on cues of reciprocation; greatest happiness derived from the love object's approval and attention; and several other parallel conceptualizations. Research in the area of love-as-attachment has focused on application of a model of three types of infant-mother attachment to romantic love between adults[24]—secure, anxious/ambivalent, and avoidant.[25]

Another important theoretical contribution to the psychology of love has been Stemberg's triangular theory of love.[26] This theory holds that "love can be understood in terms of three components: intimacy (close, connected, bonded feelings of warmth), passion (romantic, sexual, physical drives), and decision/commitment (short- and long-term intentions to love and to maintain love for another). Similar to Lee's[16] love-styles, these three components of love, alone or in various combinations, describe a larger set of the kinds of loving. These include liking (intimacy alone), infatuation (passion alone), empty love (decision/commitment alone), romantic love (intimacy plus passion), fatuous love (passion plus commitment), compassionate love (intimacy plus commitment), and consummate love (intimacy plus passion plus commitment).

Other scholars have proposed definitions, conceptual models, taxonomies, and theories of love, with an emphasis on romantic and passionate love between spouses or (potential) lovers. Early work includes Solomon's[27] psychoanalytic and developmental theory of the stages of love (self-love, projected love, romantic love, and mature love), and Benoit's[28] differentiation of adoration (or emotional love), appetitive (or physical) love, and benevolent (or intellectual) love. Later theoretical work includes Fromm's[29] distinction between genuine love and pseudo love; Maslow's[30] distinction between being love and deficiency love; Rubin's[31] contrast of love and liking; and, differentiations of romantic love and conjugal love[32] and of passionate love and compassionate love.[33] A creative empirical synthesis of the above work yielded a five-factor model comprising romantic dependency, communicative intimacy, physical arousal, respect, and romantic compatibility.[34] Other approaches have been based on behavioristic reinforcement theories;[35] on a theory of love as a set of correlated romantic, familial, and friendship bonds;[36] and, on relations common to both love and liking when certain clusters of feelings are added to friendship.[37]

MEASUREMENT OF LOVE

Development and validation of instruments to assess aspects of love began in the early 1970s. Since then, many reliable and valid scales and multidimensional indices have appeared, with most of them addressing the romantic expression of love. A few approaches have been enduring, and they are summarized in this selective review.

The Erotometer is an inventory of 50 items measuring 18 components of heterosexual love.[38] These items were derived empirically from a larger list of 82 items, itself reduced from an original list of 500 items. Measured on a 3-point Likert scale (0 = absent, 1 = weak, 2 = strong), these items are brief statements affirming "your own actual feelings, attitudes, desires, wishes, and the like regarding only a specific person of the opposite sex."[38] Examples include "A desire to be together forever," "Making the other person secure," "Sharing the partner's opinions," "Enjoying just being together," "Lifting the other person's ego," and "Expressing my feelings openly." Scores range from 0 ("no love") to 100 ("strongest love"). Test-retest reliabilities from .78 to .86 have been reported, as well as corrected split-half reliabilities ranging from .88 to .95.

Another influential approach is the 13-item Love Scale developed by Rubin[31] as a measure of the "social-psychological construct of romantic love ... [as] an interpersonal attitude." Scale items are simple statements selected in such a way as to "be grounded in existing theoretical and popular conceptions of love."[31]

The most popular multidimensional measurement approach to love is based upon Lee's theory of love styles.[15] Despite his assertion that "the best assessment of your preference of love-style is a review of your experience, not a paper-and-pencil test,"[16] efforts have been made to operationalize the love-style schema as a self-response instrument. An early effort was the SAMPLE profile,[39] a list of 50 agree/disagree items, each tapping a respective love-style.[40]

Many attempts have since been made to refine and revise the SAMPLE for use in various settings, with mixed results.[16] More successful has been the work of Hendrick and Hendrick[41] to develop and validate a new multidimensional scale based on Lee.[15]

In both its original and revised versions,[42] the Love Attitudes Scale has been a popular instrument over the past decade.

LOVE, HEALTH, AND HEALING
Review of Empirical Findings

Several studies have examined the association between love, broadly defined, and health outcomes. Love received from one's wife was associated with reduced risk of morbidity in terms of the 5-year incidence of angina pectoris[43] and duodenal ulcer.[44] The perception of having received parental love 35 years earlier was found prospectively to be related to reduced risk of morbidity for several chronic diseases diagnosed in midlife, including coronary artery disease, hypertension, duodenal ulcer, and alcoholism.[45] Likewise, reporting a loving relationship with one's parents also was associated with subsequently lower rates of cancer mortality.[46] Holding little love for one's parents was associated with higher levels of psychological distress in a cross-sectional study of adolescents.[47] Experiencing love (defined as positive affect plus absence of social isolation) was the strongest correlate of self-esteem in a sample of multiple sclerosis patients.[48] Reporting loss of love was among the most common antecedents of completed or attempted suicide or suicidal behavior.[49]

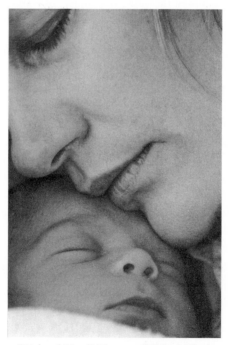

"Mel and Nate." (Courtesy Michael Eller.)

Other, more unusual research has identified potentially salutogenic or therapeutic effects of love through unconventional experimental protocols. A now-famous study examined the effects of watching a documentary film about the work of Mother Teresa of Calcutta on the concentration of salivary immunoglobulin A (S-IgA), a marker of immune function; S-IgA concentration rose significantly in study subjects, and remained high an hour after the film ended in those subjects who took part in an exercise in which they "recalled times in their lives when they had loved or been loved."[50] The author concluded that "dwelling on love appears to be important for strengthening this aspect of immune function."[50]

Researchers also have discovered that "sincere love, appreciation, and care cause the heart rhythms to have a smooth, regular, coherent pattern which results from a nervous system in balance."[51] One remarkable study found several electrophysiological correlates of intentional heart focus on the feeling state of love.[52] Subjects shifting to a mentally and emotionally intentional state of appreciation, and then from appreciation to love, produced changes in heart rate variability (HRV) (i.e., the beat-to-beat variation in heart rate controlled by the parasympathetic nervous system) indicating states of greater "internal coherence." The researchers concluded that, for their subjects, these findings represent "an indication of exceptional self-management of their mental and emotional natures... [and thus] a state of deep peace and inner harmony."[52]

There has been some speculation that such a state may be "potentiated by a relative inhibition of the left hemisphere's critical analytic brain functions"[53] such as may occur during a "cognitive-sensory inhibitive state (like *samadhi* or *satori*)," or through hypnosis or during self-reported paranormal experiences, brought about by a projection of feelings of love onto a love object. This state of physiological coherence and spiritual-like entrainment resulting from loving intentions has been implicated in both self-healing and the healing of others,[54] through enabling one in a state of "resonance" to balance, release, and reform subtle-energetic "holoforms" that can induce illness in the physical body.[55] This state also has been linked to high serum levels of oxytocin, secreted by the hypothalamus, and it is said to be "the altruistic love hormone."[56] It has further been proposed that love may take the form of a "subtle energy" generated within a healer and able to be sent and received across space and time.[57] According to Dossey,[58] these sorts of findings suggest that "the capacity for empathy and love ... is written into our biology."

TOWARD AN EPIDEMIOLOGY OF LOVE

Research on supportive relations seldom has attempted to measure love per se.[59]

Study of the epidemiology of love requires a substantive knowledge not just of the variable or exposure in question, but of how the epidemiologic triangle comes into play in disease causation and of the concepts and mechanisms of epidemiologic theory. The course, spectrum, or career of a given disease or health-related condition from its subclinical, presymptomatic phase through morbidity, recovery, or death can vary considerably across populations and individual people.[60] A first step in investigating the health effects of love should be to carefully consider how love might fit into epidemiologic models of disease/health causation.

Epidemiologists typically conceive of psychosocial factors as host factors, whereby exposure is measured according to single items and scales often developed and validated by behavioral, social, or health psychologists or by medical sociologists (e.g., social support, Type A behavior, health locus of control, life events stress, coping). The factors that either increase or decrease the risk of subsequent morbidity (illness) or mortality (death) are known, respectively, as risk factors and protective factors. For example, tobacco smoking is believed to be a risk factor for lung cancer incidence, and Type B behavior is (or once was) believed to be a protective factor against myocardial infarction incidence. In both cases, the orientation is toward prediction of a deleterious outcome "downstream" along the natural history of disease. Antonovsky[61,62] has suggested focusing on factors that promote "salutogenesis," or the production of health, through facilitating adaptation and fostering a "sense of coherence." Such salutary factors may benefit health through bolstering host resistance, or the ability of individual people or populations to successfully resist the effects of particular exposures that would be pathogenic in hosts with weaker constitutions. Salutogenic factors thus serve to hold back the tide of expected illness in at-risk populations (disease prevention), elevate normal populations toward a higher state of wellness (health promotion), or lead clinical populations to a state of recovery (healing).[63]

According to Pitirim Sorokin,[64] a noted sociologist who wrote extensively on this topic, love is "contagious"; is an "energy"; can be "accumulated or stored," as in the epidemiologic concept of a reservoir; can undergo "release" to be "distributed," as in the epidemiologic concepts of vector- and vehicle-borne transmission; and, finally, exhibits a "curative power." In his conceptualization of a "mysterious energy of love," Sorokin[65] essentially argues for a view of love not just as a host factor—a psychosocial characteristic of individual people, dyads, or groups—but as an agent. Furthermore, according to Sorokin's description, love is an agent of salutogenesis.

Characteristics of Love-as-Salutogenic-Agent

In describing the characteristics of an agent, epidemiologists begin with certain intrinsic properties, such as physical dimensions and structure, growth and survival requirements, life cycle, host specificity, and antigenic stability.[66] From the perspective of love as an agent, several questions might be posed: What is the latent factor structure of love? Is love a multidimensional construct? Do certain types of love more easily flourish within particular hosts? How long can a given exposure to love last in particular hosts? Are multiple exposures to love necessary to maintain its sequelae? Are some people or types of people more or less impervious to love? Do the presumably salutary effects of love last indefinitely, or do they wear out at some point? Do these effects vary according to the type or amount of love to which a given host is exposed?

Next, epidemiologists consider the biological properties of agent-host interaction, namely, infectivity, pathogenicity, virulence, and immunogenicity.[66,67] Infectivity has to do with how well a given agent succeeds in invading and proliferating within a given host following exposure. Pathogenicity is an agent's ability to cause clinical signs of disease within infected hosts. With a view of love as a salutogenic agent, additional questions might be asked: How easily does love "take" in some hosts? Does love grow more or less easily in certain hosts? What host characteristics, psychosocial or otherwise, and what environmental circumstances are required for love to flourish within and among people?

How much love is required for a salutogenic reaction to be initiated? How often does love-initiated salutogenesis lead to complete healing or self-actualization? How much love is required to induce host resistance, and how long does this last?

In addition, there are other considerations in describing the activity of a given agent. There may be a gradient of infection, whereby particular hosts have subclinical (i.e., presymptomatic) infections but are still capable of infecting others.[68] These hosts are known as carriers.[67] When not infecting hosts, agents may reside in reservoirs, living organisms or inanimate objects that serve as a temporary or permanent home in the natural environment.[67,69] With respect to love, again, certain questions arise: Is the amount of love necessary to create an effect in the life of a host the same or different across hosts? Are there people who, although seemingly unloving, can induce loving feelings in others? Do certain people or social institutions act as "storehouses" of love—bottomless cisterns of love-energy available in a never-ending supply to those who interact with the reservoir? Sorokin,[64] for example, spoke of how love may accumulate and be stored in individuals (such as great saints and masters), in social institutions (including their structures, functions, agencies, and vehicles), and in culture (in its ethos, worldview, and attendant ideologies).

Transmission of Love-as-Salutogenic-Agent

There are many ways that an agent may be transmitted to a host.[67-69] These mechanisms of transmission are divisible into direct and indirect transmission—that is, transmission that is respectively immediate and through close person-to-person contact (e.g., through sexual contact), on the one hand, and through vehicles (inanimate objects), vectors (biological organisms), or airborne particles, on the other. Indirect transmission serves to convey an agent from a reservoir through the environment to a host. When the agent resides in an animal reservoir, transmission is termed *zoonotic*.[70] Thinking in terms of love as an agent, several questions come to mind: Are certain kinds of love only transmissible through close-up contact? Can love be vehicle-borne (e.g., through heirlooms, architectural structures, toys, poems, songs, photographs)? Can love be vector-borne (e.g., through plants, pets, meals, flower arrangements)? Does love reside in pets or wild animals, available for transmission to human hosts? Are the effects of love a "sexually transmitted disease"?

In addition, epidemiologists are concerned with the modes of transmission of an agent, whether via a common source or through serial propagation.[67,71] Common-source (or -vehicle) transmission results from exposure of a host population to an agent through a single common source. Exposure can be a one-time event (called *point-source transmission*), or may be repeated or continuous. Serially propagated (or progressive) transmission results from transmission from host to host, whether directly or indirectly (i.e., involving a vehicle or vector). Important considerations are the incubation period (the interval between exposure and onset of pathogenesis [or salutogenesis]), generation time (the interval between onset of infectivity in a host and maximum communicability of the host), and portals of entry and exit (the agent's ways in and ways out of a host). From the perspective of love as an agent, several more questions can be raised: Does all love originate from one or more common sources (e.g., God, acts of loving kindness) or, like the occultists' "ether," is it everywhere? Can love be passed along from person to person without losing its potency? How many exposures to love are required to transmit love to others? Can love be passed from people to things and back to people again? How long after exposure to love does salutogenesis begin? Does this incubation of love vary across different people or groups? How long after love-induced salutogenesis in a host is that host best able to spread love? How is love received in a host (i.e., through the gross senses, through intuition, through the "subtle" bioenergy fields, through the heart *chakra*, mentally, emotionally)? How is love released from a host (e.g., through words, through actions, through appearances, through interpersonal interaction)?

Another consideration regarding transmission of an agent is emergence, which refers to newly apparent or rapidly increasing agents, infections, or diseases.[72] Agents are classifiable according to factors related to their emergence, including ecologic and economic change, population and demographic shifts, international travel, technological change, and adaptation by the agent.[72,73] Human behavior "plays a critical role"[72] in emergence, and with sufficient involvement can precipitate outbreaks, or epidemic transmission in a limited geographical area. Here, determination of contact patterns becomes especially important.[70] With respect to love, more questions can be asked: Have there been recent outbreaks of behavior change or salutary effects in people attributable to love (e.g., the "Toronto blessing"[74])? Can sudden and unexplainable epidemics of healing events subsequent to absent or distant prayer be attributable to "nonlocal" transmission of love, as has been suggested?[75] Has the spread of love been enhanced or suppressed throughout the twentieth century by rapid advances in global telecommunications, facilitation of world travel, urbanization, and destruction of natural habitats? Can love mutate; can one type of love become another, or can love be transformed into something else that is then transmissible to and among human hosts? How is love spread among people and groups? Are there different sociometric patterns of transmission of love in families, non-kin networks, religious fellowships, communities, and ideological and geopolitical groupings? As Kark[2] has noted, "The social structure and functioning of a population group influence transmission of the agent." The implications of this maxim for the epidemiology of love are clearly far-reaching.

This idea of love as a salutogenic agent is just one possible approach to an epidemiology of love. In the case of love, certain great mystics, avatars, and saints have been described as being so full of love that they actually become love. Those who come into contact with such self-realized beings describe feeling as if they are in the presence of love itself. Descriptions of this phenomenon are found among such twentieth-century figures as Mother Teresa, Paramahansa Yogananda, Rebbe Schneerson, Peace Pilgrim, Corrie ten Boom, Ramana Maharshi, Pope John Paul I, and the fourteenth Dalai Lama. It is no surprise that study of the lives and works of such individuals was seen by Sorokin[64] as a window to the ultimate manifestation of "supreme love" and as an incomparable font of ideas to help us frame expectations as to how love influences health and well-being. Perhaps such lives can serve as source material for new theoretical perspectives and hypotheses to guide development and growth of the epidemiology of love.

References for this essay are located on the DVD accompanying this book.

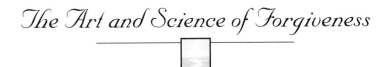

The Art and Science of Forgiveness

FREDERIC LUSKIN

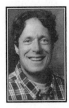

I WORK AS A CLINICAL SCI-
ence research associate at the Stanford
University School of Medicine, where I teach people ways to manage
their stress and reduce their risk of heart disease. About 6 years ago
I started to research the effect that forgiveness had on physical and emotional well-being. I was interested in forgiveness because of personal
hurts and the enormous cost of unresolved anger that I had seen in my
psychotherapy practice. Toward that end I developed a process of teaching people to let go of the grudges and grievances they carried around.
As I started to teach forgiveness, I discovered that an unexpectedly large
number of people responded to this work with fascination, confusion,
enthusiasm, and mistrust, and almost no one knew for certain exactly
what forgiveness was and why it might be useful to study.

I have learned many things as a forgiveness researcher and teacher.
First, learning to forgive has allowed me to release some of the baggage
that I have been carrying. I learned how easy it was for me to react with

anger or frustration when people did not behave the way I thought they should. I learned how to change much of that pattern and am the better for this. More remarkably, I have been given the opportunity to prove just how valuable forgiveness can be. Through my research projects and teaching, I have helped thousands of people understand what forgiveness is and is not and where it fits in the cycle of hurt, grievance, and healing.

My work as director of the Stanford Forgiveness Projects has demonstrated that learning to forgive has both emotional and physical benefits. Our first study was a randomized controlled study that recruited Stanford students as participants. The intervention group received six sessions of a 50-minute group training that guided people through the steps of forgiveness. The treatment group showed significant reductions in hurt, state, and trait anger and significant increases in forgiveness, hope, self-efficacy, and spiritual connection. As the students learned to forgive, they become more forgiving in general, not just toward one particular person who did them wrong. Follow-up assessment showed the gains were maintained 10 weeks after the end of the intervention.

The second research project recruited volunteers who had an unresolved interpersonal hurt and were between the ages of 25 and 49. The only hurts that we excluded were acts of physical and sexual violence perpetrated within the last 5 years. In this randomized controlled design, participants again showed significant improvement in hurt, state and trait anger and optimism, but also reported significantly less stress and a significant reduction in the physical symptoms of stress. These included physical problems such as dizziness, stomach pains, back ache, and/or muscle tension. This study is the largest forgiveness study to date, with 269 participants who had a follow-up assessment 18 weeks after the end of the intervention. At that time the treatment group's forgiveness of the offender continued to rise while the other indicators continued to show significant improvement relative to the control group.

The next two research projects we initiated were uncontrolled pilot studies on the effect of forgiveness training with people from Northern Ireland who had lost immediate family members to the sectarian violence. For the first study we brought a handful of mothers, from both the Catholic and Protestant communities, who had lost sons to murder.

The murders occurred between 2 and 20 years prior to the week of forgiveness training. The women spent 1 week at Stanford and received daily 120-minute sessions in forgiveness training. The women were assessed both at the end of the week and then 6 months after returning to Northern Ireland. At the 6-month follow-up, the group showed a 40 percent decrease in depression, significant decreases in stress and hurt, a significant increase in optimism, a 20 percent reduction in anger, and a 100 percent increase in forgiveness.

The second Northern Ireland project brought 17 people from both sides of the conflict to Stanford again for a week of forgiveness training. We recruited people who had any immediate family member murdered. This group was heterogeneous, where we had men and women of varying ages who had lost siblings, parents, or children. This study did not obtain sufficient follow-up data because of the unrest in Northern Ireland at the time we sent the questionnaires. At the end of the forgiveness training, participants showed significant improvement in stress, depression, and hurt. Participants in this study also reported significant improvements in physical vitality, which includes appetite, sleep patterns, energy, and general well-being.

I have collaborated on two other research projects where forgiveness training was given to volunteers who did not have a specific interpersonal hurt. In the first uncontrolled pilot project we worked with a group of financial advisors from American Express who wanted to improve their emotional competence, with the goal of increased sales. This was a year-long study conducted through a one-day workshop and ongoing individual conference calls with each advisor. In the workshop we presented some simple strategies for aligning goals feelings and behavior along with a half-day presentation on forgiveness.

For this group, forgiveness was presented as a healthy response to the normal difficulties of business, such as complaining clients, uncertain financial markets, uncooperative business associates, and the mistakes of co-workers. At the end of the year we had access to the advisors' sales reports and saw an improvement in gross sales of 18 percent, along with a 24 percent reduction in stress and a 20 percent increase in the ability to experience positive states such as rest, productivity, attention, caretaking, and pleasure.

Finally, a project conducted at a cardiology clinic at a Florida hospital researched the effect of an 8-week forgiveness intervention on blood pressure in mild/moderate hypertensive patients. This research project again demonstrated a significant reduction in anger among all participants but also showed that those people who were particularly angry at baseline also showed a decrease in mean arterial pressure at post-test.

The $64,000 question is, If forgiveness is so good for us, why do so few of us choose to forgive when people hurt us? First, we do not really understand what forgiveness is, and, second, no one has taught us how to forgive. Most people are confused about what forgiveness is and is not. The biggest misconception I face is from people who think that forgiving an offense, such as an adulterous affair, means that you condone the offense. I am reminded often that we can only forgive that which we know to be wrong. Your partner's affair was wrong, but you do not have to suffer indefinitely because you were betrayed. If you can say that an act was OK, then you have no need to forgive the offender.

Secondly, forgiveness in no way means you have to reconcile with someone who treated you badly. I see this confusion over and over in the work that I do. For example, if you were the recipient of childhood abuse or are in a harsh relationship, you can forgive the offender and, as part of that choice, make the decision to end or limit contact. Forgiveness is primarily for creating your peace of mind. It is to create healing in your life and return you to a state in which you can live and be capable again of love and trust. Forgiveness does not have to lead to reconciliation. For example, many people forgive an abusive parent but sever contact with that parent. In contrast, many married couples reconcile after an affair but do not forgive. It can also be helpful to remember we can change our minds, and a decision to sever contact in the present is often revisited in the future.

Another misconception concerning forgiveness is that it depends on whether or not the abuser or lying person apologizes, wants you back, or changes his or her ways. If another person's poor behavior was the primary determinant for your healing, then the unkind and selfish people in your life would retain power over you indefinitely. Forgiveness is the experience of finding peace inside and can neither be compelled nor stopped by another. In another vein, you can forgive your ex-spouse for his or her insulting speech and even for abandoning you and your children, but forgiveness in no way means you do not take the ex to court to make sure your children get the support payments to which they are entitled. Forgiveness and justice are not the same. You can seek justice with an open heart just as well as with a bitter one.

Lastly, forgiveness does not mean that we forget what has happened to us in our urge to move forward and get on with our lives. It is ludicrous to expect anyone who has been badly hurt not to remember the wound. That does not, however, suggest that people need to dwell on their wounds or craft life stories in which the wounds play a central role. Painful events can be life-enhancing experiences when we grieve and learn from them. What we suggest is that people remember their common humanity and focus on what they have done to learn from their experiences.

What I see over and over again from my research and teaching is that people have the capacity to make peace with their past. They regain their ability to trust and love and stop blaming other people for their emotional distress. They take more time to count their blessings and less to complain about what went wrong. They understand that they need to look more at who they become and less on what has happened, and they grasp that each day they wake up with a fresh start, no matter what happened to them yesterday. They learn to forgive and heal in both body and mind.

The most important lesson I have learned is that forgiveness can be taught. Forgiveness is a skill that can be presented through education, guided instruction, and practice. Because of the lack of role models and the lack of good education, people think forgiveness is harder than it may be. They are also generally unaware of forgiveness' benefits. The religious traditions usually tell us to forgive but do not offer the practical steps as to how. We live in a culture that prizes the expression of anger and resentment more than the peace of forgiveness. Because of this, too many do not take the opportunity to heal themselves, sometimes from great emotional pain and the physical consequences that result. What follows are my nine steps for training in forgiveness.

1. Know exactly how you feel about what happened, and be able to articulate what things about the situation are not OK. Then, tell a couple of trusted people about your experience.

2. Make a commitment to yourself to do what you have to do to feel better. Forgiveness is for you and not for anyone else. No one else even has to know about your decision.

3. Understand your goal. Forgiveness does not necessarily mean reconciliation with the person who upset you or condoning his or her actions. What you are after is to find peace. *Forgiveness* can be defined as the peace and understanding that come from blaming that which has hurt you less, taking the life experience less personally, and changing your grievance story.

4. Get the right perspective on what is happening. Recognize that your primary distress is coming from the hurt feelings, thoughts, and physical upset you are suffering now, not what offended you or hurt you 2 minutes—or 10 years—ago.

5. At the moment you feel upset, practice stress-management techniques to soothe your body's fight-or-flight response.

6. Give up expecting things from other people, or your life, that they do not choose to give you. Recognize the "unenforceable rules" you have for your health or how you or other people must behave. Remind yourself that you can hope for health, love, friendship, and prosperity and work hard to get them. However, you will suffer when you demand that these things occur when you do not have the power to make them happen.

7. Put your energy into looking for another way to get your positive goals met than through the experience that has hurt you. Instead of mentally replaying your hurt, seek out new ways to get what you want.

8. Remember that a life well-lived is your best revenge. Instead of focusing on your wounded feelings, and thereby giving the person who caused you pain power over you, learn to look for the love, beauty, and kindness around you.

9. Amend your grievance story to remind yourself of the heroic choice to forgive, and focus your conversation on what you have learned about yourself and life.

Gratefulness

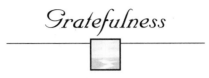

BROTHER DAVID STEINDL-RAST

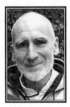

HOW WE CAN WE BE GRATE- ful in troubled times? This is an extremely challenging question, for which there is a short answer and also a long answer that can be given only in an overview. I have found that there are three tools—three pliers, so to speak—that can help pry open this question.

First, what do you really mean? This question invites us to be very explicit about the terms of our inquiry. When I speak to groups on this subject, I invite them to raise their hands whenever they encounter a term that is unclear or unfamiliar. It's important to speak the same language, because it is too easy to talk past one another unknowingly, believing that we share the same definitions and assumptions when, in fact, we bring very different meanings to the discussion.

Second, how do you know? This question points in the direction of epistemology, the branch of philosophy that studies the nature of knowledge—in particular, its foundations, scope, and validity. For practical purposes, I can answer this second question right from the start: We should always speak from direct experience. Of course, I will also extrapolate from sources beyond my own experience, for interpretations also have their place. But it is most important to be able to say: "Yes, I know this from experience. Or at least I have experienced something that makes it possible for me to understand to a greater degree. I can have access to true knowledge based on experience as a territory." For something to be true to us as individuals, it must be true for our very own experience.

Third, so what? This is a crucial question because it is the one that gets asked least often. Let me paraphrase: Why do you find it so important to raise the first two questions? Why even raise the first two questions?

To explore our original question, how to be grateful in difficult times, it is important to ask, When we are grateful, what are we grateful for? In the last analysis, we are always grateful for opportunity. It may be the opportunity to enjoy, to interact, to create, to act in a new way. The gift within every gift is opportunity. In troubled times, the opportunity is to do something about it.

Of course, there are many things we cannot be grateful for in the normal sense. Here language is important. Notice my phrase "in the normal sense." This reminds us that 99 percent of the time, the opportunity that is offered us by this given world is the opportunity to enjoy. But we tend not to think of that. In fact, we find ourselves effectively sleeping through the opportunities we are given, in countless situations. We only wake up when something comes around that jolts us into awareness of something that is hard to be grateful for. "How can I be grateful for that?" is our question. But if we had been grateful all the time before, we would be perfectly in practice and more able to respond, "There is always opportunity in each moment; what's the opportunity at this moment?"

And what might pop out is that the opportunity is to do something new at that moment. At the very least, in troubled times we can ask the question: What is my opportunity to act in this moment? What can I do? If you don't know, you might ask someone else. That person may not know either. So you keep asking, and if everyone asks everyone else, it becomes possible to think and act in new ways in response to the question of what we can do at this moment. It surely would be a different world if we asked this question in trying times.

So, the short answer to how we can be grateful in difficult times is: We can always be grateful, at any time and in any place, for opportunity. The only task in troubled times is to find what opportunity this very trouble offers us to act with gratefulness.

Now to the longer answer: How can you truly *be* and not be grateful? After all, *to be* means to be grateful. *To be* means more than simply to exist, more than just to hang around. It means to be alive, to be creative, to be responsive, to experience depth and meaning in our lives. When we take being seriously, inevitably we are driven to ponder the very ground of existence, the deep basis of what we mean by being at any level, at all levels.

Gratefulness is a house with many rooms. In a moment of true gratefulness, we find ourselves experiencing many things at once. If you pause to recollect an instance where you felt deep and profound gratitude, you may remember a deep calmness, a marvelous stillness in your being. That is one room. But you may also remember that you visited another room, which you might call *fulfillment*. You feel full with gratefulness, a fullness that is not always present in other experiences. Another aspect you may find is the experience of being uplifted—we stand taller in moments of gratefulness. And, moments of gratefulness very often bring a sense of being connected—acknowledged, recognized, present to existence in a richer sense.

Each of these realms—calm, fulfillment, fullness, being uplifted and feeling connected—has an opposite that you can always also feel when you are grateful. Going back to your experience of gratefulness, it may surprise you to realize that when you feel calmest, you may also feel highly energized. The greater the calm, the greater the sense of vitality. There is a joyful excitement in deep gratefulness, and it is perfectly compatible with enormous calm. You feel fulfilled, yet also receptive. The two are perfectly compatible—as if the capacity to receive a gift also makes it possible to give something back to the invisible source or ground of all experience.

And while gratefulness characteristically makes you feel uplifted, you also feel humbled. The world *humble* comes from the word *humus*, or *earth*. So, you are down to earth at moments of deep gratefulness, as opposed to flying around proudly in the sky. That sense of connection with the earth, and with the very ground of your being, makes it possible to stand tall.

So it's a paradox: When you're calm, you're also energized. When you're fulfilled, you're receptive. When you're uplifted, you're humbled—glad to be "small" or childlike. Remember when you were small? We were happy to be children; we didn't want to grow up. We're perfectly happy to be little. In gratefulness we feel connected with all; we feel acknowledged and recognized. And yet, again paradoxically, we are totally unconcerned about ourselves. There's a self-forgetfulness that is enhanced with gratefulness. And with this experience of gratefulness that unites yet transcends seeming opposites comes something new: thankfulness.

We can distinguish gratefulness from thankfulness. Gratefulness is like holding a bowl that is brimming with goodies, and if you tip it ever so slightly it will overflow. Thankfulness is that overflowing, the sheer exuberance of gratefulness. Does that ring true with your experience? There are two phases to being grateful—the first pertaining to its fullness, and the second finding expression in true thanks.

Thanks is always an expression. *Thank* and *think* come from the same root. The gratefulness that comes before the thankfulness may involve little more than a split second and has nothing to do with thinking. It's simply a state of being. Then comes the overflow, expressing itself in conscious thanks. In religious terms, gratefulness is very Buddhist; thankfulness reflects more elements of the Abrahamic traditions, including Christianity and Judaism. These two are not contradictory; it's where you choose to put the emphasis that matters.

For instance, gratefulness plays an important role in Buddhism. Practitioners at Buddhist centers and retreats continuously bow at every possible opportunity. Every moment is a reason for gratefulness. Yet there is very little emphasis on expressions of thanks, because the very idea of thanking immediately introduces the idea of someone to whom you are grateful. Gratefulness, however, is simply a state of being. In the religions of Abraham—Judaism, Islam, and Christianity—verbal expressions of thankfulness are far more common.

Whenever we are dealing with paradox as I have described it, we can be pretty sure we are dealing with the Ultimate. If it's not paradoxical, you haven't reached the Ultimate. Now of course there are some paradoxes that can just be created by stupidity; every paradox does not mean you are approaching the Ultimate. But if you reach the Ultimate, it must be paradoxical because the territory involves the coincidence of opposites. All opposites coincide in the Ultimate.

So with gratefulness and thankfulness, we are dealing with the Ultimate. And we are dealing with a realm of experience that is profoundly integral. The sense of paradox we experience in gratefulness and thankfulness is a giveaway of their integral nature, which is to say their wholeness and completeness, beyond the mind's habit of dividing experience into parts.

Where do we encounter that reality that some call God, or the Divine? On one level, we experience it as that mysterious ground from which we come, from which all arises, the source of everything and nothing. We live in a world that has no bottom. You have probably heard the story about the teacher who said the world rested on a turtle, and the turtle rested on yet another turtle: "It's turtles all the way down." For us, mystery is all the way down. We know some things about that mystery—that it is the source of everything, for instance. It is the source of everything that is, and it is the source of ourselves.

This is because everything is given. Most of the time, we don't even want what is given to us; it's just there whether we like it or not. If we have the right attitude, gratefulness is the only appropriate attitude toward everything that is given, which is to say toward everything, because everything is a gift. So mystery is that from which everything arises and that to which everything returns.

Another area in which we may experience this mystery is in ourselves. You are a mystery to yourself. Some might say, "Of all the mysteries I encounter in this life, I am the most mysterious!" We discover ourselves only by living, by making choices; it is not as if we first know ourselves, and then we act. We discover ourselves in making choices—and not only yourself, but you discover others, through relationship. And the more intimately you come to know another person, the more mysterious they become to you. "We have been married for 50 years, and now we have discovered how little we know one another."

Everything that we can experience with our senses is an expression of that same mystery that brings forth everything. In this sense, the Ultimate is not only the mysterious source from which everything comes up but also as expressing itself in everything you see. And when you catch on to that, your spirituality gains a completely new dimension. You see the divine in everything that you see, whether an object is made by human hands or it is part of nature. Why do so many people say, "I meet the divine most when I go into nature"? Because you are divine and you walk into the divine, and you experience the Ultimate made visible.

A health challenge or healing crisis opens for many people to the realm of the spiritual. When the gift of good health is interrupted, we have the opportunity to realize that the well-being we so take for granted is a gift. And the loss of good health is very often experienced as a gift, because it can be a doorway to new understandings of self in relationship to others. I have spoken to so many people for whom a healing or medical crisis was eventually experienced with gratitude. The same people described feeling anger, frustration, fear, and similar familiar feelings; yet I have often heard people say that these feelings were not contradicted by a simultaneous sense of gratefulness and thankfulness.

How can this be so? If we very carefully feel our way into our own experience, we can discover that our very life—our living, our thinking, our loving—is again totally mysterious to us, for we meet the divine mystery again and again. What does knowing mean? What is consciousness? Our being conscious is the contact with the ultimate mystery. And now you can look at this life we are given—the dimensions of mystery, manifest and unmanifest—as being embedded in the divine.

You can look at this in terms of gratefulness like this: The ultimate Source, unmanifest, gives itself totally into the manifest, created world. And the manifest returns to the Ultimate in each act of gratefulness and thanksgiving. Because when you really give thanks, you're not giving a donation or tip. To give thanks fully is to acknowledge that I have nothing and I give back all the nothing I am to the Source from which it arises. That giving, itself, is again mysteriously divine. Gratefulness and thanksgiving are themselves a divine movement because before those expressions, existence is just static. The divine movement of the manifest coming out of the Source is repeated in gratitude and thanksgiving, which then become acts of returning to the Source.

The result is what might be called a "circuit dance of gratefulness." And again, this dance is fundamentally integral, in that it joins together realms that the mind so often breaks asunder. And this is a view of our spiritual embedding of our relationship to the divine that is based on universal human experience. And it is compatible with all the spiritual traditions that exist; all spiritual traditions place gratefulness at the heart of their teachings. Even many people who do not wish to identify with a religious tradition can be heard to say gratefulness is at the heart of their spiritual sense of the world.

Let me close with a marvelous passage from Christopher Fry's play *A Sleep of Prisoners*:

> Dark and cold we may be, but this
> Is no winter now. The frozen misery
> Of centuries breaks, cracks, begins to move;
> The thunder is the thunder of the floes,
> The thaw, the flood, the upstart Spring.
> Thank God our time is now when wrong
> Comes up to face us till we take
> The longest stride of soul men ever took.
> Affairs are now soul size.
> The enterprise
> Is exploration into God.

The Contemplative Mind in Society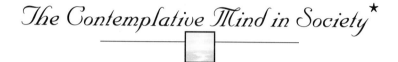*

JON KABAT-ZINN

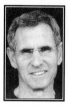

THE TELEPHONE, THE TRANsistor, and the home computer transformed the society by quantum leaps, driven by the extraordinary power of the enhanced connectedness made possible through the controlled channeling of electric current and by the market forces such possibilities generated. Before that, it was the steam engine, the railroad, and the automobile, the harnessing of chemical and mechanical power.

The transformative effects on society of large numbers of people purposefully cultivating a more mindful and contemplative life are potentially as powerful, if not more so, than such technological advances in power and connectivity and the capabilities to which they give rise.

However, widespread adoption of contemplative "technologies" and their associated shifts in worldview will be very different, given their inner orientation and use of more subtle energies. For one thing, they offer scant opportunities for economic exploitation, which would be highly undesirable in any event. This does not mean that a widespread

---

*Adapted from Kabat-Zinn J: The Contemplative Mind in Society, *The Center for Contemplative Mind in Society*, 1996.

adoption of contemplative values and practices would not have profound economic and political benefits. I believe it certainly would.

In the past 150 years, human beings have learned to interface comfortably with machines and, in the past decade or so, with emerging information/digital technology. Many people are becoming "computer literate" on an operational level, and this skill is now being taught in the schools as a fundamental aspect of economic survival in the job market.

But we have yet, as a society or a culture, to come to grips with the profound and irreversible implications of such technological changes and their effects on the pace of life, or the rate, amount, and quality of information and images that human beings, even children, have to "process" in a day. We have yet to fully appreciate the impact of these technologies on the quality of our individual and family lives, on the meaning and quality of our work lives and environments, as well as on our greater political and cultural goals and social values—to say nothing of our tremendous capacity for self- and eco-destruction. All this technology, although itself potentially enhancing of connectivity and communication, is also alienating, intrusive, and isolating.

I would suggest that it is now time for society to turn its attention to developing what we may call "inner technologies." The untapped potential of the human mind for individual and collective creativity and wisdom has to be intentionally cultivated. It needs training of a certain kind (for example, as found in many contemporary consciousness disciplines) if it is to keep up with the precocious challenges of our technological advances without losing all sense of value and meaning in our individual and collective lives.

An "inner technology," of which meditation in its most generic sense and most basic form (mindfulness) is the cardinal element, has the capacity to elevate our consciousness up to and beyond the challenges posed by our technological advances and to harness them, as well as the power of the mind, for the greater good and harmony of all people and the planet. This capacity is built into a "universal grammar" of human psychology, I believe, just as our capacity for speech is built into our brain structure through a universal grammar/language instinct. And just as with language development, it needs exposure and some training to fully develop this capacity. What is involved is basically a deep familiarity and intimacy with the activity and reactivity of one's own mind and some competency in navigating through our mind and emotions with equanimity, clarity, and commitment.

From my work in the field over the past 20 years, I see that more and more people are taking up or coming back to the practice of meditation and making it an integral part of their daily lives in a nonmechanical way. As they do this, and as they communicate about it more freely, they tend to develop a deepening understanding of its potential uses and transformative value, one that is grounded in their own direct experience. Personal values tend to change subtly or not so subtly, as well as behaviors, each in uniquely personal but describable ways. I see this inner process as an expanding view of what it means to be fully human and a planetary adult—both as an individual and embedded within a collectively shared, conscious, and continually interacting network (society, *sangha*).

I hold an optimistic, if somewhat radical, scenario of the transformative possibilities for our era. I like to think that we are facing and are already unwittingly engaged in a very real opportunity for seeding a second Italian/European Renaissance in the United States, if not worldwide. I believe we need to at least attempt to formulate a large vision of the possible and then work toward it incrementally; we should be careful, however, not to delude ourselves about potential problems with ambition or power, or about the potential resistance to any efforts to further a contemplative orientation in our society and its institutions. A collective, continuously evolving vision of what we think we are doing and why will serve us well as a resource of deepening clarity and motivation. Then, by paying careful attention to the details and making sure that our efforts reflect the wisdom and compassion the topic of the contemplative mind represents in the first place, we will be building the inner counterparts of the telephone, transistor, or computer. I believe that the rest will, in some profound way, take care of itself.

POTENTIAL FOR A SECOND RENAISSSANCE

As I see it, a profound social/cultural revolution, or what I prefer to think of as a second Renaissance, is possible, at least in first- and second-world countries, if not globally. It is driven by strong currents of desire for greater meaning and fulfillment, health and well-being, leisure and comfort, and the expectation of relative longevity that the past several centuries of technological progress in first-world countries have generated. The power of this strong inward longing in our society for well-being, meaning, and connectedness should not be underestimated.

The Italian Renaissance emerged out of a thousand years of relative cultural and social "darkness" and was fueled by a renewed appreciation for the sacred and a strong desire to integrate it into the domain of the human through new forms of art and architecture. And, of course, it was fueled by a scientific method based on confidence that careful direct observation and measurement could help elucidate the mystery of the work of God, as well as by explorations to discover new worlds (for plunder, trade, subjugation, and religious imperialism). On the artistic and architectural side, it was driven in large measure by the creative impulse and genius of individuals such as DaVinci and Michelangelo, whose work was well-funded by a small number of wealthy and enlightened patrons.

One might argue that conditions are ripe, at least in the United States, for the beginning of a new and more enlightened and broad-based Renaissance, one that may well last more than a few hundred years and whose emergence may be far more rapid than its predecessor of 500 years ago, given the time acceleration of our day and our speed-of-light communications technology. The question for us now is how to further the emergence of such a profound and complex cultural transformation, which in some ways is already unfolding.

We will also need to ask, since the contemplative and the sacred have always been undercurrents of life in our society, why it is that such an emergence has not happened before. We will need to think about and anticipate what present and future obstacles to such an undertaking might be. These are large historical questions that no one person can give complete answers to. However, refining our thinking about them through dialogue that honors the work of scholarship but goes beyond the scholarly will be essential to developing new models for social learning and social action along contemplative lines.

Up to this time, the subject of how to live consciously (or religiously, in the old terminology) has been an arcane, age-old scholarly debate.

The challenge, I believe, is to make it real within the conduct of our own lives through personal engagement and experimentation. It will also be important not to hide our personal involvement but to let our efforts become known and resonate in larger circles of the society on all levels. In order to do this, our vocabulary and our thinking and our efforts must transcend religion as we know it, with its historically parochial and sometimes evangelical and messianic interests, ideologies, and hierarchies, so as to be a truly universal expression of the direct experience of the numinous, the sacred, the tao, god, the divine, nature, and silence in all aspects of life and not conflict with our healthy affirmation of the need to keep church and state separate, given what both church and state represent.

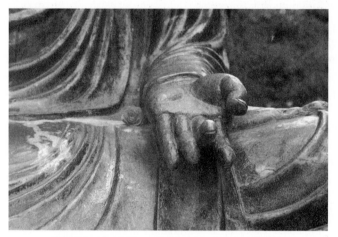

"Buddha Hand Flower." (Courtesy Michael Eller.)

Moreover, strange as it may sound, such a movement needs to avoid the human impulse to let this come about through the emergence of one particular person who takes on the role of avatar, savior, messiah, charismatic leader, or spokesperson, tempting as this is for many people. This has been the historical pathway by which the mega-emergences of the path of the sacred have manifested, through the major world religions and various cults. But the framing of a single person as the encapsulation of our understanding takes it out of the domain of direct experience and inevitably introduces a dualism and a lack of personal responsibility and engagement that create more problems than they solve. The same is true for the predominance of a single idea, ideal, belief system, or view of truth or an us/them, enlightened/unenlightened, meditator/nonmeditator mentality.

Part Four

HONORING MULTIPLE WAYS OF KNOWING

MARILYN SCHLITZ
TINA AMOROK

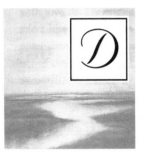

ifferent ways of knowing are called for by science on one hand, and religion on the other. As we hold this tension, we become increasingly aware of the call to go more deeply into the epistemological pluralism that now epitomizes contemporary health care. Adding alternative and complementary practices from the world's traditions answers this call to embrace different ways of knowing and understanding healing and curing. In this section we examine the philosophical and practical implications of diverse worldviews and belief systems, as they co-exist in American medicine today. We also hear from a small sample of the incredibly rich and abundant perspectives that inform integral medicine.

EPISTEMOLOGICAL PLURALISM

We begin with an essay on the implications of alternative and complementary medicine for science and the scientific process by medical anthropologist Marilyn Schlitz and philosopher Willis Harman, the former president of the Institute of Noetic Sciences. They argue that new findings in the areas of complementary and alternative medicine (CAM) research have profound implications for science and its application in the biological and medical domains. In particular, many alternative epistemologies involve a worldview in which human experiences, including thoughts, feelings, and intentions, are believed to interact in causal ways with subtle forms of "energies," "forces," or "spirits" to create a healing response. Such beliefs currently have no place in the Western scientific paradigm. Rather than treating them each piecemeal, the authors ask how an integral approach may help to solve the kinds of problems that are presented in simple reductionism.

Dr. Stanley Krippner, a cross-cultural psychologist, examines the epistemology and technologies of shamanic states of consciousness. The practice of shamanism, he writes, involves "a group of techniques that enable its practitioners to enter the 'spirit world' to obtain information that is used to help and to heal members of their social group." Today we have the opportunity to include and learn from shamanism and the shamans' "sources in imagination, intuition, visions, dreams, the senses, and the body." Krippner suggests that these ways of knowing may complement intellect and reason to construct cooperative and collaborative lifestyles for the pluralistic world in which we live—"a world that shamanic epistemology would appreciate and enjoy, a world that shamanic technology would strive to honor and protect."

Dr. Frances Vaughan, a pioneer in humanistic and transpersonal psychology, continues to expand our appreciation of multiple epistemologies in her essay exploring multiple ways of knowing. She asserts the need for an integral theory of consciousness to understand the fullness of being—one that honors objective, subjective, and intersubjective perspectives at the same time. She goes on to say that many of the world's wisdom traditions teach that an intelligent, self-organizing consciousness animates and sustains nature, and it is a virtue to relate to all of life as sentient, and to all beings as possessing subjectivity. In so doing, Vaughan states, "we will then recognize the connection that exists between each one of us and the whole of nature."

INTEGRATING THE WISDOM OF THE WORLD'S WISDOM TRADITIONS

Our next collection of essays speaks to the integration of the wisdom of the world's healing systems. Nancy C. Maryboy and David H. Begay, both Dine cosmologists, consider the restoration of dynamic balance in the traditional ways of healing expressed through Navajo consciousness. Living and working as teachers on the Navajo reservation themselves, the authors explore traditional Navajo healing as it has been handed down through the generations in the American Southwest. In order to discuss Navajo healing processes, they note, "it is necessary to explore the context in which traditional healing is understood and in which it takes place, since the very processes are holistic and interrelated with all that exists in the universe."

Speaking from the heart of the Tibetan healing tradition, Sogyal Rinpoche, a master of the Dzogchen tradition and one of the most revered interpreters and teachers of Tibetan Buddhism, writes about the spiritual heart of Tibetan medicine. Following the teachings of Buddha and speaking of what he has found to be most effective in the West, he writes, "The mind is both the source of happiness and the root of suffering. At the same time it possesses an extraordinary capacity for healing, it also plays its part in making us ill. The whole thrust of Buddhist practice is precisely to eliminate these negative states of mind and to cultivate the positive ones, transforming our mind and its emotions and thereby healing our entire being—body, speech, mind, and heart." Sogyal Rinpoche goes on to say that to recognize the true nature of the mind is the ultimate healing experience and practice.

Finally, we have a chapter by neuroscientists Garret Yount, Ph.D., and Yifang Qian, M.D., Ph.D., together with Honglin Zhang, M.D., the director of the Office of Qigong Research at China's Academy of Traditional Chinese Medicine. In this review of the subtle energy medicine of Qigong, the authors touch on both the cultural history of traditional Chinese medicine and the research that has addressed its efficacy. While many formal studies have been conducted in China, they note, the standards of proof are significantly different in Western science. Again, we are reminded of the need to hold multiple epistemologies as we work toward the development of a model of medicine that is integral and inclusive.

Ultimately, an integral approach to medicine will be facilitated by the weaving together of traditional healing practices with more contemporary medical systems. In this process, we need to examine the ways in which a common current of healing philosophy links these otherwise differing approaches. What is the common ground? And what are the barriers and stumbling blocks that need to be acknowledged and overcome so that the best possible approach to the patient and the patient's care may be made available? Our responsibility as healers and as patients largely begins with these questions and a deep inquiry into their possible answers.

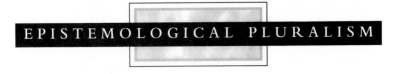

The Implications of Alternative and Complementary Medicine for Science and the Scientific Process*

MARILYN SCHLITZ
WILLIS HARMAN

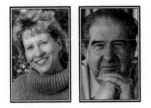

PRIOR TO THE MODERN period in which we now live, health care was characterized by a pluralism of choices. Indeed, during the eighteenth and nineteenth centuries, various types of alternative and complementary medicines co-existed with the fledging, allopathic, science-based medicine throughout Europe and North America. The 1910 report on North American medical schools by Abraham Flexner,[1] commissioned by the Carnegie Foundation, changed this situation by supporting the growing movement that used a dogmatic definition of science to judge medical options. Alternative approaches such as homeopathy,

---

*Adapted from Lorimer BD: *Thinking Beyond the Brain,* Edinburgh, 2001, Floris Books.

midwifery, and chiropractic were essentially forced out of the official medical system.[2]

Today, alternative and complementary medicines are experiencing a revitalization. New developments include a growing professionalization, the creation of several professional journals, the establishment of the Office of Alternative Medicine at the National Institutes of Health, the reimbursement of selected alternative treatments by some insurance providers, a proliferation of books and conferences concerning research and clinical practice, and survey data suggesting that Americans are spending billions of dollars per year on alternative treatment options.[3]

Despite these advances, alternative and complementary medical practices remain marginalized relative to the dominant bio-medical model. One important factor in this situation is the form of science that has shaped modern medicine, a form that has evolved with a certain passion and worldview about the nature of reality. Indeed, modern Western science fundamentally entails three important metaphysical assumptions that limit its ability to integrate alternative medicines:

1. *Realism* (ontological—leads to epistemological conclusion). There is a real material world independent of mind that is, in essence, physically measurable (positivism). We are embedded in that world, follow its laws, and have evolved from an ancient origin. Mind or consciousness evolved within that world; the world pre-existed before its appearance and continues to exist and persist independent of consciousness.

2. *Objectivism* (epistemological and ontological). A form of materialist realism that says that the world is knowable and persists as a domain of objects unaffected by perceiving subjects. That real world therefore can be studied as object—that is, it is accessible to sense perception and can be consensually observed and validated.

3. *Reductionism* (epistemological). Knowledge is attained by a process of analyzing, explaining, or validating data in terms of the constituent parts of objects and/or the laws that determine their behavior. The real world is described by the laws of physics, which are believed to apply everywhere. The essence of the scientific endeavor is to provide explanations for complex phenomena in

terms of the characteristics of, and interactions among, their component parts.

These assumptions, and the methods they require, currently dominate biomedical science. The present situation in American medicine involves a deepening understanding of such factors as the role of DNA in determining the nature of the organism, an expanding reliance on advanced and expensive technology, and a growing faith in the power of modern biomedical theory. To some extent these metaphysical premises have been reevaluated through an understanding of the relativistic views of science recently explicated by works in the history, sociology, and philosophy of science.[4-7] More central to our concern here, however, are the new findings in the areas of alternative and complementary medicine that have profound implications for science and its application in the biological and medical domains. In particular, many alternative epistemologies involve a worldview in which human experience—including thoughts, feelings, and intentions—is believed to interact in causal ways with subtle forms of "energies," "forces," or "spirits" to create a healing response. Such beliefs currently have no place in the Western scientific paradigm.

A fundamental difficulty appears to be that Western science continues to be caught in a basic dualistic trap—that of considering the subject doing the mapping as separate from the map. Getting a more accurate map (based more on modern physics, more "holistic," more "systems") does not seem to solve this problem. Rather, it may be useful to reflect on the possibility that thoughts are not merely a reflection on reality but are also a movement of that reality itself. The map-maker, the self, the thinking and knowing subject may actually be a product of and a participant in that which it seeks to know and represent.[7,8] The critical epistemological issue is whether we humans have basically one way of contacting reality (namely, through the physical senses) or *multiple* (the other senses, including intuition, somatic feelings, and direct apprehension).[9]

The importance of the issue shows up in a central ontological question: Is consciousness caused (by physiological processes in the brain, which in turn are consequences of a long evolutionary process) or is it causal (in the sense that consciousness is not only a causal factor in present phenomena but also a causal factor throughout the entire evolutionary process)? Western scientific method urges toward the former choice, whereas some of the phenomena of alternative and complementary medicines (e.g., placebo effects, psychosomatic trauma and healing, intentionality) suggest the latter choice.

There is in the medical world much faith that explanations of some of the claimed results in alternative and complementary medicine (as well as debunking of some other claimed results) will be forthcoming from this strengthening biomedical science. At the same time, much of complementary and alternative medicine does not fit even with accepted new views of science, such as quantum mechanics and complexity theories. It seems to be true that, taken together, these diagnostic, therapeutic, and health-promoting practices pose a fundamental challenge to the metaphysical foundations of Western science, which is based on assumptions of materialism, objectivism, reductionism, and physical determinism. We wish to explore the extent and implications of that challenge.

INCOMPATIBILITIES BETWEEN THE ALTERNATIVE MEDICINE AND SCIENTIFIC WORLDVIEWS

There are areas of alternative and complementary medicine in which not only do we lack scientific models that would help explain the "mechanisms" of healing, but the models that do arise from the various complementary medical systems (e.g., subtle energies, mind-body-spirit holism, intentionality) do not seem compatible with the Western scientific worldview. Examples include homeopathy; acupuncture, *qigong*, and traditional Chinese medicine; *ayurvedic* (Indian) medicine; Tibetan medicine; and various practices utilized by Fourth World peoples. Even herbal therapies, nutritional supplements, aromatherapy, meditation and biofeedback, guided imagery, body work, and so on may be of questionable compatibility to the extent that they involve holistic models that include causal consciousness.

Subtle Energies

Many alternative healing practitioners associate healing with what are commonly referred to as "subtle energies," or "fields." This concept may include electromagnetic and other energy fields throughout, and in the space surrounding the body, but it may also involve factors that are, at least so far, not physically measurable.[10] The admitted ambiguity allows a co-convening of those who believe all phenomena will eventually be understood in terms of energy fields that fit within the known models of science, together with those who find psychological and spiritual phenomena to involve aspects of reality not representable in terms of measurable fields.

There are many cultural instances of such "subtle fields." In the Eastern cultures, we find such concepts as prana, *ch'i, or ki*, concepts that find no easy place in our scientific lexicon. Traditional chinese medicine (TCM), for example, is a comprehensive professional discipline, based on a complete system of thought. Within this epistemology the human body is seen as a reflection of the natural world—a whole within a larger whole. Energy and fluids in the body are spoken of as flowing like channels and rivers. A medical diagnosis describes the body in terms of the elements—wind, heat, cold, dryness, dampness—concepts that have no place in current Western diagnostic categories.

The complementary terms *yin* and *yang* are used by the TCM practitioner to describe the various opposing physical conditions of the body. *Yin* refers to the tissue of the organ, while *yang* refers to its activity. TCM also introduces a major component of the body, *ch'i*, that Western medicine does not acknowledge. This "vital life energy" flows through the body following pathways called *meridians*, which move along the surface of the body and through the internal organs. According to this view, organs can be accessed for treatment through their specific meridians, and illness can occur when there is a blockage of *ch'i* in these channels. TCM incorporates a wide range of methods of treatment, including herbal medicine, acupuncture, dietary therapy, and massage. These have all become more or less acceptable in Western medicine; however, the conceptual model including the central *ch'i* concept is by no means compatible with the assumptions of Western science. While the medical model makes use of the body's energy using electroencephalography, electrocardiography, and electromyography for diagnostic purposes, it has yet to incorporate "subtle energies" for the purpose of healing.[11]

For another example of subtle energies within the framework of alternative medicine, we turn to homeopathy, which was founded in the late eighteenth century by the German physician Samuel Hahnemann.[12] It remains reasonably acceptable in continental Europe, where in one sense it is more or less integrated with conventional medicine. Within the current scientific medical paradigm, however, the underlying principles comprise a challenge to conventional medicine's concepts of illness and healing. These basic underlying principles are:

a. Like cures like; the same substance that in large doses creates symptoms like those of the disease, in minute dosage can be used to cure it.

b. Dilution increases potency; potency is greatest after dilution has reduced the amount below chemical detection.

c. Illness is specific to the individual; an illness generally defined will be treated in homeopathy only after finding the symptom pattern unique to the patient.

Like TCM, homeopathy is a complete self-contained alternative system of medicine that reportedly can have a therapeutic effect on almost any disease or health condition. On the other hand, the implied formal causality in homeopathy does not fit the efficient causality of Western science.

Intentionality

The role of the mind and intentionality represents one of the key features of most alternative medical systems and is an important challenge to Western scientific epistemology.[13] Broadly defined, intentionality involves the projection of awareness, with purpose and efficacy, toward some object or outcome. It includes ways in which a person's mind is able to interact with his or her own body, such as in self-healing; ways in which people's intentions can influence others through direct or indirect communication, such as in placebo and "nocebo" effects; and, more difficult to reconcile with our current scientific worldview, ways in which intentions may influence others through some "nonlocal" means.

While psychological approaches that assume intentionality, including imagery techniques, have been used by alternative practitioners for centuries in order to help mobilize the healing process, such concepts as psychosomatic illness, stress disorders, placebo effect, dissociation, and mind-body medicine have met with considerable resistance. This is due, in large part, to the fact that consciousness as a causal factor is excluded from the scientific worldview. Today, guided imagery is widely used for relief of chronic pain and other symptoms and for accelerating healing and minimizing discomfort from injuries and illness symptoms.[14-19] Imagery has been used to bring about healing from serious illness; spontaneous patient imagery has been used to better understand the meaning of symptoms or to access inner resources. Intentionality is not only implicit in all of this; a connection between imagery and real physiological effects is assumed.

As of now, we have no clear understanding of how this healing effect works within the context of our bio-medical models. The influence of a healer's or patient's intentions (including expectations) on the physical state of the patient puzzles or disturbs some medical professionals and is a troubling artifact for many researchers. But it can also be viewed as an untapped resource in healing. Although the typical view of placebos is that they should be controlled or eliminated, the phenomenon may in fact turn out to be a powerful agent in linking intention, belief, expectations, and bodily responses.[20] The challenge of delineating all significant variables is considerable and may be one reason that so little has been done to integrate placebos into clinical practice. More research could be done to analyze nonspecific factors including rapport, anticipation, and hope in a way that begins to clarify their roles in healing. At the same time, we must develop reliable holistic methods and approaches that allow us to understand the healing relationship in other than reductionistic terms.

More difficult conceptually are the claims made by healers that they can use intentionality to access some form of "transpersonal" consciousness—consciousness that seemingly originates from a "higher source," passes through one person, the healer, to another, the patient—at a distance. The idea of transpersonal or "nonlocal" healing has widespread support in many cultures. Further, it is widely believed that people can obtain information about the world around them without any direct sensory contact. So we find, for example, that in the Spanish folk medicine of *curanderismo*, or in the *obeah* practices of the southern Caribbean, or among the Kaluli peoples of the Papua New Guinea rainforest, healers believe that they are able to physically affect other people at a distance through some kind of direct mental or spiritual interaction. What's more, they say they can heal this way without other people necessarily knowing about the effort—presumably eliminating any direct placebo effect. According to the Western scientific paradigm, such phenomena are impossible; nevertheless, increasing data support the claims.[21-25] But there is currently no explaining such results with accepted scientific concepts.

Intuitive Diagnosis

With regard to medical diagnosis, many alternative practitioners and physicians utilize their consciousness in a fashion that is not understood by Western science. Frequently this is described as a hunch or intuition that the practitioner had no reason to assume would be helpful but that turned out to be exactly what needed to be done. The physician Oliver Wendell Holmes described the intuitive process by saying that "all of us have a double who is wiser and better than we are and who puts thoughts into our heads and words into our mouths."[26] Despite this, most Western-trained physicians have been taught to rely on objective tools of science for diagnostic insights, excluding their own subjectivity except in some very marginalized way.

The most startling evidence of remote diagnosis is in the form of anecdotal data. Perhaps two of the best known cases are Edgar Cayce and Caroline Myss. Cayce (1877-1945) discovered this apparent ability accidentally. Hundreds of times, in an altered state of consciousness and after being given by hypnotic suggestion the name and location of an ailing person at some remote location, he would come up with a detailed diagnosis, apparently accurate in the vast majority of cases.[27] The work of Myss is similar, except that she remained in a state of conscious awareness. By telephone call from her partner, C. Norman Shealy, a Harvard-trained neurosurgeon and researcher, she would be given a patient's name and date of birth. According to Dr. Shealy's data, her diagnoses were "93 percent accurate."[28] In spite of such anecdotal data on successes, however, little research has been done on the role of intuition in diagnosis. As Daniel Benor[21] writes, "Intuitive diagnosis has received less attention than healing. This neglected modality has much to offer modern medicine."

Fulfilling this potential, however, will require some radical alterations in the basic assumptions of modern scientific medicine.

POSSIBLE ALTERNATIVE ONTOLOGICAL ASSUMPTIONS

At a fundamental level, these alternative approaches imply pictures of reality that are not in accord with the Western scientific worldview. They pose both an epistemological and an ontological challenge. It might seem more reasonable to take up the challenges one by one—the possibilities of subtle energies, the role of the mind in healing, the puzzle of intentionality, the mystery of remote diagnosis, and so on. Science has often progressed by focusing on the simplest and most tractable case first and later proceeding to the more complex.

However, there is an alternate strategy that also has precedent in the history of science. Consider the origin of the evolutionary hypothesis. In the mid-nineteenth century there was much to be learned from studying separately the great variety of microorganisms, plants, and animals with which the planet is populated. But Charles Darwin boldly turned his attention to the synthesizing question: How can we understand *all of these together?* The result was the concept of evolution, around which practically all of biology is now organized.

There would seem to be an analogous situation in the multifaceted challenge posed by alternative and complementary medicine. We appear to need some sort of conceptual framework within which to understand a broad range of phenomena and experiences. As noted by medical historian Marc Micozzi,[11] "When homeopathy or acupuncture is observed to result in a physiologic or clinical response that cannot be explained by the biomedical model, it is not the role of the scientist to deny this reality, but rather to modify our explanatory models to account for it. In the end, there is only one reality." What sorts of conceptual frameworks and organizing metaphors could be used to help us understand the many facets and dimensions of Western medicine and complementary medicine *all considered together?*

A step toward resolving this long-standing impasse may be the recognition that it is, in a sense, a historical accident that physics was taken to be the root science. That led naturally enough to such ideas as seeking objectivity through separating observer and observed; taking reality to be essentially that which can be physically measured; and seeking explanations of the whole in terms of understanding the parts.

But what if the study of living systems had been taken to be the root science, rather than physics?[29] Had this been the case, science would undoubtedly have taken a more holistic turn. It would have recognized that wholes are self-evidently more than the sum of their parts and would have adopted an epistemology more congenial to living organisms. It might well have adopted a different ontological stance in viewing reality.

Such an alternative ontological stance was proposed, following Arthur Koestler[30] by American philosopher Ken Wilber,[7,8] that of considering reality as composed of "holons," each of which is a whole and simultaneously a part of some other whole—"holons within holons" (for example, atom-molecule-organelle-cell-tissue-organ-organism-society-biosphere). Holons at the same time display agency, the capacity to maintain their own wholeness, even as they are also parts of other wholes. A holon can break up into other holons. But every holon also has the tendency to come together with others, resulting in the emergence of creative and novel holons (as in evolution). The drive to self-transcendence appears to be built into the very fabric of the universe. The self-transcending drive produces life out of matter and may be the basis of consciousness.

Holons relate "holarchically." (This term seems advisable because "hierarchy" has a bad connotation, mainly because people confuse natural hierarchy [inescapable] with dominator hierarchy [pathological].) Thus cell-holons are parts of organ-holons, which in turn are parts of organism-holons, which are parts of community-holons. For any particular holon, *functions* and *purposes* come from levels higher in the holarchy; *capabilities* depend upon lower levels.

In the holarchic picture of reality, the scientist-holon seeking to understand consciousness is in an intermediate position. Looking downward in the holarchy (or to the same level, in the social sciences) and exploring in a scientific spirit of inquiry, it is obvious that the appropriate epistemology is a participative one. Looking upward in the holarchy, it is apparent that the appropriate epistemology involves a holistic view in which the parts are understood through the whole. This epistemology will recognize the importance of subjective and cultural meanings in all human experience, including some religious or interpersonal experiences, that seem particularly rich in meaning even though they may be ineffable. In a holistic view, such meaningful experiences will not be explained away by reducing them to combinations of simpler experiences or to physiological or biochemical events. Rather, in a holistic approach, the meanings of experiences may be understood by discovering their interconnections with other meaningful experiences.

If this ontological stance is accepted, a good many seemingly opposing views in Western thought become reconciled. From the level of the human-holon, the scientist looks mainly downward in the holarchy; the mystic looks mainly upward. Science and religion are potentially two complementary and entirely congenial views; each needs the other for more completeness. In Western philosophy there have been three main ontological positions: the materialist-realist, the dualist, and the idealist. Again, the materialist looks downward, the idealist upward, and the dualist tries to reconcile fragments of the two—all represent but partial glimpses of the holarchic whole.

This new ontological stance takes some living with to fully appreciate how successfully it helps resolve many of the time-honored puzzles of Western philosophy—the mind-body problem, for example, and free will versus determinism. Since everything is part of the one holarchy, if consciousness or purpose is found anywhere (such as at the level of the scientist-holon), it is by that fact characteristic of the whole. It can neither be ruled out at the level of the microorganism, nor at the level of the Earth, or Gaia. Nor need we be nonplussed by evidence of alternative and complementary medicine concerned with experiences that don't fit with a materialist, reductionist ontology.

IMPLICATIONS FOR SCIENTIFIC EPISTEMOLOGICAL ASSUMPTIONS

As within the presently dominant concept of medical science, the epistemology implied by this ontological stance, and to some extent defensible even without it,[31] will insist on *open inquiry* and *public (intersubjective) validation* of knowledge; at the same time, it will recognize that these goals may, at any given time, be met only incompletely. Taking into account how both individual and collective perceptions are affected by unconsciously held beliefs and expectations, the limitations of intersubjective agreement are apparent.

This epistemology will be "radically empirical" in the sense urged by William James[31] in that it will be *phenomenological* or experiential in a broad sense. In other words, it will include subjective experience as primary data, rather than being essentially limited to physical-sense data. Further, it will address the totality of human experience—no reported phenomena will be written off because they "violate known scientific laws." Thus consciousness will not be conceptualized as a "thing" to be studied by an observer who is somehow apart from it; research on consciousness involves the interaction of the observer and the observed or, more accurately, the *experience* of observing.

This adequate epistemology will be, above all else, humble. It will recognize that science deals with *models and metaphors representing certain aspects of experienced reality*, and that any model or metaphor may be permissible if it is useful in helping to order knowledge, even though it may seem to conflict with another model that is also useful. (The classic example is the history of wave and particle models in physics.) This includes, specifically, the metaphor of consciousness. Perhaps this sounds strange?

Indeed, it is a peculiarity of modern science that it allows some kinds of metaphors and disallows others. For example, it is perfectly acceptable to use metaphors that derive directly from our experience of the physical world (such as "fundamental particles," or acoustic waves), as well as metaphors representing what can be measured only in terms of its effects (such as gravitational, electromagnetic, or quantum fields). It has further become acceptable in science to use more holistic and nonquantifiable metaphors such as organism, personality, ecological community, Gaia, universe. It is, however, taboo to use nonsensory "metaphors of mind"—metaphors that tap into images and experiences familiar from our own inner awareness. We are not allowed to say (according to the dominant scientific paradigm) that some aspects of our experience of reality are reminiscent of our experience of our own minds—to observe, for example, that some aspects of animal behavior appear as though they were tapping into some supraindividual nonphysical mind, or as though there were in instinctual behavior and in evolution something like our experience in our own minds of *purpose*.

The expanded epistemology we seek will recognize *the partial nature of all scientific concepts of causality*.[32,33] (For example, the "upward causation" of physiomotor action resulting from a brain state does not necessarily invalidate the "downward causation" implied in the subjective feeling of volition.) In other words, it will implicitly question the assumption that a nomothetic science—one characterized by inviolable "scientific laws"— can in the end adequately deal with causality. In some ultimate sense, there really is no causality—only the Whole evolving.

It will also recognize that prediction and control are not the only criteria by which to judge knowledge as scientific. As the French poet Antoine de Saint Exupéry put it, "Truth is not that which is demonstrable. Truth is that which is ineluctable." Here we find that the unquestioned authority of the objective and detached observer is challenged. In particular, the double-blind controlled experiment, considered the gold standard of clinical research, is thrown deeply into question if the consciousness of the experimenter or the clinician is causal.[34] An engaged epistemology will involve recognition of the inescapable role of *the personal characteristics of the observer*, including the processes and contents of the unconscious mind. The corollary follows that to be a competent investigator, the researcher must be *willing to risk being profoundly changed* through the process of exploration. Because of this potential transformation of observers, an epistemology that is acceptable now to the scientific community may in time have to be replaced by other, more satisfactory new criteria, for which it has laid the intellectual and experiential foundations.

BROADER IMPLICATIONS

Research on perception, hypnosis, dissociation, repression, selective attention, mental imagery, sleep and dreams, and memory and memory retrieval all suggests that the influence of the unconscious on how we experience ourselves and our environment may be far greater than is typically taken into account. Science itself has never been thoroughly reassessed in the light of this recently discovered pervasive influence of the unconscious mind of the scientist or the healing practitioner. The contents and processes of the unconscious individually and collectively influence perceptions, "rational thinking," openness to challenging evidence, ability to contemplate alternative conceptual frameworks and metaphors, scientific interests and disinterests, scientific judgment—all to an indeterminate extent. What is implied is that we must accept the presence of unconscious processes and contents, not as a minor perturbation but as a potentially major factor in the construction of any society's particular form of science. Again, we may have to re-evaluate the role of the experimenter effect in outcome studies, as well as our firm reliance on double-blind control studies and other assumptions about objectivity, materialism, and reductionism.

The implications of research in these areas go even further. They suggest holistic interconnection at levels yet to be fully recognized by Western medical science. The ontological stance of the universe as holarchy appears to have great promise as the basis for an extended science in which consciousness-related phenomena are no longer anomalies but keys to a deeper understanding—a science of medicine that transcends and includes the science we have. The most important thing is not to accept a particular answer but to open the dialogue about the metaphysical foundations of Western science and their relationship to understanding mind-body-spirit health and healing.

CONCLUSION

Science and society exist in a dialectical relationship. The findings of science have a profound effect on society; none of us has any doubts about that. But science is also a product of society, very much shaped by the cultural milieu within which it developed. Western science and medical science have the forms they do because science developed within a culture placing unusual value on the ability to predict and control.

What assumptions underlie the attempt to marry alternative and complementary medicine to the U.S. allopathic, science-based medicine? On the one hand, these approaches encourage openness to whatever has seemed to work in the past; diversity of approaches for a diversity of persons; empowerment of the individual to choose their own medical options and hence be more highly motivated in their own health care. On the other hand, if alternative medicine in the United States and elsewhere is to be fitted into the fee for services, power of the professional, managed care, and scientific assumption structure, it is likely to be subtly shaped by that structure so that its effectiveness may not be the same as in its original cultural context.

Besides the choice to ignore or adapt to the existing structure, there is a third choice—whole-system change.[35] We need to look at the forces that might make this plausible. How might society move toward a really integral system of healing?

References for this essay are located on the DVD accompanying this book.

The Technologies of Shamanic States of Consciousness[*]

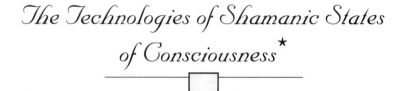

STANLEY KRIPPNER

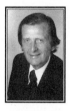

A LTHOUGH THE TERM *shaman* is of uncertain derivation, it is sometimes traced to the language of the Tungus reindeer-herders of Siberia, where the word *saman* translates into "one who is excited, moved, or raised."[1] An alternative translation for the Tungus word is "inner heat," and an alternative etymology is the Sanskrit word *śaman,* or "song."[2] Each of these terms applies to the activities of shamans, past and present, men and women who enter what are often described as "shamanic states of consciousness" in order to engage in spiritual practices that benefit their community.[3] Although Siberia is the site of original usage of the term *shaman,*[4]

---

[*]This study was supported by the Saybrook Graduate School and Research Center Chair for the Study of Consciousness. An earlier version of this paper appeared in *The Journal of Consciousness Studies* 7:93-118, 2000.

practitioners of shamanism appear around the world, not only in hunter-gatherer and fishing societies, but in centralized societies and urban centers as well. Shamanism can be described as a group of techniques that enables its practitioners to enter the "spirit world" to obtain information that is used to help and to heal members of their social group. This technology involves various types of mental and physical self-regulation; hence it is relevant to noetics, the scientific study of phenomena classified under such descriptors as "consciousness" and "mind."

THE *VELADAS* OF MARÍA SABINA

Mental and physical self-regulation can be observed in shamanic rituals, especially the healing rituals that afforded them an opportunity to express their community's conceptions of reality in a social setting. Shamanic rituals were essential to the career of the Mazatec Indian María Sabina, who lived in the state of Oaxaca, Mexico. Since childhood, María Sabina had been interested in herbs and worked for a period of time as a *curandera,* or herbalist. Later, she felt that she had been called to become a *sabía* (i.e., "one who knows") and ingested psilocybin mushrooms as a way of "knowing" the condition and treatment of her clients.

As a *sabía,* or shamanic healer, María Sabina manifested considerable self-control during her *veladas,* chanting liturgies containing an overlay of Roman Catholic imagery that cloaked the odes used by the Indian priests who had been overthrown by the Spaniards in the 1520s. The Spanish Inquisition outlawed the *veladas,* but the Mazatecs took them underground for 4 centuries.

One night, María Sabina dreamed that it was her mission to share this sacred knowledge with the world. Soon after this dream, on June 29, 1955, a group of U.S. investigators headed by R. Gordon Wasson arrived. Eventually, doña María and the psilocybin mushrooms were featured in *Life* magazine, and the field of ethnomycology was born.[5,6]

Doña María's reported dream is unique for several reasons: It ran counter to the attempts of male elders to keep their practices secret, and its egalitarian and universal motive violated the political power of her society's male hierarchy. She paid dearly for this action; her grocery store was burned to the ground, and her son was murdered.

María Sabina's worldview is expressed in her chants; in one, she apparently alludes to her shamanic journeys:

> I am a woman who flies.
> I am the sacred eagle woman, [the mushroom] says;
> I am the Lord eagle woman;
> I am the lady who swims;
> Because I can swim in the immense,
> Because I can swim in all forms.
> I am the shooting star woman,
> I am the shooting star woman beneath the water,
> I am the lady doll,
> I am the sacred clown,
> Because I can swim,
> Because I can fly.[5]

Doña María's feelings of unity with nature and with the spirit world are revealed by another set of chants; the lyrics also portray her active role in attaining knowledge:

> I have the heart of the Virgin,
> I have the heart of Christ,
> I have the heart of the Father,
> I have the heart of the Old One,
> It's that I have the same soul,
> The same heart as the saint, as the saintess;
> I am a spirit woman,
> A woman of good words, good breath, good saliva,
> I am the little woman of the great expanse of the waters,
> I am the little woman of the expanse of the divine sea.
> I am a woman who looks into the insides of things,
> A woman who investigates, Holy Father,
> I am a woman born, I am a child born,
> I am a woman fallen into the world.[5]

In other words, María Sabina employed an investigative way of knowing; she looked "into the insides of things." She and other shamans learn from "the spirits," "the waters," and "the divine sea." Tradition and holy writ might provide source material for the shaman, but it is the life experiences mediated by his or her "heart" and "soul" that are the final arbiters of knowledge.

SHAMANISM AS A BIOLOGICALLY DERIVED SPECIALIZATION

Winkelman[7] proposed that María Sabina and other shamans represent a "biologically derived" human specialization and that these potentials are actualized through social adaptations. This proposition could be used to explain the ubiquitous appearance of shamans as well as the fundamental role of altered conscious states and/or heightened perception in shamanic healing and divination practices.

These potentials can be described as "neurognostic" because they involve neural networks that provide the biological substrate for ways of knowing[8] (i.e., an epistemology). I would add that these neurognostic potentials are not the exclusive domain of shamans; primordial humans performed healing and divinatory functions themselves before specialization established a hierarchy. Evidence for this position can be found in fairly egalitarian tribal societies such as the Kung of southwestern Africa, where about half the males and a sizable number of females shamanize, producing the "boiling energy" (i.e., sweat) used in their healing rituals.[9]

Neurognostic potentials provide the basis for those patterns of perception, cognition, and affect (i.e., "consciousness") that are structured by an organism's neurological systems. They are probably reflected in what Jungians call an *archetype*, a term that can be conceptualized as a predisposition that provides organizing principles for the basic modes of consciousness and elementary behavior patterns, including the intuitive capacity to initiate, control, and mediate everyday behavior.

Stevens[10] suggests that "from the viewpoint of modern neurology, Jung's work stands as a brilliant vindication of...the value of intuitive knowledge." When ritualized shamanic performance is described as archetypal, the activity reflects biologically based modes of consciousness, a replacement of the ordinary waking state through discharge patterns that produce interhemispheric synchronization and coherence, limbic-cortex integration, and integral discharges that synthesize cognition, affect, and behavior.[11]

In this regard, Shweder[12] found that Zinacanteco shamans in Mexico possess cognitive capacities that distinguish them from non-shamans, such as having available a number of constructive categories, imposing these forms onto ambiguous situations; these integrative capacities may have facilitated the development of shamanic epistemologies over the millennia.

A variety of procedures, agents, and other technologies are available to evoke limbic system slow wave discharges that synchronize the frontal cortex.[13] In addition, shamans—as a group—can be characterized as "fantasy-prone,"[14] endowed with capacities, genetic to some degree, that facilitate their use of imaginative processes. Fantasy-proneness exists on a continuum; most humans engage in fantasy, imagination, and play (especially "pretending" and "role-playing") periodically, but shamans draw upon this trait for their specialization.

Many of the early shamans may not have been dependent on transient consciousness alteration but manifested a heightened perceptual style that was part of their everyday state of consciousness. Berman[15] suggested that "heightened awareness" may be a more accurate description of shamanic consciousness than "altered states" because their intense experience of the natural world is described by them in such terms as "things often seem to blaze."

Paradoxically, shamans are characterized both by an acute perception of their environment and by imaginative fantasy. These traits (the ability to construct categories, the potential for pretending and role-playing, and the capacity to experience the natural world vividly) gave shamans an edge over peers who had simply embraced life as it presented itself, without the filters of myth or ritual.[15]

All of these traits may be related to the evolution of the human brain—namely the development of specialized subsystems that are activated during shifts in consciousness. The hallmark of cortical evolution is not the ever-increasing sophistication of specialized cortical circuitry but an increasing representational flexibility that allows environmental factors to shape the human brain's structure and function.[16]

Pinker[17] proposed that the "mind" is made up of many modules, each honed by aeons of evolution, and shamans may have learned to integrate these modules.[18] If so, shamanic technologies represent the initial institutionalized practices for this integration, both through shifts in consciousness and community bonding rituals.[7] These practices became codified in the form of myth, ritual, and ceremony, providing for social solidarity and specialization. Shamanic healing practices could be identified as the initial "integrative medicine" because they helped reconcile individuals with their community, provided internal integration (e.g., between "mind" and "body," between internal attitudes and external behavior).

SHAMANIC TECHNOLOGIES

Eliade[19] wrote about the "technologies of the sacred," and shamanism can be described as a collection of these technologies. In psychological terms, shamans are socially designated practitioners who self-regulate their attentional states to obtain information unavailable to other members of their social group. Shamans were probably humanity's original specialists, combining the roles of healers, storytellers, weather forecasters, performing artists, ritualists, and magicians.

The oral traditions that preserved the myths that structured a culture's identity and worldview may not have been originated by shamans but appear to have been passed down by them.[20] For example, María Sabina and her fellow shamans preserved, in their chants and rituals, Mazatec mythologies for more than 4 centuries, preserving their cultural identity in the face of Spanish oppression. To facilitate this societal function, many shamans developed techniques to assist the elicitation and movement of "inner heat," to enable their shamanic journeys, and to facilitate their contact with the "upper" and "lower" worlds. This technology allowed them to encounter spirit entities, ancestral spirits, the tribe's animal totems, and other resources that had found their way into mythological songs and stories.

Epistemology is concerned with the nature, characteristics, and processes of knowledge, and I am suggesting that shamanic epistemology drew upon perceptual, cognitive, affective, and somatic ways of knowing that assisted early humans to find their way through an often unpredictable, sometimes hostile series of environmental challenges. Not only did early humans have to become aware of potentially dangerous environmental objects and activities, they needed to have explanatory stories (enacted as mythic rituals) at their disposal to navigate through the contingencies of daily encounters and challenges. The acute perceptual abilities of shamans, in combination with their intuition and imagination, met their societies' needs.

Postmodernists hold that there can be many viable worldviews, depending on who is asking the question and the methodology used in answering it.[21] Tribal people did not necessarily insist that their mythic worldview was applicable to the lives of their neighbors. Therefore the case can be made that postmodernists have returned full circle to certain premodern shamanic perspectives, regaining valuable aspects of an epistemology that was denigrated as a result of colonization and conquest.

Shamanic eclecticism and syncretization was apparent in my interviews with María Sabina, who put her epistemology into concrete terms. At the time of our interviews, doña María had retired from active shamanizing, but she told me, "When someone came to me for help, we would eat the mushrooms together. Jesus Christ is in the mushrooms, and he revealed to us the solution to the problem." Wasson[22] observed that the mythical origin of doña María's *veladas* dates back to the time when Piltzintecuhtli, the "Noble Infant," received the sacred plants as a gift from Quetzalcoatl. Doña María's references to Jesus represent a synthesis of the Christian and the pre-Conquest religions.

SHAMANIC STATES OF CONSCIOUSNESS

The word *consciousness* is used in various ways, but I define it as the pattern of an organism's perceptual, cognitive, and affective activities and/or experiences at a given moment in time. An alteration of consciousness is a significant shift or deviation in an organism's customary pattern, as experienced by that organism and/or as observed by others. Some of these shifts have been considered "states" of consciousness because they are marked by behaviors and experiences that typically cluster together; each society has its own conception of what constitutes an "ordinary" state of consciousness and what may be considered "changed," "alternative," or "altered" states of consciousness. According to Wade,[23] "virtually all shamanic experiences occur in an altered state, which cannot be regarded as a naturally-occurring developmental stage."

On their arrival in North America, Jesuit priests were shocked by the behavior of Ojibway Indians during their traditional healing procedures. It was customary for Ojibway *wabeno* (shamans) to heal by means of drumming, rattling, chanting, dancing erotically (while naked), and handling live coals. The *wabeno* then rubbed their heated hands over the client while chanting the songs previously learned in their vision quests.[24] Among the Dieguenos and Luisenos Indians of southern California, potential shamans were selected at as early as 9 years of age on the basis of their dreams. It was important that a prospective shaman in these tribes also had visionary experiences that resulted from ingesting such mind-altering plants as datura, or jimson weed, during their ceremonials. During these altered states, the novice received a guardian spirit in the form of an animal totem as well as healing songs and other knowledge about cures and dream interpretation.[25]

Symbolic manipulation is apparent in shamanic rituals, and altered states often help to access these symbols. Symbols are more than ritual markers that denote the beginning, middle, or end of the process; they serve as keys that unlock the door to a full participation in the ritual, taking participants into another order of reality, where spirits come to life and healing dramas unfold.[26] The drum often symbolizes the "World Tree" that the shaman needs to climb so as to reach the "upper world" (or descend to the "lower world") during the altered state. What they find in these realms differs from society to society; in some, the "upper world" is the home of ancestors, but for others, they reside in the "lower world."

The ritualistic blowing of smoke in four directions symbolizes an appeal to spirits in the "four quarters" of the universe. Directionality is apparent in the elaborate Navaho sand paintings that the shamans destroy after they have served their purpose. Symbolism is also evident in the reports from those vision quests of the Plains Indians that helped future warriors contact their guardian spirits. Dobkin de Rios[27] describes these quests as attempts at "personal ecstatic learning" in the service of eliciting biochemical changes in the body that would enhance the altered state. Hence, tribal shamans played an important role in preparing, instructing, and guiding their initiates, as well as interpreting their visions.

Since the time of Goethe, many scholars have proposed that the epistemology of primordial people began with their sensorimotor experiences.[28] According to these scholars, mythmaking, a basic propensity of humankind, has its referents in bodily functions as well as in observable nature. Sansonese[29] notes, "The more ancient the myth, the more often do parts of the human body play an explicit role in the myth"—for example, Adam's Rib and the Egyptian myth of Set and Isis.

It will be recalled that one of the possible derivations for the term "shaman" is "one who is excited, moved, or raised" while another is "inner heat"; both refer to bodily processes and the appreciation of the sensory world. In addition, they both are examples of politicized talents (along with fire mastery, symbolic death, and entering "trance" states) that privatize shamanism and restrict its membership.

THE EVOLVING MIND

In his account of the evolution of the human mind, Mithen[30] describes the emergence of general intelligence as well as of four specialized "cognitive domains"—namely, technical intelligence, social intelligence, natural history intelligence, and language. It is likely that these "domains" share information in what Baars[31] refers to as a "global workspace." Consistent with Newton's[32] emphasis on language as a tool for communication, Mithen[30] holds that language was originally social.

Once the capacity for language was present, it was highly adaptive, eventually providing early humans with the ability to reflect on their own and other people's mental states. In this way, it began to interact with social intelligence and, still later, early humans were able to talk about tool-making (technical intelligence) as well as hunting and plant-gathering (natural history intelligence). Such capacities were advantageous because they could construct more accurate, hence more adaptable, models and descriptions of external events.[33]

Once these intelligences became linked across their respective domains, the resulting "linkage" enabled the production of symbolic artifacts and images as a means of communication. It also led to the essentially human tendency to attribute personality and social relationships to plants and animals, a result of the integration of social intelligence and natural history intelligence. Artifacts indicating human body decoration (e.g., pieces of ocher) date back 80,000 years or more[34]; other artifacts demonstrating the capacity for visual decoration (e.g., beads, pendants) date back 40,000 years,[30] to the time after the Cro-Magnon people emerged. A human-shaped ivory statuette from Hohlenstein-Stadel in southern Germany is the earliest existing statuette and has been dated at 30,000 to 33,000 years.[30] The origins of shamanism are often traced back at least 30,000 years.[19] In Western Europe, the Upper Paleolithic era began some 35,000 years ago, and is best known for its remarkable efflorescence of image making.[35] For example, the paintings in the Lascaux caves of southern France date back 17,000 years.

There are a plethora of geometric forms thought by some to be signatures of the artists; if so, this convention was not revived until the Renaissance. Some animals have been cleverly painted so that they share body parts, while other figures are superimposed on each other and are distinguished by color shading.[36,37] And, for some observers, the most exceptional feature of the drawings is their narrative form; they appear to tell a story.[38] I agree with Tattersall's[39] comment that upon leaving Lascaux, one is overawed by the magnificence of what these remote ancestors wrought many millennia ago. However, Hughes[40] noted that the rock paintings in the sacred cave sites scattered across northwestern Australia "are as impressive as anything in the caves of Lascaux or Altamira, and tens of thousands of years older. As far as we know, The Australian Aborigines stood at the very dawn of human image-making." To some, these features in the European caves suggest a search for spirit animals that could become "allies" if they could be drawn by shamans through a permeable "membrane" that separated the ordinary and the nonordinary worlds.[40] In the Niaux cave, for example, the shadows cast across the rock can represent, to the expectant eye, the outline of a bison; then only a few deft strokes were needed to add the rest of the body. If the light is moved, the animal disappears back through the "membrane." The person has thus mastered the spirit animal; he or she can make it come and go at will. Once more, Berman[15] cautions that there are other explanations for the profusion of animal images, one of them a simple desire to execute a naturalistic portrayal. Sometimes, grazing deer are simply grazing deer.

Symbolic or not, Winkelman[18] points out that neuropsychology provides a basis for these rock art motifs; hardwired, neurologically structured perceptual constants are the structural basis of these motifs, reflecting perceptions obtained through shamanic states of consciousness. The animal images reflect "the importance of neurognostic perspectives in understanding shamanism."

Clottes and Lewis-Williams[35] have stated that "all shamanic activity and experience necessarily take place within a particular kind of universe, or cosmos. [But] the ways in which this shamanic cosmos is conceived are generated by the human nervous system rather than by intellectual speculation or detached observation of the environment." For me, neurognostic potentials and social construction operate in tandem, and the ensuing dance produces a phenomenon that needs to be examined from the vantage point of both perspectives.

Commenting on the paintings themselves, Mithen[30] deduces, "There is nothing gradual about the evolution of the capacity for art: the very first pieces that we find can be compared in quality with those produced by the great artists of the Renaissance.... All that was needed was a connection between these cognitive processes which had evolved for other tasks to create the wonderful paintings in Chauvet Cave," which date back some 30,000 years. Also predating Lascaux was the extraction of decorative red and black pigment from Bomvu Ridge, in South Africa, some 40,000 years ago.[41]

The magnificent distinctiveness of these works is noteworthy in view of Ludwig's[42] proposition that "the visionary or magic function of these media...was more important than esthetics":

> The shaman artist...employed carved masks, music and art for the purposes of healing, negotiation with unseen spirits, exerting magical influences on creatures, and depicting his [or her] adventures in the spirit world.[42]

Again, neurognostic structures can be hypothesized to have formed the basis for these creative products; Clottes (as cited in Gore, 2000[43]) asserts, "People can no longer say art evolved from crude beginnings."

The sepia, black, and red ocher used in the Chauvet, Altamira, and Lascaux paintings might be symbolic. However, Berman[15] offers an alternative: The experience of these early humans was direct and immediate. This epistemology runs through many postmodern writings; for example, Globus[44] remarks, "We do not know reality, according to postmodernism, by means of any representations of reality. We know reality directly and immediately; there is nothing that gets between us and the reality we always and already find ourselves in."

Modernity, in contrast, relies on representations of reality—mental and neural representations that mediate between humanity and the world. In other words, modern epistemologies assume that an investigator can provide a near-identical match between words and the phenomena they attempt to describe. Postmodern epistemologies assume that this type of representation is impossible, and that symbolism, metaphor, and allegory provide better descriptions of outer and inner experience; several descriptions, some of them paradoxical, frequently are used to "deconstruct" a phenomenon in an attempt to creatively fathom it.

THE SEARCH FOR "REALITY"

Western science is characterized by a search for satisfactory explanations of "reality." This search is achieved by statements of general principles; these can be tested experimentally or through repeated observations.[45] Shamanic epistemology also attempts to explain "reality," employs repeated observations, and makes statements about general principles. However, credence is given to revelation and inspiration from the "spirit world," from plant and animal "allies," and from "journeys" associated with changed states of consciousness. A provocative example is the complex brew *ayahuasca,* which goes by many other names, depending on the part of the Amazon where it is used. Shamans have imbibed *ayahuasca* for hundreds of years, but its origin remains a mystery to Western investigators. Some tribes attribute this knowledge to spiritual beings from subaquatic realms, others to the intervention of giant serpents.[46]

Narby[47] comments,

> Here are people without electron microscopes who choose, among 80,000 Amazonian plant species, the leaves of a bush containing a...brain hormone, which they combine with a vine containing substances that inactivate an enzyme of the digestive tract, which would otherwise block the effect. And they do this to modify their consciousness. It is as if they knew about the molecular properties of plants and the art of combining them, and when one asks them how they knew these things, they say their knowledge comes directly from [the] plants.

For three decades, I worked with an intertribal medicine man and shamanic healer, Rolling Thunder. When I asked him how he was able to identify the curative power of plants he had never used previously, he told me, "I ask the plant what it is good for. Some plants are only meant to be beautiful. Other plants are meant for food. Still others are to be used as medicine. Once a healing plant has spoken to me, I ask its permission to take it with me and add it to my medicine pouch." Rolling Thunder's epistemology was remarkably similar to that of the Amazonian shamans who work with *ayahuasca*.

Reports reminiscent of shamanic epistemology and technologies appear from time to time in first-person descriptions regarding technical and creative accomplishments. Robert Louis Stevenson wrote that ideas for some of his short stories came from the "little people" who influenced his dreams. Giuseppe Tartini dreamed that a devil composed a piece of violin music for him, which he later transcribed. Sriniwasa Ramanujan noted that the Hindu goddess Namakkal provided him with original mathematical insights while he dreamed. Herman Hilprecht attributed an archeological discovery to a Babylonian priest who visited him in a dream. Francisco Candido Xavier's prodigious literary output was supposedly made possible by discarnate "spirits" who dictated his poetry, plays, and best-selling novels. Johannes Brahms confided that his best symphonic work was divinely inspired (e.g., Krippner & Dillard[48]).

In a world beset by quandaries and crises, survival no longer depends upon the process of natural selection or chance mutations but rather on intentional deliberations and conscientious decision-making. Western modernity has failed to build a universal human culture upon a foundation of abstract rational thought.

Humanity cannot repeat the past, but postmodernity would do well to reconsider the personal, metaphorical language that the Royal Society of London deliberately scuttled in its attempt to produce a universal language of objective and unequivocal symbols.[49] The failure of this project ignored one of the points permeating this essay: Language makes use of the same structures as those involved in sensorimotor activity; these structures take the form of analog models of reality, and the resulting images ground humankind's concepts, constructs, and intentions.

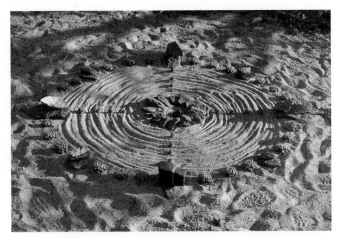

"Circle in the Sand." (Courtesy Michael Eller.)

Shamanic technologies first and foremost were devoted to finding game animals, locating and using medicinal plants, determining the best time to plant and harvest crops, and other matters of daily survival. Shamanic technologies also had spiritual uses, but contemporary Westerners often emphasize the transcendental side of shamanism to the neglect of its practical aspects.

Vandervert[50] proposes that so-called "image-schemas" are not tantamount to the organism's storehouse of images, but the space-time representations that co-exist with perceptual processes, both of which precede mental imagery. These space-time simulation structures are genetic in origin and are responsible for the state-estimating functions that are connected to the cerebrum's mapping systems. The resulting image-schemas are whetted by experience as well as by developmental processes.

Vandervert's proposal that image-schemas represent "foundational meanings" is reminiscent of Jung's description of archetypes, the structural predispositions that allegedly provide the organizing principles for consciousness and behavior. These image-schemas collectively represent what Vandervert considers to be a "calculus" of archetypal processing.[50]

The nervous system evolved in ways that enabled it to foresee many future events, and rapid simulation was the basic approach to survival-conducive prediction.[51] The nervous system's ability to produce such simulation structures as image-schemas permitted anticipatory, feed-forward processing.[52] For Vandervert,[50] image-schemas represent the foundational structures needed "for modeling/mapping functions conducive for survival." Without this ability to make estimates of future conditions, vertebrate organisms could not have survived to reproduce. According to Vandervert, the auditory-vocal sharing of image-schematics eventually led to language.[50]

I would propose that the image-schemas of those men and women whom a community held to be shamanic practitioners were especially adept when prediction was demanded. Game needed to be located, weather patterns needed to be forecast, enemy movements needed to be anticipated, and escape routes needed to be discovered. These tasks required feedforward processing, and the shamanic fine-tuning of image-schemas through heightened perception and/or changed states of consciousness may have assisted this assignment.

Such neurognostic frameworks are needed to integrate human neurophysiology with human epistemology and to explore what Chalmers[53] refers to as "the hard problem": how consciousness arises from physical systems. "While evolution can be very useful in explaining why particular physical systems have evolved, it is irrelevant to the explanation of the bridging principles by virtue of which some of these systems are conscious."

One final example from the life of María Sabina demonstrates these image-schemas. When she was called to shamanize, doña María received the image of an open book that grew until it reached the size of a person. She was told, "This is the Book of Wisdom. It is the Book of Language. Everything that is written in it is for you. The Book is yours, take it so that you can work." In accepting this call, doña María became a "woman of language" and what Rothenberg[54] calls a "great oral poet."

Now may be the time to reconsider the ways of knowing exemplified by doña María and their sources in imagination, intuition, visions, dreams, the senses, and the body. Perhaps these ways of knowing can enter into tandem with intellect and reason to construct cooperative and collaborative lifestyles for the pluralistic world in which we live, a world that shamanic epistemology would appreciate and enjoy, a world that shamanic technology would strive to honor and protect.

References for this essay are located on the DVD accompanying this book.

Multiple Ways of Knowing[*]

FRANCES VAUGHAN

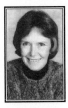

CONNECTING THE INNER world of mind and spirit to the outer world of action is our "common work"—yet each of us approaches it from our own unique perspective. What is common is our search for connections that are meaningful. What is different is the variety of viewpoints.

Professionally (as scientists, philosophers, and therapists) and personally (no matter what our career may be), all of us are engaged in "consciousness work." The greatest danger in this work is to mistake what a single viewpoint reveals as though it were the whole.

The task facing us is this: How do we build those bridges that enable us, with mutual respect and understanding, to expand the dialogue so we

---

[*]Adapted from "Essential Dimensions of Consciousness: Objective, Subjective, and Intersubjective," presented at the conference "Toward a Science of Consciousness," Tucson, Arizona, April 1998. In *Noetic Sciences Review* 47:34, Winter 1998.

can come to appreciate a wide variety of points of view? What's called for is the ability to hold different perspectives at the same time.

To move toward a more integral theory of consciousness—one that includes a variety of perspectives—we need to distinguish between the objective, subjective, and intersubjective approaches. Each contributes in its own way to the exploration of consciousness. Standard science has a lot to say about objective approaches, so I won't say much about objectivity here, except that it tends to describe the world and our experience in terms of separation between the observer and the object observed. It's about "I-it" relationships. The problem with the objective approaches is that they don't address questions of value, meaning, and purpose.

When we explore subjectivity, we're talking about our own experience, our own internal sense of meaning. This is how we connect our inner life with our outer work in the world. This is as true for scientists, philosophers, and humanists as it is for transpersonal psychologists. We all need to acknowledge and attend to our subjectivity when we speak about consciousness. We know, for example, that all our perceptions are filtered through our own subjectivity. Our emotions, our feelings, our worldviews all color what we perceive in the world. Not only that, but we tend to find what we look for. And we know that our experience tends to reinforce our beliefs—but our beliefs also shape our experience.

Furthermore, we also know that our beliefs and concepts are embedded in cultural contexts—and so we need to be attentive to intersubjective perspectives as well. We may think we have an independent, objective point of view, but in fact we are the product of social conditioning. So even though the objective approach often claims to be meaning-free, it may contain meaning all the same. Perhaps it's just that science cannot apprehend it.

Meaning is essential to our lives, and it is important to recognize that, subjectively, we overlay meanings on our actions in the world. When we overlook the fact that we attribute meaning to what we do (otherwise we wouldn't be doing it), then we are likely not to recognize our blind spots, our own misperceptions.

Intersubjectivity can help fill in our perceptual and cognitive "blind spots" by revealing to us aspects of the world that we might otherwise miss or distort. We know we can be fooled by our senses; that's quite clear.

What is often more difficult to realize is that we can be just as easily fooled by introspection. Subjectivity, like so-called objectivity, is fallible. In sorting out what we know, I think it is important that we differentiate how we know. For instance, using our senses (sensory empiricism) differs from rational analysis (rationalism), and contemplative knowing (transcendental intuition) is further distinguishable from both sensory empiricism and rationalism.

Most of the work in science is based on sensory and rational ways of knowing. But expertise in one area doesn't mean we understand or have access to knowledge derived from another. Thinking rationally about consciousness is very different from observing events going on in the brain, and both of these are very different from our subjective experiences of consciousness in contemplative practice.

Sometimes all of us—scientists, philosophers, humanists—suffer from a kind of narrow vision: We get so engrossed in a particular field, and each field has so much to learn and so much to understand, that we forget there are other domains and other ways of knowing that also require training and attention.

Appropriate discipline-specific training is needed in all domains. If you are going to explore consciousness as a brain function, you will train to be a neuroscientist; if you are going to study consciousness as a metaphysical phenomenon, you will train in philosophy; if you are going to study consciousness through "inner empiricism," you will train in one of the contemplative disciplines. An integral approach to consciousness studies will recognize that each domain has its own limitations.

The different modes of knowing, such as using the senses, reason, and contemplation, can take different perspectives—first-person subjective, second-person intersubjective, and third-person objective. The three modes of knowing do not map neatly onto the three perspectives, though we may say, roughly, that contemplation is subjective, verbal reasoning or language is intersubjective, and the senses are objective.

Whichever perspective we engage, and whichever way of knowing we use, a common procedure underlies any worthwhile approach to the common work of relating inner experience to outer action. It's useful to remember that every domain of knowledge—whether it's objective, subjective, or intersubjective—follows a three-phase way of knowing, outlined by Ken Wilber: First, there's an injunction (to follow this or that procedure), then there's the apprehension (of data observed or experienced as a result of that procedure), and then there's the confirmation or verification (of the data by comparing observations/experiences with a peer group who have likewise followed this process). Whether our work is in the hard sciences, in the so-called soft sciences, or in spiritual development, we still need to be willing to follow the injunction, do the training, learn from our own experience—really have a direct experience—and then have that confirmed, by checking it out with others who are also knowledgeable in that area of understanding. I think that's probably one of the most fundamental areas of common ground underlying all these three perspectives.

If we are to move toward a more integral approach to consciousness, we will acknowledge all perspectives, all the different ways of knowing, and include all the different ways of investigating and talking about this topic.

It's often been said that humanity, even the world, is now in a race between consciousness and catastrophe (a new twist on "the human race"). That's why I think it is so vitally important that we acknowledge that whatever we're doing as individuals is only a very small piece of the puzzle. Instead of being caught up in academic politics or competitiveness, we need to find ways of collaborating—it's vitally important for the human race. Consciousness exploration is definitely a joint effort.

We do not exist as separate and isolated beings. We all exist in an intricate network of mutually conditioned relationships (the domain of transcendent intersubjectivity or trans-subjectivity)—and, to me, this is clearly the context we need to hold as we pursue our interest in consciousness studies. As we explore intersubjective consciousness, we will recognize the difference between what Martin Buber called "I-thou" relationships and "I-it" relationships—the difference between relating to others as centers of vital subjectivity like ourselves, or as vacuous objects, mere "things."

If, as many spiritual traditions tell us, consciousness pervades nature through and through, then we can, and should, relate to nature—both terrestrial and cosmic—as consisting of vital, sentient, subjective beings, not as dead, objective things. We will then recognize the connection that exists between each one of us and the whole of nature.

What is real to one person may be an illusion to another. We need a community of peers to validate and confirm our experiences, and we need to remember that, to a great extent, we do create the world that we inhabit by the way we think. The Buddha said: "With our thoughts we make the world." And from a Christian tradition: "The concept of the self stands like a shield, a silent barricade before the truth. When concepts of the self have been laid by, is truth revealed exactly as it is.

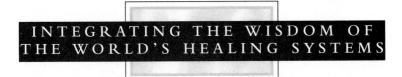
Restoration of Dynamic Balance: Traditional Ways of Healing Expressed Through Navajo Consciousness

NANCY C. MARYBOY
DAVID H. BEGAY

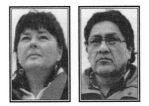

IT HAS BEEN SAID THAT there is more written about the Navajos than almost any other indigenous peoples. Countless books have been focused on traditional Navajo ceremonies: the process, symbolism, sandpaintings, chants, and other aspects of traditional Navajo healing. The majority of these books and articles portray multiple aspects of Navajo healing as seen and interpreted through the perceptions of the (primarily non-Indian) authors themselves, but seldom as seen and understood through the minds of the Dine, the Navajo people. In this chapter we will address aspects of traditional Navajo healing as understood and lived for generations in the American Southwest. In order to discuss Navajo healing processes, however, it is necessary to explore the context in which traditional healing is understood and in which it takes place, since the very processes are holistic and interrelated with all that exists in the universe.

AUTHORS' EXPERIENCE ON THE NAVAJO NATION

The authors both live and work on the Navajo Nation, a reservation that occupies a sizeable area of the states of Arizona, New Mexico, and Utah, comparable in size to West Virginia. This area is a small reflection of the greater area that was once roamed by the nomadic and later pastoral Athabaskan peoples, including the Navajo and Apache.

The authors have worked at Dine College, the Navajo tribal college, and at a K-12 BIA Grant/Charter school located in the far western section of the Navajo Reservation. They provided field research for the Navajo Healing Project, sponsored by the National Institute of Mental Health and Case Western Reserve University during the 1990s, conducting 8 years of interviews with Navajo patients and healers. Dr. Begay is a full-blooded Navajo, and Dr. Maryboy is Cherokee and Navajo. Both come from families of ceremonial practitioners.

TRADITIONAL NAVAJO WAYS OF KNOWING

Among the Navajos living on the Navajo Nation, the largest indigenous sovereign nation in the United States today, there might be little consensus as to what Navajo "religion" or Navajo healing is. There are three major arenas of belief that compete and, in some cases, exist in harmony that are most active today. Most Navajo people live in accordance with tenets of faith of traditional Navajo ways of knowing or those of Christianity or the Native American Church, which can incorporate aspects of Christianity or be wholly indigenous to areas of the southwest and Mexico. However, for the purpose of this chapter, we will concentrate on the traditional Navajo ways of knowing, as expressed through the complexity of the ancient Navajo language, and how these ways of knowing inform and address aspects of healing.

TRADITIONAL NAVAJO HEALING PROCESS: HOLISTIC AND COSMIC

Outside the Navajo Reservation little is understood of how the body, mind, and spirit are perceived through the traditional Dine (Navajo) consciousness, especially as the interconnections relate to the Navajo healing process, a holistic and dynamic process with immense cosmic interrelationships. It is extremely difficult to describe an indigenous holistic healing process through a nonholistic language such as English, especially when the worldviews are so dissimilar and so few people possess the detailed linguistic and ceremonial knowledge in both English and Navajo languages.

LANGUAGE AS A REFLECTION OF CONSCIOUSNESS

Language is a reflection of consciousness and is reflected in worldviews, ways of viewing and being in a world surrounding and acknowledged by a people. The English language, being a language of separatism and reductionism that depends on static entities, is heavily reliant upon the domination of nouns. Most indigenous languages, on the other hand, are composed of verbs, process and motion concepts, ways of being and living in the universe. As indigenous cultures have been (forcibly and in some cases willingly) exposed to what have become dominant cultures in local areas, the indigenous peoples have been required to express Euroamerican concepts of separatism and static entities through traditional thought processes of movement and interrelationship. This has not always led to true communication and understanding and is true for both cultures in what we might call borderland areas.

IMPACT OF CHRISTIANITY ON NAVAJO LANGUAGE

Writers of standard academic English have used words such as religion, God, spirit, art, and healing to describe traditional Navajo processes, yet the translations are imperfect and in most cases provide only superficial or actually misleading meanings of significance. Missionaries to the Navajo during the last century and a half have translated the Bible into the Navajo language, transforming an oral language into a written word. This same process occurred in many native communities across the United States. The translations were primarily facilitated in order to further the process of Christianization, the dark underside of which was to eliminate the native ways of knowing.

Some religions, such as Catholic and Episcopalian, retained enough cultural aspects of the indigenous ways as to impart a native and inclusive flavor to the services of worship. Other groups, primarily Pentacostal in nature, actively sought to destroy any vestiges of traditional native practices, as completely incompatible with the new religion. Even today you will hear of Pentacostal families destroying medicine bundles and other traditional items by fire, despised as symbols and labeled as actual tools of the devil.

The process of translating the Bible involved the use of standard academic linguistic skills, transforming oral sounds into written phonemes and morphemes, leading to a complex system of writing and a written dictionary. In an academic sense it is said that the Navajo language is one of the most difficult languages in the world, comparable in difficulty to Basque, Hungarian or Saami.

DIFFERENT LANGUAGES CARRY DIFFERENT WORLDVIEWS

Academic translations, however, do not begin to do justice to the richness, complexity and cosmic aspects of an oral language based on process and motion, relationship and interrelationship. It may be difficult for a non-native to understand the strong emphasis placed on language. From a monolingual English point of view, it seems that different languages are just different labels for the same things in the world. From the native consciousness, however, language is of extreme importance, carrying a worldview that is rich and different from the Cartesian world.

What do we mean by "carrying a worldview?" A culture's worldview cannot be expressed in its richness and complexity without the thoughts and words needed to articulate and support it. When you lose a language, you lose the intellectual and spiritual complexity of a way of being in the world. Among indigenous peoples, language is far more than a way of expression; it is also an internal manifestation of one's essence, life, and consciousness.

INDIGENOUS LANGUAGES REFLECT A DIFFERENT COSMOVISION

There is an enormous difference between an English speaker learning French, for example, and a Navajo speaker learning English. In the first case, one is remaining within the IndoEuropean linguistic family and expressing the Western worldview. In the second case, one is making a transition to an entirely different language stock and an entirely different non-native cosmovision. The indigenous speaker is naturally thinking and talking as a participant in his or her universe, whereas the English speaker is thinking and talking as a nonparticipant, one who is separated from and dominant over nature. As we will see, these differences have tremendous ramifications in discussing the nature of consciousness and healing.

Every language has its own characteristics, beauty, aesthetics, and ability to express what the speaker desires to say. Each language can discuss certain ideas more eloquently and specifically than others. Leanne Hinton, who has written widely on California Indian languages, points out that "our language does not limit us to certain viewpoints, but it does guide us strongly along particular mental pathways. And from this perspective, languages are far more than words and arbitrary rules of grammar, they are windows to whole systems of beliefs and values."[1]

INDIGENOUS KNOWING IS ONGOING FLUX-OF-BEING

Knowing is consciousness. Native knowing is native consciousness expressed as a holistic, integral way of living. Native ways of knowing are native ways of being human as manifested through living. This includes concepts of reciprocity, within a context of dynamic balance and harmony. Also included are social concepts of kinship and communal relationship, within a pragmatic ecological consciousness. Deep knowing is grounded in the native language. Because the native language is expressing a native consciousness that is holistic, both direct and indirect means of knowing are utilized. Means and knowing are intrinsically connected in the Navajo language. In Navajo one could say that knowing is not a static state of being but rather an ongoing state of being or ongoing flux of being.

Perhaps the closest approximation to indigenous holistic thinking today is occurring in the subatomic realm of quantum physics, wherein scientists are learning that the English language has no words to describe what they are finding. As they enter further into the subatomic realm, they are seeing that life is a process, a flux. They are finding entities that cannot be clearly defined as waves nor particles, that are neither nouns nor verbs. The Navajo worldview has ancient terms for these scientific discoveries; in other words, the Navajo language can contain both seemingly polarized concepts of being as one indivisible entity, as the language is holistic and inclusive.

BASIC METAPHYSICAL CONCEPTIONS ARE DISSIMILAR

Author Gary Witherspoon, who has lived years on the Navajo Reservation, writes of the difficulties inherent in the translation of cross-cultural metaphysical concepts by illuminating the very different foundations of reality between Navajo and Western consciousness.

> An example of the kind of underlying metaphysical premise to which I am making reference would be the Western conception of the relationship between mind and body, or mind and matter. Especially since the Cartesian age of natural and mental philosophy and possibly even before, Western thought has been dominated by the basic and complete separation of mind and matter, idea and entity, and subject and object. To Western thinkers what goes on in the mind is subjective, while that which occurs in the world of matter and energy is objective....These basic metaphysical notions, which are taken for granted by most Western intellectuals, are denied in Navajo thought. Navajo philosophy assumes that mental and physical phenomena are inseparable, and that thought and speech can have a powerful impact on the world of matter and energy...Navajo interpreta-

tions of the constitution of reality and the causation of events are all based on an unbreakable connection between mind and matter.[2]

EVERYTHING IS PART OF A SACRED, NONHIERARCHICAL WHOLENESS

In almost all native languages, there is no one word that means "religion." The concept of religious as separate from nonreligious simply does not exist in traditional Navajo thinking. Everything is part of a sacred wholeness, everything is *Diyin*, in the traditional Navajo consciousness. There is no literal translation for *Diyin*; trying to describe it is like asking someone to define something holistic through reductionistic terminology. Many translations of the concept of *Diyin* carry Hebraic/Christian connotations, such as a translation of *God*. Even using words such as *holy, sacred* or *divine* are misleading, as they imply that there is another class of being that is separate, not holy, not sacred, not divine. This separation is not what Navajos mean by *Diyin*. *Diyin* is a nonhierarchical, sacred process of life; therefore *Diyin* is not a noun. Dan Moonhawk Alford expressed this concept when he wrote, "God is not a noun."[3]

DYNAMIC ORDER AND BALANCE OF INTERRELATED PROCESSES

Diyin is an organic process, with life and movement implicit in the meaning. This life process is universal. It is an extremely complex order of relationships with multiple recursive processes within processes and patterns within patterns, somewhat similar to a visual fractal matrix. It is an orderly process with a dynamic and never-diminishing, never-ending self-organizing order. The order is tremendous and cosmic, and the order itself is *Diyin*. Implicit in this process is a complex dynamic balance, *as'ah naaghai*. The balance is achieved through the interaction of negative (*sa'ah naaghai*) and positive (*bik'eh hozhoon*) relationships. Notice the order: The negative is expressed before the positive, in comparison to Western thinking. The interaction and relationship is *Diyin*. It is not separate from the human being nor from the human life experience, which is the process. The process generates the order, which is *Diyin*, and the order is the process.

COSMOLOGY OF COMPLEMENTARITIES

Probably the most central and seminal concept in Navajo cosmology is expressed through the term *nanit'a sa'ah naaghai, nanit'a bik'eh hozhoon,* which provides the cultural essence and ideological matrix that binds the human with all cosmic forces and energies. Implicit in this concept is a cosmic male-female complementarity expressed as *sa'ah naaghai* (male life energy) and *bik'eh hozhoon* (female life energy). Where the two complementarities intersect, there is a central dynamic balance where equilibrium and harmony are continuously germinated. Navajos refer to this vital central life-giving process primarily through the term *as'ah naaghai.*

This process is diametrically opposed to the Cartesian division between mind and matter, upon which much allopathic medical practice is based. In accordance with traditional Navajo thinking, the interrelationships of physical, mental, and spiritual processes of the human being are embodied through the tremendous cosmic movement that provides the balancing order. Navajos call this movement *alilee as'ah naaghai.* The human is a natural participant in this systemic order, self-regulated by natural forces and phenomena. Human consciousness evolves through this process, and the process itself is *Diyin.* Ultimately *Diyin* needs to be contemplated at a very deep level of thought in order to understand the reality of the indigenous mind.

A PARTICIPATORY WORLD OF SUBJECTIVE, DYNAMIC RELATIONSHIPS

Traditional Navajos understand embodiment through *Diyin,* a completely natural organic process. The indigenous definition is quite different from the anthropomorphic descriptions of embodiment, as described in almost all published literature on Navajo philosophy. The traditional Western conception of embodiment involves placing physical characteristics (body) onto an existing spiritual form. In contrast, traditional Navajos closely observe and experience the totality of the natural process of which they are an integral part through a language of interrelationships, expressed through sacred oral narratives, which are often referred to as *mythology,* in a somewhat denigrating manner.

Classic Cartesian-based science adulates the objective mind. Traditional Navajos think from both an objective and subjective consciousness, separately or simultaneously. Increasingly, more contemporary scientists, especially in areas of quantum physics and other wholeness sciences (e.g., chaos, complexity, systems, networks) emphasize the participatory (implying subjectivity) and relational aspects of subatomic phenomena and systems research. Traditional Navajo language already exists within a participatory world of subjective dynamic relationships and furthermore can naturally articulate these phenomena.

Gregory Bateson is one of a handful of Western philosophers who have understood and articulated the vital importance of relationship thinking. "Relationships should be used as a basis for all definition,"[4] he argues. Fritjof Capra, another relational thinker, paraphrases Bateson when he writes, "Anything, he [Bateson] believed, should be defined, not only by what it is in itself, but by its relations to other things."[5] Traditional Navajo knowledge in its widest context is a dynamic process of relationship similar to Bateson's conception. Traditional ways of knowing are themselves an impetus to connect to further processes and relationships. Learning is thus never complete. It is a constant process of becoming. Knowing, too, is never complete. It is also an ongoing state of being.

HEALING IS A LIFELONG PROCESS, HOLISTIC AND COSMIC

Healing too, according to traditional Navajo understanding, is never complete. One never reaches a static plateau of perfection, a completely healthy state. Healing is a process, often a lifelong process. A healing, as differentiated from a symptomatic cure, can be temporary or more permanent. It can be a temporary alleviation of pain or a cluster of pain symptoms, or it can be a more permanent elimination of symptoms. However, a weak spot or mark may remain, and the illness can remanifest in another guise, sometimes years later.

In a discussion of Navajo healing, the English word *healing* itself must be clarified. In English the words *healing* and *curing* are somewhat interchangeable. They most often imply a cessation of symptoms. The origins of the word *healing* are similar to those of the word *healthy,* which in turn are related to *hol*, or *whole*, *wholeness* (and even *holiness*). The way we use the word *healing* in the context of Navajo healing is based on these ancient definitions, implying wholeness and health. Thus when we say *healing*, in relation to Navajo healing, we mean a holistic and dynamic process, interrelated with cosmic energies, that is never-ending and deals with far more than idiopathic symptoms.

TRADITIONAL HOLISTIC HEALING IS ROOTED IN NATURAL COSMIC ORDER

Traditional Navajo healing can be examined in terms of onset of symptoms, diagnosis, and therapeutic restoration (a restoration to a dynamic state of harmony and balance). Traditional holistic healing is rooted in the natural cosmic process and order. Healing can occur across time and space. Symptomatic illness can manifest in an individual, in generations of a family, or as in the case of multigenerational grief, in a longitudinal post-traumatic stress of an entire people (coming from harrowing historic events such as the Navajo Long Walk or Cherokee Trail of Tears).

Traditional Navajo healing is a therapeutic and efficacious process emphasizing the importance of diagnosis, followed by corrective treatment to initiate restoration of balance (healing) within a holistic curative perspective. The process may be instantaneous, but most healings require time and some effort of the part of the patient after the initiation of healing by ceremonial means. Navajo healing is associated with concepts of nonlocality, and it is said that a prayer or offering can have instant effect, both locally and to the furthest reaches of the universe.

TRADITIONAL NAVAJO HEALING INVOLVES CEREMONIAL RESTORATION

To many non-Navajos who have some familiarity with Navajo healing, the most outstanding and unique aspects of this indigenous practice contain some version of ceremony, with rituals such as elaborate sandpaintings, song, and prayer. Most healing takes place through proper diagnosis and ceremonial restoration. Song in the ceremonial language is an integral part of the ceremony. When traditional Navajos put emphasis on song, they are actually articulating and singing the creative activity and workings of the universe. The Navajo knowledge and transferral of the universal forces that are expressed through song are expressions of vibration in tune with universal healing energies. The cosmic order provides processes and organizational principles inherent in ceremonial song. Thus songs must be sung properly and in order. Mistakes in songs can negate an entire ceremony.

A HOLOGRAPHIC UNIVERSE WITH MULTIPLE DIMENSIONS

The cosmic order is a cyclical experience. The dynamic order within the cyclical movement of the cosmos is a universal occurrence based on natural recursive systems and immutable energies. Traditional Navajos perceive the universe as all-inclusive, each element being a holographic component of a self-organizing holistic system. The traditional organization is somewhat similar to concepts utilized in contemporary system and chaos theory.

Within this traditional paradigm, the number four is an important directional component of the holistic order, often expressed as the four cardinal directions, the four sacred mountains, the four seasons of the year, to name but a few. There are many additional natural phenomena embodied in the four directions, each being necessary for completeness and balance. Four is not the only number of special significance. With increasing complexity, one can discuss cosmological phenomena in terms of other numbers, such as six, twelve, twenty-four and so on. Three-dimension worlds can become worlds of four, five, six, and seven dimensions.

Traditional Navajo healing enfolds the above mentioned dimensions and directions into relational processes. There are distinct yet interrelated processes that occur as healing is facilitated and as a patient gains a therapeutic restoration of harmony through what may be termed a cosmological therapy, which contains an experience of (re)connection with the universe.

COSMOLOGICAL THERAPEUTIC PROCESS

One might say that the initiating process of healing is a mental process, in which symptoms of disease are illuminated. The entire process is stimulated by an internal and/or external stimulus that initiates the thinking process or consciousness. Thus a symptom of imbalance occurs, which can become conscious or can remain at a subconscious level. A gradual, or in some cases immediate, dawning of awareness occurs, as a sense of discomfort or pain may manifest through internal sensory perception.

As a more conscious realization occurs, through a growing sensory perception, one begins to realize that something is out of order and begins an assessment of the situation. The symptom becomes a conscious manifestation of mental and physical imbalance. The imbalance begins to take on additional implications. Certain environments may make the symptom feel worse. The irritation may be intensified by a natural process. In fact natural processes will provide clues, if only one can sense them. The wind, the sunlight, the pollens, and environmental pollution may intensify a condition.

Other physical symptoms may attach themselves to the original imbalance. One becomes aware of a multiplicity of invisible interconnections within the organic system. These complex alignments are visible and understandable to Navajo diagnosticians. However, they are most often invisible and discounted by Western allopathic physicians who have been trained to deal with causality-factored diagnoses.

RELATIONSHIPS WITH BOHM'S "IMPLICATE ORDER"

The complex linkages of what David Bohm terms the "implicate order" between mental, physical, social, cosmic, and spiritual realms provide the holistic phenomena that Navajo refer to as *indigenous medicine*. Bohm's notion of holistic order, in which any given element contains the totality of the cosmos enfolded within itself, pertains to both consciousness and the Navajo healing process. "Parts are seen to be in immediate connection," explains Bohm, "in which their dynamical relationships depend, in an irreducible way, on the state of the whole system.... Thus one is led to a new notion of unbroken wholeness which denies the classical idea of analyzability of the world into separately independently existing parts."[6] Bohm's notion of unbroken wholeness, as expressed in the previous quotation, is of course very close to the native version of holistic thinking.

TREATMENT OF MANIFESTED IMBALANCE

To return to the process of healing, the assessment that one has begun points out an imbalance of manifested discomfort or disease that is out of synchronization with the desired balance of what Navajos would call *hozhoo*, loosely glossed as *harmony*. This imbalance is evaluated in terms of a relationship to an earlier, more desirable state of being, the state of the well-balanced person. A rebalanced state would be a lessening of discomfort, or cessation of pain. At the same time, an understanding of the spiritual connection to holistic healing may develop, providing conscious guidance for restoration of balance.

There are natural movements to all things, or *hoogaal*. In the Navajo way, one must be aware of these movements and properly acknowledge them. If one inadvertently gets in the way of these natural cosmic movements, harm may result. The proper ways by which to live life are reflected in the cultural prohibitions and authorized procedures of the Navajo. Things that happen in accordance with an improper order can often be ceremonially corrected and rebalanced. This is a traditional perspective of the process of healing.

In the Navajo way of thinking, the causes of imbalance (disease) and healing (restoration of balance) are intrinsically interrelated. Reconnection and restoration of balance with the natural environment need to be facilitated. The restoration of balance becomes an initiation process in and of itself, giving the patient spiritual authority along with increased understanding. Through the spiritual and ceremonial assistance of a traditional practitioner, healing may occur.

OPTIONS WITHIN CULTURAL CONTEXT

The next part of the healing process is an articulation of the cognitive process through communication. The pain or symptom is communicated to others, usually to members of one's family, who will assist in assessing the proper procedures to be followed. There are many choices. One can go to a clinic for consultation with a physician. One can go to a traditional Navajo diagnostician. Dreams can be interpreted. Many options are available but the thinking is generally set within a Navajo cultural context, spiritually connected to the natural and cosmic forces. For traditional Navajos, options of going to different ceremonial practitioners are weighed in terms of location, relationship, financial cost, and time available.

Navajo healing focuses on the use of natural forces and meditation for diagnosis. This may include the use of starlight and crystals, the use of animal and plant powers, and cosmic energies, all of which are seldom if ever used in allopathic medical diagnosis. In Navajo healing, much emphasis is placed on the diagnosis, which in turn provides the foundation for the initiation of healing. There is a concentration on the total person, including effects from past generations and emotional, social, psychological, and spiritual imbalances, as well as the physical symptoms.

ILLNESS AS MANIFESTATION OF HOLISTIC IMBALANCE

According to traditional Navajo healers, sometimes referred to as *medicine men* but more correctly today referred to as *practitioners of the healing arts*, the physical ailment is merely a manifestation of a deeper, more holistic imbalance. Rather than treating the physical symptom alone, through what can be termed a Band-aid approach, the entire holistic system must be evaluated before a comprehensive healing can be initiated. The use of herbal remedies is widespread. Herbs are normally acquired with extreme care and proper spiritual protocol. Remedies related to animals are often used for treatment. Some of these methods are similar to traditional *Ayurvedic* and Chinese medicine approaches.

NAVAJO DIAGNOSTICIANS

There are many types of Navajo diagnosticians. One can go to a traditional hand trembler, who diagnoses through personal connections with vibrations of natural forces. Hand tremblers utilize the energies of certain stars as well as the energy and wisdom of the horny toad and thunder. The vibrations that come to the hand trembler in response to questioning lead to diagnosis of the cause and potential resolution of the patient's problem.

Another type of diagnostician is the crystal gazer, or star gazer, who diagnoses problems through crystal and starlight. Just as the Western astronomer speaks of the ancient light from the stars that is just reaching the earth, so too do star gazers speak of the stars as "my ancient relation from whence I came" (*sitsooi yoo*). Stars are light. Crystals are stars. Crystals are light. Light is consciousness, according to traditional Navajo thinking. Just as the hand trembler will identify the cause and probable restoration of balance for the patient, so will the crystal and star gazer. These types of diagnostic ceremonies are very popular today on the Navajo Reservation.

Diagnosis can also be done by means of listening or use of charcoal, fire, water and plants. Prices and procedures are variable. The fee for a diagnostic process can range between $5 to $300 or more. The length of time is also variable, ranging from a few minutes to 1 or 2 entire nights.

Traditional diagnostic ceremonies are very different from medical diagnostic procedures. In the first place, the patient usually does not volunteer any information about his symptoms. The traditional diagnostician does not usually ask any questions of the patient. The diagnosis comes from natural and cosmic information sources. There is no probing exploratory surgery, nor extensive, invasive testing.

CEREMONIAL HEALING

After the diagnosis, a plan for ceremonial healing is usually set. There are many types of ceremonies; however, most of the ceremonies are classified as either protectionway or blessingway. Practitioners specialize in certain ceremonies and often take lifetimes to learn them. Today some ceremonies are going extinct, either from lack of apprentices to learn the ceremonies or lack of the appropriate herbs. Ceremonies can last 1 hour or up to 9 nights. Some ceremonies will involve just the patient, and some will involve entire families and communities, such as Enemyway or Nightway (*Yei Bi Chai*) ceremonies.

Many ceremonies involve a transference of spiritual healing essence through creation of elaborate sandpaintings (dry paintings) and oral narration of cosmological mythologies. The narrations and ceremonial materials are emphatically not symbols of bygone eras; the patient actually becomes the one who undergoes the cultural healing, a re-creation and a reconnection with age-old energies and beings.

The process that takes place after a healing is effected through ceremonial means and procedures are often overlooked by non-Navajo scholars. Patients must often observe 4 days of "holiness" following prescribed behaviors, such as not bathing, not cutting meat, not chopping wood, no sexual relations, not observing anything violent, and so on. This demonstrates a seriousness on the part of the patient and a deep desire for healing to occur. There is a traditional way to wash up after the 4 days have been observed. After this time, one does not discuss the healing or symptoms; one behaves as if the healing has occurred.

For traditional Navajo, the emphasis is on the entire healing process that allows a revitalization to continue. Growth is implicit and intrinsic to this process. Healing thus implies natural growth, consequently providing a regenerative process.

INTEGRATIVE HEALING APPROACHES

Today more and more doctors on the Navajo Reservation are learning about the native ways of healing. Ceremonial hogans are being built at Indian Health Service hospitals to accommodate and respect the native healing ways. It is not unusual for families to bring traditional healers into the patient's room.

At the same time, medical doctors such as Larry Dossey, Andrew Weil, and Deepak Chopra are integrating medical and alternative healing approaches through discussions of holistic healing and ancient approaches of Chinese and *Ayurvedic* medicine. Their work, along with that of David Bohm on the implicate order and holoverse, shares striking similarities with Navajo philosophy in the area of healing arts.

"Healing is holistic," states Dr. Beulah Allen, native traditionalist and chief of staff of the Indian Health Clinic, Tsaile, Arizona. "It doesn't matter whether you utilize Western medical services or the traditional healing methods, the most important thing is that you are a participant in your own holistic healing. Both processes can only initiate healing, but the ultimate restoration of your health and harmony has to come from you."[7]

References for this essay are located on the DVD accompanying this book.

The Spiritual Heart of Tibetan Medicine: Its Contribution to the Modern World*

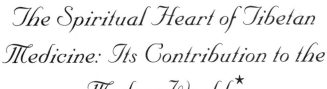

SOGYAL RINPOCHE

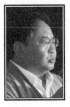

YOUR HOLINESS, EMINENT doctors and scholars, ladies and gentlemen, it is a great honor for me to address you today at this International Congress on Tibetan Medicine. What I shall endeavor to do is to explore, very briefly and with my limited understanding, the spiritual and mental dimensions of healing within the Buddhist tradition of Tibet. I will speak from my own experience of what I know to be effective in the West. Of course, whatever I do understand I owe to the infinite kindness of my masters, especially Jamyang Khyentse Chokyi Lodro,

---

*Originally presented at the First International Congress on Tibetan Medicine, November 7, 1998; Washington, D.C. In Rinpoche S: The Spirit of Buddhism. San Francisco, 2003, Harper San Francisco.

Dudjom Rinpoche, and Dilgo Khyentse Rinpoche, who embody so perfectly the wisdom and compassion of the Buddhist path. The ancient science of Tibetan medicine is rooted in the teachings of Buddha, and the essence of these teachings is the central importance of the mind. The Buddha[1] said, "Commit not a single unwholesome action,/Cultivate a wealth of virtue,/To tame this mind of ours—/This is the teaching of the Buddha." He also said, "We are what we think./All that we are/Arises with our thoughts./With our thoughts we make the world./Speak or act with a pure mind—/And happiness will follow you."[1] The mind is both the source of happiness and the root of suffering. At the same time it possesses an extraordinary capacity for healing, it also plays its part in making us ill.

But how exactly can the mind provoke physical illness? The *Four Tantras*, the authoritative sources for Tibetan medicine, are quite explicit:

> Here is an explanation of the *general* cause of all illness. There is but one single cause... and this is said to be ignorance due to not understanding the meaning of "selflessness"....
>
> Now for the *specific* causes: from ignorance arise the three *poisons* of attachment, hatred and closed-mindedness, and from these, as a result, are produced disorders of wind, bile and phlegm.[2]

The basic source of sickness is diagnosed as "ignorance"; in other words, attributing a false sense of a lasting and independent self to ourselves and the phenomena around us. This, the Tibetan medical tradition tells us, arouses the following:

- Craving and desire, which are responsible for disorders of the "wind" (lung)
- Hatred and pride, causing disorders of the "bile" (*tripa*)
- Bewilderment and closed-mindedness, provoking ailments of the "phlegm" (*beken*)

For years now, around the world, there has been a growing understanding of the correlation of mind and body and the link between ill health and the way we cope with stress and our emotions. In his book *Emotional Intelligence*, Daniel Goleman summarizes data from a number of studies indicating the significance of emotions in medicine. He writes:

People who experienced chronic anxiety, long periods of sadness and pessimism, unremitting tension or incessant hostility, relentless cynicism or suspiciousness, were found to have double the risk of disease.... This order of magnitude makes distressing emotions as toxic a risk factor as, say, smoking or high cholesterol are for heart disease—in other words, a major threat to health.[3]

Just as distressing states of mind can cause disorders, so can positive, uplifting states promote good health—states such as peace of mind, optimism, confidence, humor, companionship, love, kindness, compassion, and devotion. Again, this has also been observed countless times in the West and more recently, for example, with Norman Cousins, who laughed his way back to health, as well as in the findings of Dean Ornish,[4] whose *Love and Survival* discusses the effects of emotional support and love on physical health and life expectancy.

TRAINING THE MIND

The whole thrust of Buddhist practice is precisely to eliminate these negative states of mind and to cultivate the positive ones, transforming our mind and its emotions and thereby healing our entire being—body, speech, mind, and heart.

The Buddhist approach to transforming the mind begins by working with our *attitudes* toward life, using the power of reason to analyze our delusions, disturbing emotions, and even our basic assumptions, so as to find, simply speaking, a way of being happy. The Tibetan master Dodrupchen Jikme Tenpe Nyima spells out the link between peace of mind, happiness, and health (see note):

> Whenever you are harmed by sentient beings, or anything else, if you make a habit out of just perceiving only the suffering, then when even the smallest problem comes up, it will cause you enormous anguish in your mind. This is because the nature of any perception or idea, be it happiness or sorrow, is to grow stronger and stronger by being repeated. When the power of this repetitive experience gradually increases, after a while most of what you perceive will become the cause of actually attracting unhappiness towards you, and happiness will never get a chance....
>
> When you are *not* at the mercy of the suffering caused by anxiety, then not only will all other kinds of suffering evaporate like weapons dropping

from the hands of soldiers, but even illnesses will normally disappear on their own.

The saints of the past used to say, "When you are not unhappy, or discontent about anything, then the mind will not be disturbed. If the mind is not disturbed, the inner air [wind] will not be disturbed. That means the other elements of the body will not be disturbed either. Because of this your mind will remain undisturbed, and the wheel of constant happiness will turn.

Such a contemplation forms part of the Buddhist training of the mind in loving kindness and compassion, which is called *Lojong*. When the ultimate cause of all our suffering and sickness is our holding onto a false view of self, our constant selfish grasping and the negative emotions it provokes, then nothing can be more effective or skillful as a remedy than to steep the mind in love, compassion, altruism, and thinking of others.

The Buddhist practices of compassion and love are immensely powerful at transforming the emotions and healing ourselves and others. One practice that has had an enormous impact among Western people is *Tonglen*, the practice of "giving and taking." In their imagination, practitioners summon all of their resources of positive emotion and train in taking through compassion the suffering and illnesses of others—giving, with love, every source and kind of happiness and well-being.

Tonglen practice reduces and eliminates the grasping ego while enhancing our concern for others. As a result, what has been discovered is that it is deeply therapeutic, especially for those who feel the sense of lack in their lives or unfulfillment or even "self-hate" that are so prevalent these days. This is why I have developed a series of practices applying *Tonglen* to help bring about such healing.

In Tibet the healing power of *Tonglen* was legendary. Today, in the West, the potential of such practices remains largely unexplored, though I feel they could have astounding results if applied more widely in cases of mental and physical illness.

MEDITATION

The other practice I would like to mention—one that so many who are working with the sick have in one context or another found to be a

profound source of healing—is meditation. The spirit of Buddhist meditation is captured so beautifully by Nyoshul Khen Rinpoche:

Rest in natural great peace
This exhausted mind
Beaten helpless by karma and neurotic thought,
Like the relentless fury of the pounding waves
In the infinite ocean of samsara.
Rest in Natural Great Peace.[5]

Through the practice of "calm abiding," or tranquility meditation, our restless, thinking mind subsides into a state of deep inner peace. The warring, fragmented aspects of ourselves begin to settle and become friends; negativity and aggression are disarmed; frustration, tension, and turbulent emotions are defused; and the unkindness and harm in us is removed, revealing our inherent "good heart." So meditation is real *inner disarmament.*

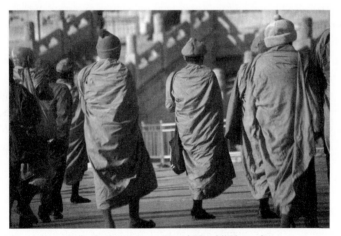

"Monks." (Courtesy David "Dudi" Shmueli.)

From this state of "calm abiding" comes the expansive clarity and insight of "clear seeing": Duality dissolves; ego dwindles, and confusion evaporates; the whole way we look at ourselves changes; and we give space to emotions, learn from them, and become free from their sway.

As this "clear seeing" progressively deepens, it leads us to an experience of the intrinsic nature of reality and the nature of our mind. When the cloudlike thoughts and emotions fade away, the skylike nature of our true being is revealed and, shining from it, our Buddha nature—*bodhicitta*—like the sun. And just as both light and warmth blaze from the sun, wisdom and loving compassion radiate out from the mind's innermost nature. Grasping at a false self, or ego, has dissolved, and we simply rest, inasmuch as we can, in the nature of mind, this most natural state that is without any reference or concept, hope or fear, yet with a quiet but soaring confidence—the deepest form of well-being imaginable.

One oral instruction from the great masters of the past resonates this innermost nature of mind: *Chu ma nyok na dang/Sem ma cho na de.* Nothing could be simpler yet more powerful: Water, if unstirred, will become clear—that's a fact. In just the same way, the very nature of mind is such that if you do not alter, fabricate, or manipulate it with needless thinking, it will by itself find its own natural state of peace and well-being. So many have found that even a glimpse of the nature of mind is utterly transforming, nourishing, and purifying. For if "dis-ease" is due to our losing sight of our true nature, to recognize the nature of our mind must be the ultimate healing.

Padmasambhava, who introduced Buddhism into Tibet in the eighth century, clarifies this even further: "Don't regard illness as a hindrance, or consider it a virtue. Leave your mind unfabricated and free...cutting through the flow of conceptual thoughts...old illnesses will disappear by themselves and you remain unharmed by new ones."

CONCLUSION

Healing practices generally fall into three different approaches: prevention, applying antidotes, and transformation. Using an everyday example, they could be compared to avoiding your enemy, facing him and dealing with him, or turning him into a friend. Today I have touched only on meditation and on training the mind in loving kindness and compassion, but there is a vast range of healing practices, especially within the *Vajrayana* Buddhist tradition, in which healing is achieved through trans-

formation. Some of these will be presented during this Congress. They employ every kind of skillful means—visualization, mental imagery, sound, mantra, movement, and yoga—and embrace every facet of the human mind—imagination, intellect, and emotion. A number of these methods have been used to great effect to help combat illnesses such as cancer and AIDS.

Finally, I feel that the real power and strength of the lineage of Tibetan Buddhism is seen most clearly in its great practitioners and masters, whose mere presence is deeply healing in itself. Our good fortune is that someone such as this is here with us today, in the person of His Holiness the Dalai Lama. It is largely due to His Holiness, I believe, that Tibetan medicine has endured and thrived in the way that it has. I would like to salute here the Tibetan Medical and Astrological Institute in Dharamsala, India, which was one of the very first Tibetan institutions to have been established by His Holiness in exile. At the same time, let me also pay tribute to all the other Tibetan physicians and centers of Tibetan medicine around the world.

To see a major conference like this on Tibetan medicine, attended by so many eminent doctors, scientists, and scholars from all over the globe, gives me enormous pleasure; I applaud it and congratulate the organizers with all my heart. It presents us with an exciting opportunity, and I hope that, in the wake of this Congress, the dialogue will continue. The holistic approach of Tibetan medicine, which deals with both mind and body, holds tremendous promise, but so far we have only skimmed the surface of what it has to offer the world. As we enter the twenty-first century, we can and should imagine research of many kinds. For example, we might delve into how to make these amazing Buddhist healing methods available alongside Tibetan medicine—in the right environment and to patients who would be receptive—thereby exploring their combined power of healing.

Yet for the Tibetan medical tradition to be more effective in serving people's needs, two things will be required: (1) a greater understanding and communication between Tibetan doctors themselves, and (2) a greater exchange and collaboration between Tibetan physicians and Western doctors and scientists that never compromise the integrity of Tibetan medicine. As His Holiness says,

Tibetan medicine is an integrated system of healthcare that has served the Tibetan people well for many centuries and which, I believe, can still provide much benefit to humanity at large. The difficulty we face in bringing this about is one of communication, for like other scientific systems, Tibetan medicine must be understood in its own terms, as well as in the context of objective investigation.[2]

Then, I feel certain, Tibetan medicine will take its rightful place as a universally respected, major system of medicine and healing and prove itself to have more and more to offer—in a world increasingly beset by diseases and disorders—toward the relief of suffering everywhere.

NOTE

Quoted from *sKyid sDuf; Lam Khyer* by Dodrupchen Jikme Tenpe Nyima (1865-1926) in his *Collected Works*, volume 5, pp. 351-366, published by Chorten Gonpa, Gangtok, Sikkim. Also translated as "Instructions on Turning Happiness and Suffering into the Path of Enlightenment" by Tulku Thondup in *Enlightened Living*, Boston, 1990, Shambhala pp. 117-129.

References for this essay are located on the DVD accompanying this book.

Changing Perspectives on Healing Energy in Traditional Chinese Medicine

GARRET YOUNT
YIFANG QIAN
HONGLIN ZHANG

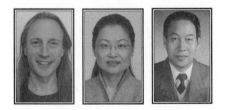

IN TRADITIONAL CHINESE medicine (TCM) a universal healing energy is called *Qi*, a "vital energy of life." Regulating *Qi* is the basis for all therapeutic modalities of TCM, including acupuncture, herbal therapy, moxibustion, massage, meditation therapy, and so on. In a broad sense, all of TCM is a form of "energy medicine" because the goal is always to correct an imbalance of some aspect of the vital energy *Qi*. The current Western phrase *energy medicine* correlates more narrowly, however, to one specific TCM treatment modality: meditation therapy. This modality is more commonly referred to as *Qigong* in recent years. In this chapter, we describe the concept of *Qi* in TCM, the basis for self-meditation therapy, historical legends of "distributing *Qi*" as a form of medical treatment, the emergence and definition of *Qigong*, and modern scientific explorations of *Qigong* as a form of energy medicine.

ANCIENT TIMES TO PRESENT: CHINESE HEALTH-PROMOTING MEDITATION EXERCISES

The original concept of *Qi* came from the ancient Chinese philosophical theory of primordial energy (*Yuan Qi Lun*).[1] At the center of this theory is the concept that all things are formed from *Qi* (*Wan Wu Jie Sheng Yu Qi*). It is an abstract recognition formed from observations of natural phenomena, such as ice changing to water then to vapor, that, although becoming invisible, still exist. Other examples include wood burning to ashes and smoke and giant rocks eventually transforming to sand. Ancient people concluded that all things in the universe—with or without life—are made up by an ultimate, invisible, yet ever-existing *Qi*. This *Qi* can be indefinitely divided into smaller pieces, indicated by the phrase "extreme smallness without internal limit" (*Zhi Xiao Wu Nei*). Things formed by *Qi* can also be indefinitely large in size, indicated by the phrase "extreme largeness without external limit" (*Zhi Da Wu Wai*).

In accordance with the concept that all things are formed from *Qi*, ancient medical theory posits that the human body is formed by *Qi* and that the body correlates with nature (*Tian Ren Xiang Ying*). This is clearly reflected in what is believed to be the first complete TCM textbook, *The Yellow Emperor's Classic of Internal Medicine*,[2] originally published in China more than 2,000 years ago. The book is believed to be a collective work written and repeatedly edited by multiple medical experts and scholars during the period of the late Warring States, *Qin* and *Han* Dynasty (around 400 B.C.–200 B.C.). It was written under the name of the ancient saint Yellow Emperor, and it systematically recorded the basic theories of TCM that had been collected through oral tradition. In the chapter titled "Treasure the Life and Preserve the Form," it is stated that the human body is born by heavenly and earthly *Qi*. Ancient TCM theory summarizes that the sources of such *Qi* are from Innate *Qi* of Parents, Acquired *Qi* of Water and Grain, and Breathed-in *Qi* of Nature. The function of

Qi in the body is reflected in the physiology of the different organ systems. The Spleen and Stomach *Qi* (*Pi Wei Zhi Qi*) represents digestive function; the Defense *Qi* (*Wei Qi*) represents immune function; the *Qi* as the General of the Blood (*Qi Wei Xie Shuai*) represents circulation; the Lung *Qi* (*Fei Qi*) represents respiration; the Kidney *Qi* (*Shen Qi*) represents reproduction; and *Qi* of Transformation (*Qi Hua*) represents metabolism.

As diseases are believed to be caused by deficits and imbalances of *Qi* in the body, different TCM treatment modalities have the common objective of regulating *Qi* and restoring the balance. Acupuncture is a physical regulation of *Qi*, for example. Meditation therapy is based on the belief that a person's mind is capable of regulating *Qi*. As with the other TCM modalities, the *Qi* is directed along the meridians of the body and moves the blood. The blood supplies different organs with vital nutrients and energy. When *Qi* and blood are regulated and maintained in harmonic balance, the body stays healthy. It is important to note that aside from the concept of *Qi*, TCM also has other basic concepts that are part of therapeutic principles, including *Essence, Meridians, Five Elements, Yin and Yang, Zang Fu Organs,* and more. As with *Qi*, these concepts guide the various treatment modalities. This chapter focuses on *Qi* because it is most relevant to the topic of energy medicine.

Health- and longevity-promoting exercises involving meditation have existed under many names throughout Chinese history. What they are called varies—*Dao Yin, Fu Qi, Zuo Chan, Tu Na,* and so on—based largely on the origin of the exercises and on their different emphasis on movement, breathing, or intentionality.[3] In the first chapter of *The Yellow Emperor's Classic of Internal Medicine,* the emperor states, "I have heard that in early ancient times, there were the Enlightened People who could master the Yin and Yang in the universe, breathe in the essence of *Qi*, meditate, and their spirit and body would become whole. Their longevity could therefore be endless." This quote refers to self-meditation practices generally called "life nurturing practices" (*Yang Sheng Fa*) in ancient times. These practices were based on the concept that those who know how to nourish themselves know the way to regulate *Qi*. Self-meditation practices were one of the ways to regulate *Qi*. They were performed as part of a self-healing discipline and focused on health maintenance and disease prevention.

Thousands of styles of self-meditation practice exist in China. These styles can be divided into different categories.[4] Based on movement, there are mobile styles and still styles. Based on postures, there are standing styles, sitting styles, lying-down styles, and walking styles. Based on philosophical perspective, there are Taoist styles, Buddhist styles, medical styles, Confucianist styles, martial art styles, and folk styles. Based on practice focus, there are calm-and-still styles (focusing on quieting thoughts), thought-preserving styles (focusing thought on certain things or parts of the body), breathing styles (focusing on breathing regulation), guided movement styles (focusing on thought-guided body movement), and meridian styles (focusing on guiding Qi to travel along the meridians). Whatever the style, the common objective of self-meditation practice is to achieve a trancelike state of relaxation, wherein the Qi can be regulated and directed by the mind to correct imbalances in the body.

LEGENDS OF "DISTRIBUTING *QI*"

Aside from regulation of Qi through self-meditation, there is a phenomenon called *Bu Qi* described in ancient Chinese writings, especially Taoist literature. *Bu Qi* involves the manipulation of Qi for the purpose of "attacking others' illness." The character *Bu* means to distribute or to spread. In the book *Tao Zang* there is a section on "Secrets of Fetal Breathing in Verse" that states:

> One cultivates the Tao long and refined, the fetal breathing forms in the body. When others are ill, one knows the nature. The sick child faces the one's Qi. Tell him to clear his heart and mind. Passes the Qi to the child and tells the child to swallow many times. Direct the mind to damage the illness. The illness can soon be dissipated. The evil spirits hence escape. Liberation from the illness hence is achieved.[5]

In *The New Book of Tang* (*Xin Tang Shu*) there is a section on Taoism that described The Verse of Distributing Qi (*Bu Qi Jue*). The author (anonymous, 766-779 A.D.) stated that he met a Mr. Wang in the Luo Fu Mountain, who taught him the way of *Bu Qi*:

> When using Qi to treat others, one must do so according to which of the five organs are ill. Take the Qi of that direction and distribute it into the body of the person. The patient should face the direction and calm the heart and

worries. This is distributing the *Qi*, allowing self-healing. Afterwards the patient is asked to swallow the *Qi*. When the good *Qi* is distributed, the evil wind will dissipate.[6]

Other Taoist writings document similar practices, such as the *Seven Commentaries of Cloud Bookcase* (Yun Ji Qi Qian) of the Song Dynasty (960-1279 A.C.). Volume 59 of these commentaries, titled "Tai Qing Elder Wang's Oral Traditional Description of *Qi* Intake," details the stages of internal practice that are required prior to emitting *Qi* to treat patients:

> ... The new learners of taking *Qi* always feel full under the heart around stomach. Eat little, practice long, it naturally moves down.... One can sense it move down to the Lower Dantians (Lower Cinnabar Field). Then sense the *Qi* circulating in the body. Initially it will not reach *Jiu Zhong*. When it does, one may treat others.[7]

Volume 62, *Ten Things About Taking Qi,* talked about externally taking *Qi* (*Wai Fu Qi*):

> For example someone somewhere else has swelling and pain in the left foot. One may guide external *Qi* into your own left foot, and the other person will feel the relief. This is called remote restriction ....[7]

The Taoist alchemist Ge Hong wrote in 320 A.D., "If someone far away has been bitten by a poisonous insect, exhale onto your palm and pray." [8] Examples such as this can also be found in Buddhist literature concerning prayers for the purpose of healing illnesses. An important distinction that is commonly overlooked is that these practices and legends appear in history and religious writings, not in TCM textbooks. It is not clear whether the *Qi* referred to in these ancient contexts is the same or similar to the *Qi* in TCM. The practice of *Bu Qi* is not taught in TCM institutions and is not found in modern TCM textbooks. Therefore it is somewhat misleading for advocates and practitioners of external *Qi Gong* (see next section) to claim that their practice is based on TCM principles with historical examples of *Bu Qi*.[9]

THE 1950s TO PRESENT: *QI GONG*

The term *Qi Gong* was first used in modern China in the 1950s, initially to define a type of health-promoting exercise that emphasized breathing regulation.[10] At that time, Liu Guizhen, a resident of Hebei Province, learned a meditation called the Internal Nurturing Work (*Nei Yang Gong*) from a local peasant. He taught this exercise to many other people, who claimed that they were helped by it, and the news eventually reached the Provincial Public Health Department. Prior to being sent to Beijing to report his work to the Ministry of Health, Liu gave the exercise a new name, but there is a linguistic twist. Many Chinese characters have multiple meanings depending on the context. The character *Qi* can mean "breath," "air," "the vital energy of life," and "anger," for example, depending on the context. Likewise, *Gong* can mean "work," "power," or "success," depending on the context. Liu decided to call the exercise breathing work because it involved practicing breathing to achieve a state of relaxation. The phrase "breathing work" is written as two characters: *Qi Gong*. Unfortunately, this planted the seed for future conceptual confusion because the phrase *Qi Gong* can be interpreted as "Power of the vital energy of life" when taken in a different context.

During the opening ceremony for the China Academy of Traditional Chinese Medicine in 1955, the Ministry of Health recognized Liu for his effort to spread the self-meditation practice *Qi Gong*. National media reported this event, and Liu achieved great fame. Backed by government support, he held public classes, gave talks, and even taught *Qi Gong* to some of the country's leaders. Due to such official endorsement, the use of the term *Qi Gong* was quickly expanded beyond describing just one style of self-meditation (breathing work). Other styles of self-meditation were referred to as a form of *Qi Gong*. Eventually, the term *Qi Gong* was used very generally to describe all the thousands of styles of self-meditation practices for health.

Like many Chinese folk traditions, *Qi Gong* was suppressed during the Chinese Cultural Revolution, then enjoyed a renaissance at its end in the late 1970s. Liu reemerged as an active figure in the field. This time, however, he modified the meaning of the phrase *Qi Gong* from his original "breathing work" to the following: "The *Qi* not only means breathing, but also the vital energy according to TCM theory" and "*Gong* means power."[11] This time, Liu described the exercise as a "body-strengthening technique of cultivating the primordial *Qi*." Although the Chinese characters *Qi* and *Gong* stayed the same, the new definition represented a fundamental conceptual transformation. The descriptive phrase "breathing work" became the abstractive phrase "Power of Cultivating the Vital Energy of Life." Getting away from a simple breathing exercise that helps to focus the mind and regulate *Qi* through relaxation, the new definition de-emphasized the mind-and-relaxation part. People interpreted *Qi Gong* as an exercise with the power to generate the primordial *Qi* itself. This transformation was misleading and started people speculating: If the life energy could be cultivated internally, it might be generated in large quantity and emitted to others. Indeed, the new phenomenon, external *Qi Gong*, quickly branched out from the traditional self-meditation practices and became a treatment modality.[10]

1979 TO PRESENT: EXTERNAL *QI GONG*

An important catalyst for the external *Qi Gong* phenomenon was a series of highly publicized reports by physicist Hansen Gu[12] claiming that practitioners of *Qi Gong* could emit several kinds of physical energy, including microwave and infrared radiation. Despite the fact that these effects were detected using nonstandard equipment[10] and that the claims were never replicated,[13] the reports had a profound effect on the general public. *Qi Gong* was no longer limited to the self-meditation practices of TCM. Many people now claimed that they had acquired special powers through years of cultivating the primordial *Qi* and were able to emit *Qi* to treat patients.

During the 1980s, two opposing camps began to form to attempt to explain the apparent clinical efficacy of *Qi Gong*. Both sides considered the human to be an entity imbued with the vital energy *Qi*, but they differed over their views as to whether *Qi* could be *emitted* to treat patients. Proponents of one camp believed that therapeutic effects observed in patients receiving treatment from a *Qi Gong* practitioner resulted from nothing more than the power of suggestion. Scientists from this camp claimed to have conducted experiments in which patients would report effects even when the *Qi Gong* practitioner was replaced by an actor who simply mimicked a practitioner's behavior. Results of these studies were widely publicized in the general media, and the "end of fairy-tale external *Qi Gong*" was proclaimed.[10] In the other camp, however, many enthusiastic practitioners and patients continued to believe that *Qi* could be emitted to influence health.

The emergence of "Super *Qi Gong* Masters" was another catalyst in the field, with the term *Qi Gong* used in a manner even further from the original focus on self-meditation. In 1987 a practitioner named Yan Xin claimed to have performed experiments in Qing Hua University, Beijing (a reputable education and research institution), in which his external *Qi* had the effect of changing the structure of water, as detected by laser.[14] Despite the fact that these results were never published in a peer-reviewed scientific journal and that the Qing Hua University publicly denounced the inappropriate use of its name in relation to the studies,[10] the claim made Yan Xin an overnight media sensation.[15] Promoted as a Super *Qi Gong* Master, he started the "Super Seminars of *Qi* Induction," allegedly attended by hundreds to thousands of people who received treatment as a group. These seminars triggered the emergence of many Super *Qi Gong* Masters throughout China.[16]

In 1988 an experimental nuclear physicist, Lu Zuyin, announced at the First World Conference on Medical *Qi Gong*, held in Beijing, that he had documented "sufficient evidence to declare the fact of *Qi* emission over two thousand kilometers."[17] During a 21-month period, he and other scientists at the Institute of High Energy Physics in Beijing had conducted a series of experiments examining the decay rate of an ^{241}Am radioactive source following external *Qi Gong* treatment by the famous *Qi Gong* practitioner Yan Xin. Of the external *Qi Gong* treatments, 55 were from distances over 2,000 km. Lu claimed that the rate of radioactive decay changed significantly while the source was being treated by external *Qi Gong*.[18] The amplitude of the change was reported to be, on average, about 1 percent of the total count rate; in one instance, it reached a maximum of 10 percent. The scientists were surprised to see that the largest changes in decay rate were observed following treatments delivered from the farthest distances.[17]

Later, Lu conducted additional experiments assessing whether external *Qi* emitted by Yan Xin from the United States to Beijing could cause changes in the decay rate of radioactive ^{241}Am. Lu purports to have found that distant *Qi Gong* treatment from across the globe changed the decay rate by as much as 12 percent.[19] In March 1988 the New York State

Senate issued a legislative resolution (No. 2968 by Senator Maltese) commemorating Yan Xin. The text stated, "Dr. Yan Xin was invited to present his research results at an international conference of *Qi Gong*... was warmly received as a guest in the White House by President and Mrs. Bush, who praised him as 'the Sage of our time.'"

Even more unusual claims were made, such as one that Yan Xin could use external *Qi* to put out wild fires in northeastern China from thousands of miles away[10] and another that a *Qi Gong* practitioner named Wizard of Snowland had "successfully predicted the launching of the rocket Long March 3 on Feb. 8, 1994" using *Qi*.[13] People were soon borrowing the term *Qi Gong* to name things that had nothing to do with health promotion or even with the concept of *Qi*, such as "changing water to oil" and the familiar circus acts of standing on eggs and swallowing fire.

1990 TO PRESENT: POLITICS AND POLICIES

The expanding definition of the term *Qi Gong* continued in China throughout the 1990s, with the most prominent example being the *Falun Gong* movement. *Falun Gong* is said to be a form of *Qi Gong* that aims at refining the body and mind through exercises and meditation. *Falun Gong* differentiates itself from other *Qi Gong* practices in its emphasis on moral character, incorporating Buddhist and Taoist social principles and pulling *Qi Gong* into a political arena. The tight organization of *Falun Gong* was demonstrated on April 25, 1999, when about 10,000 *Falun Gong* members besieged a government compound in the capital city of Beijing, demanding to be recognized officially as a form of *Qi Gong*. It was the largest mass gathering in the capital for a decade. The incident led to a large-scale crackdown on the group and, in July 1999, the banning of *Falun Gong* by the Chinese government. The leader of the movement now resides in the U.S., and *Falun Gong* members stage daily demonstrations in front of the Chinese consulate in San Francisco, handing out flyers condemning the Chinese government.

Fallout from the banning of *Falun Gong* has had tremendous impact on all forms of *Qi Gong*, because in the early 1990s *Falun Gong* was a member of the Chinese Qi Gong Scientific Research Association.

Although it was eventually expelled by the association in 1996, its overlap with *Qi Gong* has been problematic for external *Qi Gong* practitioners. Just as TCM practitioners accused external *Qi Gong* practitioners of hijacking the word *Qi"* earlier, external *Qi Gong* practitioners now accuse *Falun Gong* practitioners of hijacking the word *Gong*. By 2002, many practitioners in China had stopped practicing external *Qi Gong* for fear of being perceived as being associated with *Falun Gong*.

Another reason for the decline of external *Qi Gong*'s popularity in China is tightened government policies around its practice. On October 19, 1989, the State Administration of Traditional Chinese Medicine in China issued an official policy (89 *Guo Yi Yi Zi* Number 7) titled "Stipulations on Enforcing Regulations for *Qi Gong* Medical Treatment (Pilot)," which states:

> *Qi Gong* therapy is a practice of coursing through the meridians, regulating mind and balancing Yin and Yang, *Qi* and blood through self-meditation in order to dispel diseases and maintain health. It is one of the components for medical health maintenance in traditional Chinese medicine.

In recent years, due to falling behind of management, lacking of adequate laws and regulations, as well as lacking of strict enforcement of existing laws and regulations, there is a lack of orders in the area of *Qi Gong* therapy. The problem is especially prominent in terms of using "emitting external *Qi"* to treat patients. Some take advantage of the opportunity to exaggerate the effect of *Qi Gong*, even deceive the people while seeking to profit, thus creating an extremely negative impact on society.

In order to strengthen the management of *Qi Gong* therapy, to protect the interest of the people and healthy development of *Qi Gong* therapy, the following regulations are now issued:

....

4. Those who treat others by "emitting external *Qi"* must apply for permission from Traditional Chinese Medicine Agency or Health Administration Agency at or above the Regional (City) level, in addition to obtaining qualifications as medical doctor or medical practitioner. The receiving agency is to evaluate the clinical efficacy for the disease that the treatment is being applied for, by investigating the treatment in 30 cases

of such disease. The applicant may register and receive "*Qi Gong* Therapy Permit" only after the treatment has been validated as effective by pertinent experts through statistical analysis. The performance of such therapy must be limited to the specific illness.

...

6. Non-medical and non–health care facilities (including the military) may not develop *Qi Gong* therapeutic activities. Medical and health care facilities may not employ persons who do not follow these stipulations to practice *Qi Gong* therapy.

...

8. Propaganda and reports on *Qi Gong* therapy must strictly respect science, be truthful and provide proper guidance. They must not exaggerate and pursue sensationalism, especially carry superstitious flavor. Advertisements of *Qi Gong* therapy must be approved by Traditional Chinese Medicine Agency or Health Administration Agency of at or above the Regional (City) level.[20]

On July 24, 2003, the State Administration of Traditional Chinese Medicine in China[2] issued another policy: "Temporary Procedures of Examinations for Knowledge, Techniques and Capability for Therapeutic *Qi Gong*." It establishes outlines for national examinations to evaluate whether an applicant for the "*Qi Gong* Therapy Permit" (see item No. 4 in the above policy) possesses the necessary basic professional knowledge, technique, and skills for practicing medicinal *Qi Gong*. Such examinations are to contain both written and practice parts and to be held once every 2 years at the national level. To date, no applicants have come forward, and consequently no examinations have occurred. Not a single practitioner has obtained a "*Qi Gong* Therapy Permit," including the many Super Masters now practicing in the U.S.

BRIDGING THE SCIENTIFIC CULTURAL GAP IN *QI GONG* RESEARCH

As interest in *Qi Gong* in general is declining in China, it is on the increase in the West, and the U.S. National Center for Complementary and Alternative Medicine has responded by sponsoring numerous research programs on the topic. Scrutiny of the existing Chinese scientific literature on *Qi Gong* revealed that a significant scientific cultural gap existed.[22] Clinical trials of *Qi Gong* as a self-meditation practice typically did not follow randomized, double-blind protocols, for example. In a review of "Medicinal *Qigong*"[4] that described clinical observations following multiple illnesses (e.g., hypertension, arrhythmia, stroke, asthma, chronic obstructive pulmonary disease, pulmonary tuberculosis, peptic ulcer disease, diabetes, glaucoma), most studies followed protocols that measured changes before and after a period of *Qi Gong* self-meditation exercise. Presentation of results were generally casual, such as: "Among 107 asthma cases who had integrated *Qi Gong* treatment for three months, 71 had significantly effect, 32 had effect, 4 had no effect. Total effective rate was 96.2%." In studies incorporating placebos, the placebos were always medications.

Poor design and lack of adequate controls also plague the external *Qi Gong* research field. Such flaws are easily found in all of the commonly referenced benchmark studies. No control conditions or statistical analyses were used in Gu's experiment measuring microwave and infrared radiation generated by a *Qi Gong* practitioner, for example. In Yan Xin's experiment on laser detection of an external *Qi* effect, tap water was used as a sample rather than double distilled water or deionized water (standard in biomedical experiments), and no quantification or statistical analysis was used; the results were simply presented as "Result: change? Yes."[16] In Yan Xin's experiments on radioactive decay of ^{241}Am, the protocol lacked appropriate blinding and calibration of equipment.[13] In a highly publicized experiment involving *Qi Gong* treatment of bacteria, a conclusion that external *Qi* can inhibit *Escherichia coli* growth was based on only four trials that lacked blinding, controls for experimental conditions, and statistical analysis.[9] Another general weakness in the field has been the lack of replication of experiments. A critical review that assessed a sample of 58 in vitro studies of *Qi Gong* in the Asian literature found no independent replications on any single model.[23]

Recent international scientific exchange is just beginning to remedy the cultural mismatches in the *Qi Gong* research field. A notable example is a collaborative study by laboratories in China and the U.S. that evaluated potential benefits of external *Qi Gong* therapy on a well-designed animal model of addiction.[24] It will be interesting to discover whether guidelines described in ancient Taoist texts can inform an integral approach to mind-body medicine. Does asking a patient to swallow during energy medicine treatments make a difference in efficacy, for example? If such a technique were to influence efficacy, would it be through a more effective movement of *Qi* or through a more effective hypnotic suggestion? A new look at potential mechanisms underlying energy medicine is necessary given the realization that the nervous and endocrine systems are physically intertwined with the immune system and that psychological states can regulate immune function, even at the level of immune gene expression. A compelling question that also remains is whether a strict reductionistic science is capable of finding conclusive evidence of *Qi*.

References for this essay are located on the DVD accompanying this book.

Part Five

ENVISIONING A NEW STORY FOR HEALTH AND HEALING

MARILYN SCHLITZ
TINA AMOROK
MARC S. MICOZZI

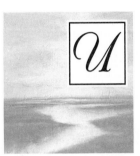 *ltimately, our vision for an integral medicine involves a new story for health and healing.* This is a multifaceted call to action. How might we reconcile the insights of consciousness studies within the complex social, political, and ecological contexts that shape our experience and practice of health care?

A central aspect of the integral model, as we develop and use it in this work, is the transformation of the health practitioners themselves. Indeed, this may be the only way to transform the practice of medicine. Health professionals today face many painful dilemmas, both personal and professional. We all struggle to maintain our integrity as whole people while having to specialize in one particular area and compartmentalize all others. We are in the midst of the tension between the scientific and spiritual forces of the profession as it undergoes change. We strive to uphold human caring in our practices while struggling with the restrictions of managed care. The technological emphasis of medicine pulls us away from building, deepening, and sustaining relationships. As noted by philosopher Ken Wilber in his forward to this book, "Integral medicine is designed, in part, to help with those dilemmas, not only as they affect the patient or client but as they affect the physician and health-care practitioner."

An integral perspective to health and healing requires a sociopolitically, ecologically, and cosmologically literate view. This kind of literacy is needed to assist in the emergence of a healthy human-earth relationship, to teach us how to survive in an increasingly fragile ecosystem and violent human civilization, and to prepare the psyches of future generations who will inherit our environmental and social legacy. The words and creative actions of people who are sociopolitically and ecologically wise can help us restore internal and external balance with our deepest sensibility of being and lifestyle.

TRANSFORMING MEDICINE

This section begins with oncologist Rachel Naomi Remen describing efforts and trends within the medical profession relating to the search for meaning in medical work and the call for a return of soul to medicine. She cites the startling statistic from one study in California that 40 percent of physicians interviewed were clinically depressed. Physicians are being challenged by problems of meaning and identity presented by the changes in the health care system and the larger social environment. The challenges in medicine represent problems but also opportunities to search for the soul of medicine.

Challenges in medicine today arise not only from the external environment but also from within the profession itself. Physician and health care administrator Tom Janisse addresses the example of the renowned Kaiser Permanente system in his chapter. He cites the alarming findings from the Institute of Medicine study in 1999 on the high frequency of medical errors as an indicator of challenges to the system. He advocates social science solutions to medical problems. His vision of the promise of integral medicine is essentially that of people working together—doctors with doctors, doctors with other members of the health care team, doctors with patients. This dynamic fosters the collective expression of spirit.

Family medicine practitioner Lawrence E. George applies Wilber's integral model to the practice of family medicine. He further develops the theme of trusting intuition in healing. George envisions a practice of primary care that moves beyond modalities to consciousness and addresses the implications for medical education. Finally, family practice provides an organizational setting that can be respectful and inclusive of these broader perspectives and a suitable institutional host for the practice of integral medicine.

Expanding our understanding of healing relationships, Jean Watson, a professor of nursing, considers the metaphysics of virtual caring communities. She explores the connections between communities of caring and examines the potential of virtual reality for transformation of the healing environment. Watson points out that while there is a technical component to these transformations, there is also a metaphysical dimension. She explores new terrain for entering virtual caring communities, providing one path toward nursing and the public's future in health care.

SOCIOPOLITICAL TRANSFORMATIONS OF INTEGRAL MEDICINE

We begin this section with an essay by James Gordon, who served as the chair of the White House Commission on Complementary and Alternative Medicine (CAM) Policy from 2000 to 2002. Gordon, a psychiatrist and expert on CAM, compares the charge of this commission with that of the Flexner Report, a document that set the standard for medical practice and licensing, as well as medical education, for the twentieth century. In Gordon's words, "the White House Commission's Report offers a blueprint for transformation based on collaboration between professionals and patients; an approach to healthcare that transcends any particular system; an appreciation that medicine and healing are in the service of mental, emotional and spiritual fulfillment, as well as physical well-being, of personal wholeness and meaning."

Dr. Sumedha Khanna worked with the World Health Organization for over 25 years and served in 60 countries. Learning from this experience, she considers the sociopolitical potentials inherent in an integral approach to medicine. She notes that a new vision of health, healing, and medicine is not only needed but absolutely imperative throughout the world. An integral model, she argues, may address the personal, social, political, national, and international issues and speak to the consumer, as well as the health-care practitioner and organization.

HEALTHY EARTH—HEALTHY HUMAN

Exploring how we may become aware of our role as conscious agents in the evolutionary process will help us enfold a healthier human story into the larger relational, ecological, and cosmological framework. Cosmologist Brian Swimme and cultural historian and theologian Thomas Berry trace the story of the universe in a dazzling blend of poetry and science, placing human consciousness at the center of our societal and planetary evolution. Their essay provides the reader with an inspired and cautionary guide into our collective planetary future.

Writing from a similar perspective, Harvard psychologist Sarah Conn offers ecopsychology as a theoretical and practical healing system that identifies the ways human beings experience themselves within the larger ecological context. She invites us to consider the idea that human "dis-ease" may be the earth speaking through our individual and collective pain and stress. Conn articulates how healthy human identity and development is constantly transforming within the Earth's ever-changing life systems, while at the same time our sense of interconnectedness and wellness deepens.

Michael Lerner, president of Commonweal and an activist for reformation in medicine, writes about the "Legend of the Great Dying," or what scientists have named our current "Age of Extinctions." Lerner further elucidates that the path to ecological sanity and sustainability lies with the emerging environmental health movement. He argues that as the science connecting the decline in human health to the decline in the health of the environment becomes more hardy, so will the environmental health movement.

William Benda, a specialist in family medicine, and Rondi Lightmark broaden our discussion of healing relationships to consider the therapeutic dimensions of human/animal bonds as a manifestation of our connection with nature. Their contribution illustrates that while people may be "horse whisperers," animals may also serve as "people whisperers." In this essay, they review evidence of the physical and mental health benefits of animal-human interactions and provide examples of the application of these approaches. Examples are provided both of companion animals in the daily living environment and animals in the wild. This chapter ends as it began, with the words of Chief Seattle (1854): "What is man without beasts? If all the beasts were gone, man would die from a great loneliness of the spirit. All things are connected...."

SOCIAL HEALING

The final section of the book begins with an essay by James O'Dea, president of the Institute of Noetic Sciences, who introduces the concept of "social healing." Social healing strives to mend present and historical wounds that have been created by conflict, collective trauma, and large-scale oppression by bringing into consciousness the areas of collective memory and experience that "remain unresolved, neglected and repressed within the psyche of groups and even nations." For O'Dea, "it requires individuals to assume the responsibility to become healing agents themselves, and, as such, it is experiential rather than ideological."

Our final essay is written by the cultural historian Thomas Berry, whose central thesis in "The Great Work" is as follows: "The historical mission of our times is to reinvent the human—at the species level, with critical reflection, within the community of life-systems, in a time-developmental context, by means of story and shared dream experience." Berry takes us through his thesis step by step, making coherent what is conceptually huge and complex. Berry ends by saying, in blessing tones, that our hope for the future lies in awakening to our participation in the dream of the Earth, carried deep within our genetic coding.

Much of modern medicine, with its high-tech and low-touch approaches, removes the healing relationship from its ground in nature. As long as we continue to hold the human relationship with nature as a backdrop to the human story, rather than at the core of our unfolding being, we will not envision a truly integral story for medicine. Experiencing ourselves as separate, rather than interrelated with other life forms and systems, including the Earth itself, is viewed by ecophilosophers and ecopsychologists alike as the most threatening pathology of our times. Restoring our lost intimacy with planet Earth then involves a healing within our deepest psychic structures to enliven our ability to perceive the beauty and sacred language of nature. This is the context in which we offer this contribution to a growing understanding of the integral role of consciousness in healing and the future of humanity.

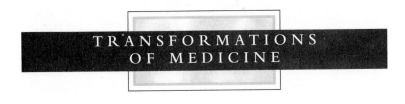

Recapturing the Soul of Medicine [*]

RACHEL NAOMI REMEN

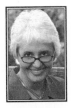

PHYSICIANS NEED TO RECLAIM MEANING IN THEIR WORKING LIVES

In the past 10 years the culture of medicine in California has changed radically. A study of 454 clinicians by the Sacramento Medical Society indicated that most had felt the effects of these changes deeply.[1] Forty percent of those interviewed were clinically depressed. Most reported that they had thought about leaving the profession at least once in the past 12 months. Even more surprising, many would not want their children to go into medicine, nor would they choose medicine as a career again.

This is not a California phenomenon. An unprecedented number of physicians nationwide, many of them young, are dropping out or seeking early retirement. Something unusual is happening among physicians, and those who care about physician well-being may need to broaden their

---

*Adapted from Remen RN: Recapturing the Soul of Medicine, *The Western Journal of Medicine* 174: 4–5, 2001.

concern from the care of impaired physicians to the care of all physicians. The future of our profession may be at stake.

There is reason to believe that our professionalism—our traditional professional stance, our attitudes, self-expectations, and indeed our training—has made us particularly vulnerable to the kind of stress we currently experience. Year after year in medical schools across the country, the first-year class enters filled with a sense of privilege and excitement about becoming doctors. Four years later, this excitement has given way to cynicism and numbness. By graduation, students seem to have learned what they have come to do but forgotten why they have come. In these times, we need to reconsider the principles by which we traditionally educate physicians. We will need to reexamine our educational goals, objectives, and Douglas Diekema strategies to help students stand up to the stresses of contemporary medical practice.

FINDING MEANING

Teaching the practice of medicine involves more than teaching its science. Medicine is in crisis, and in crisis we need to find something stronger than our science to hold on to, something more satisfying and sustaining to us as people in this work. Perhaps the answer lies in learning to cultivate the meaning of our work in the same way that we have traditionally pursued its knowledge base. We will need to learn to educate students to find meaning as skillfully as we educate them to pursue medical expertise.

In times of difficulty, meaning strengthens us not by changing our lives but by transforming our experience of our lives. The Italian psychiatrist Roberto Assagioli tells a parable about three stone cutters building a cathedral in the Middle Ages. You approach the first man and ask him what he's doing. Angrily, he turns to you and says, "Idiot! Use your eyes! They bring me a rock, I cut it into a block, they take it away, and they bring me another rock. I've been doing this since I was old enough to work, and I'm going to be doing it until the day that I die." Quickly you withdraw, go to the next man, and ask him the same question. He smiles at you warmly and tells you, "I'm earning a living for my beloved family. With my wages I have built a home, there is food on our table, the children are growing strong." Moving on, you approach the third man with this same question. Pausing, he gives you a look of deep fulfillment and tells you, "I am building a great cathedral, a holy lighthouse where people lost in the dark can find their strength and remember their way. And it will stand for a thousand years!" Each of these men is doing the identical task. Finding a personal meaning in your work opens even the most routine of tasks to the dimension of satisfaction and even joy. We may need to recognize meaning for the resource it is and find ways to pursue it and preserve it.

RESTORING A SENSE OF SERVICE

Meaning is the antecedent of commitment, and the original meaning of our work is service. Service is not a relationship between an expert and a problem; it is a human relationship, a work of the heart and the soul. Restoring a sense of service to the practice of medicine will lead us to re-examine the process by which we become physicians. Our current training furthers our expertise but not our wholeness. We are trained to value objectivity. We are taught to view a genuine human connection as unprofessional. But we cannot serve or find meaning at a distance. Learning to serve requires education, not training. The root word of education, *educari*, means to lead forth the innate wholeness of each student. Medical training often wounds and diminishes us. Restoring a sense of service in our students will require fundamental educational reform.

As professionals, we may not be fully connected to our lives. Distance may become a daily habit. In reality, most physicians lead far more meaningful lives than they realize. Proust said, "The voyage of discovery lies not in seeking new vistas, but in having new eyes." Finding meaning will require us to see the familiar in new ways.

Harry, an emergency physician, tells a story about a woman who was brought into his emergency department about to give birth. As soon as he examined her, he realized that unless her obstetrician was already on his way, he was going to get to deliver this baby himself. He had barely finished his examination when the head crowned, and, with nurses on either side of him holding the mother's legs on their shoulders, Harry delivered a little girl.

She was breathing spontaneously, and he felt a familiar sense of satisfaction at his own competence. He laid her along his left forearm with the back of her head in his left hand and began to suction her nose and mouth. Suddenly, the infant opened her eyes and looked directly at him. In that instant, Harry realized that he was the first human being this baby girl had ever seen. Deeply moved, he felt his heart go out to her in welcome from all people everywhere, and for a moment he had tears in his eyes.

All this surprised him. Harry has delivered many babies and has always enjoyed the excitement of making rapid decisions and testing his skills. But he had never before let himself experience the meaning of what he was doing or let himself know what he was serving with his expertise. He feels changed by this moment. In that flash of recognition, he felt years of cynicism and fatigue fall away and remembered why he had chosen this work in the first place. As he put it, "It all suddenly seemed worth it."

Meaning is a human need. It strengthens us, not by numbing our pain or distracting us from our problems or even by comforting us. It heals us by reminding us of our integrity, who we are, and what we stand for. It offers us a place from which to meet the challenges of life. Part of our responsibility as professionals is to fight for our sense of meaning—against fatigue and numbness, overwork, and unreasonable expectations—to find ways to strengthen it in ourselves and in each other. We will need to rebuild the medical system, not just on sound science or sound economics but on the integrity of our commitment. It has become vital to remember the essential nature of this work and renew our sense of calling to preserve the meaning of the work for ourselves and for those who will follow.

The reference for this essay is located on the DVD accompanying this book.

Through Conventional Medicine to Integral Medicine: Challenges and Promises *

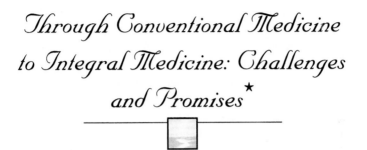

TOM JANISSE

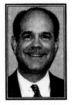

INTRODUCTORY PERSPECTIVE

Conventional medical care and the physicians practicing it are often thought both the adversary and barrier to a system of integral medicine. Although neither the widest range of complementary and alternative therapies nor their practitioners are readily included in conventional medical care, physician, group, and system proponents of integral medi-cine are working from within to enhance conventional medical care with

*Supported by Product and Service Research & Design, Northwest Permanente PC, Portland, Oregon.

these principles and practices. Kaiser Permanente (KP), the largest integrated medical care delivery system in the nation, is one of those health care systems. KP offers a large organization for a natural experiment and a progressive model to address the challenges and promises within and facing medicine. Many or all of these structures or practices may exist throughout conventional medicine across the country. The salient point is that conventional medicine today offers promise, through demonstrated current practices, of evolution toward a future integral medicine.

Two recent major events have prompted fundamental reexamination of conventional medical practice. The first was publication of the report in 1999, "To Err is Human: Building a Safer Health System," by the Institute of Medicine (IOM), a branch of the National Academy of Sciences.[1] In this report, the IOM expressed great concern for patient safety in medical care. The second event was publication in 2001 of IOM's subsequent report, "Crossing the Quality Chasm: A New Health System for the 21st Century," focusing on the broader variation and deficiency in medical practice today.[2] Their recommendations for quality improvement included patient-centered, multidisciplinary, team-based care. Although many avenues of opportunity flow from their recommendations, for me the most important promise to this report's challenge to medicine is the inspirational expectation that the patient is at the center of care. "Nothing about me without me"[3]; "We are guests in our patients' lives"; "Everything and only what the patient wants and needs, when and how they need it"[4]—all are aphorisms emerging from the work of Tom Delbanco, MD, Professor of Medicine at Harvard Medical School, and Donald Berwick, MD, President of the Institute for Healthcare Improvement in Boston and IOM member.

Some physicians immediately see technologic solutions, other physicians see disease management solutions, and others see the necessity for a true evidence base for the practice of medicine. I see social science solutions, including advances in the transpersonal nature of interaction between people, physicians, practitioners, and groups. The words of Wheatley and Kellner-Rogers, "Our behaviors change only if we decide to belong together differently,"[5] characterize the individual and collective interior of Ken Wilber's integral model, which can positively infuse objective health care work with enhanced meaning and purpose.[6] Conversations with each other, sharing experiences through stories, and working together infuses the objective practice of medicine and health care with the subjective experiences of individuals and groups.[7] Integration of all quadrants holds great promise for overcoming current challenges facing medicine.

My approach in this chapter is to explore the evolutionary changes at work in conventional medicine within KP, a large institution that I know, as a Permanente physician, from the system level through to the individual level: from field effects in the form of vision statements, leadership behavior, and subtle suggestion to individual practices of intuitive knowing and intentional healing present in private physician-patient encounters.

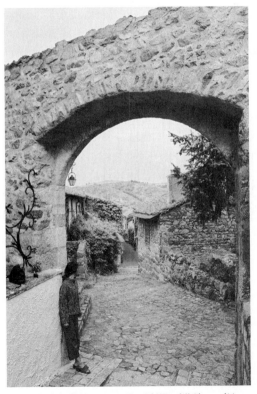

"Archadelic." (Courtesy David "Dudi" Shmueli.)

INTEGRAL VISION: A SPIRAL PROGRESSION

People, both physicians and patients, experience health care objectively in the individual exterior realm. Although people bring a subjective interior presence, this is often not evident in routine interactions. A cancer patient's subjective illness accompanies his or her physical disease into the radiation oncology unit to receive exterior radiation treatment. In the context of a consultation with a professional, little exchange may occur between the personal interiors of doctor and patient: The experience is a lonely, disconnected, objective one. The challenge for conventional medicine is to bridge this objective-subjective gap, and the promise of medicine is that when this happens practitioners and patients will find enhanced meaning and greater benefit. In the cold, impersonal moments, a fire of personal fusion will ignite.

Integrating the four quadrants of Ken Wilber's Integral Model (Figure 1) can also be viewed as a progressive journey, spiraling toward a more integral future. The following two examples show cyclic progression of evolution from polar duality to holistic integrity, the desired state in integral medicine.

A Physician

A person with a subjective intention to care for others may become a doctor. Graduating from medical school training, this person dons the

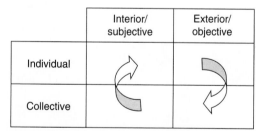

Figure 1 Ken Wilber's Integral Model shows the cyclical progression from interior (subjective) individual to interior group. (Modified by the publisher (www.shambhala.com) and author from: Wilber K: *The eye of spirit: an integral vision for a world gone slightly mad,* Boston, 1998, Shambhala Publications.)

objectivity of a professional physician, unwittingly distancing from the person within. If (s)he belongs to a medical group, however, (s)he may connect with other physician-professionals as a collective. If that group defines and shares values, then collective subjectivity emerges. To complete the cycle, if each individual physician's personal values coincide with the group's professional values, then the physicians may integrate their personal subjectivity to arrive at the place where they started, although not as the same person. This journey has occurred for many physicians in the Permanente Medical Groups.

A Health Care Team

The next growth cycle in this spiral progression toward integral medicine includes integration of the people on a health care team—physicians, associate practitioners, nurses, medical assistants, clerks, and receptionists. Team members grow from the individual/exterior (professional and staff roles) into the exterior/collective of a team. In the team's work together, they create values and a shared vision of patient care. Having decided to belong together differently, the team evolves an interdisciplinary collective interior. This collective may grow an egalitarian sensibility of contribution and fit. Finally, the group may connect further through integrating their personal subjectivity. Teams become small communities in a large organization.

INTEGRAL VISION: A HEALTH CARE MODEL

The Institute of Noetic Sciences created a vision, embedded in their name, of associating, connecting, and integrating consciousness and science. With this as reference and using an additional simple model, health care complexity can be layered into four interdependent scientific realms—medical science, systems science, social science, and economic science—with subjective consciousness emerging in the social science layer and objective consciousness pervading the other three layers (Figure 2).

Conventional medicine has historically defined and limited its scope to medical science—the anatomic, physiologic, microbiologic, and physical. For example, physicians diagnose diabetes mellitus on the basis of elevated blood glucose level and treat it pharmacologically with insulin. Two

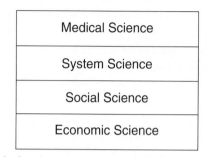

Figure 2 A simple four-layer model to represent the complex interactions of health care.

decades ago, physicians' interest expanded to systems science—describing clinical guidelines for the diagnosis and treatment of diabetes, mapping diabetic care processes, and studying the health systems in which the clinical care of diabetes is embedded. In the last decade, with direction from clinical quality groups like the Institute for Healthcare Improvement in Boston, physicians began to explore the social science of medicine. For example, KP's Care Management Institute assessed the benefit of physicians working within multidisciplinary teams to deliver medical care that had become increasingly complex with chronic disease management, consumerism, the Internet, self-care, self-management, and shared decisions. More recently, exploration has extended to study of the social structure and human interactions of those teams—how people feel about each other in their clinical work environment and development of personal and team relationships to support their health care work to serve patients.[8] In addition, understanding interdependency of systems science and social science is necessary for physicians and teams to collaborate in optimizing and managing the office practice supporting their clinical practice. Issues previously relegated to a human resources department or an office manager were worked through by the multidisciplinary teams themselves. As self-direction led to self-regulation, complex adaptive system behavior emerged.[8]

These three science layers—medical, system, and social—become intricately interwoven when the teams realize that the social sciences—the sociologic, psychologic, and anthropologic factors at work in human interactional dynamics—are critical to understanding and enhancing patient care in both small modules and large institutions.

The challenge for conventional medicine is to recognize the personal component at work in the material care provided. The promise is integration of the interior with the exterior, of subjectivity with objectivity, in the course of people working together to improve care for patients. Integrating exterior individual elements into an exterior collective can lead to developing an internal collective—the power of social science, the power of intersubjectivity.

Health Care System

KP is the largest vertically integrated health care service delivery and financing system in the country. The Permanente Medical Groups, the largest integrated multispecialty group practice in the country, exclusively contracts to deliver the medical care covered by the Kaiser Foundation Health Plan and Hospitals. Integration into a collective sets a context at an institutional and organizational level for integral medicine and creates readiness and predisposition for interinstitutional and interorganizational integral medicine.

Interorganizational Collaboration

When, in 1999, the KP Northwest (NW) Center for Health Research won one of the 12 Complementary and Alternative Medicine Research Center grants from the National Institutes of Health, it established the Oregon Center for Complementary and Alternative Medicine (OCCAM).[9] The center integrated into an executive committee the four Portland metropolitan area complementary and alternative medicine (CAM) colleges—the Oregon College of Oriental Medicine, the National College of Naturopathic Medicine, the Western States Chiropractic College, and the Oregon School of Massage—with the KP medical care delivery system, the KP Dental Care Program, and the Oregon Health Sciences University School of Dentistry.[9] This executive committee, composed of research and clinical representatives from all seven entities, ensured importing the best scientific thinking and experience in these disciplines into the rigorous research projects planned to explore effectiveness and benefit from CAM therapies. Through this exterior collective integration, researchers and practitioners began to grow an interior collective consciousness and sensibility.

Intraorganizational Collaboration

The Permanente Journal, the national medical journal of the eight Permanente Medical Groups, represents a field effect of collectivity by its mere existence, by the quality and value its visual image represents to physicians, and by the collective pride it engenders in physicians. When the journal's content creates shared practices, shared experience, and shared values, further integration of collective subjectivity is achieved.

Groups

Cooperative Health Care Clinic: Having an associated research center can be highly beneficial for people designing and developing clinical services. One new program is an example. A decade ago, John Scott, MD, a Colorado Permanente internist, developed the Cooperative Health Care Clinic concept, in which several patients with similar medical conditions gathered to have a group visit with their doctor and a multidisciplinary team.[10] More recently, in the KP Northwest Region, Charles Elder, MD, a NW Permanente internist, adapted this model to meet patients' needs for information and guidance in the area of CAM.[11] Through his association with OCCAM and as one of their first research fellows, Dr. Elder infused his referral group clinic and his research with Ayurvedic medicine principles and practices. This practice is a form of integral medicine.

In addition to the clinical benefits available from a multidisciplinary team and patient interaction, group effects extend to patients who, as a patient collective, share experiences with each other, stories, successful approaches, and empathetic intersubjectivity.

Multidisciplinary Pain Clinic: Conventional medicine has recognized the high value of collecting disciplines together to treat certain medical conditions. Cancer has been one area where the psychosocial-behavioral disciplines now constitute an important part of the treatment. Another example is the multidisciplinary chronic pain clinic established in the KP Northwest Region.[12] Initially, physicians focused on creating connections with conventional specialty departments because chronic pain was recognized as a complex, multisystem condition. Psychologic assessment and treatment was viewed as an integral part of a successful treatment program[12] More recently, value has emerged in offering CAM therapies as part of the treatment program. With a CAM research center in the KP organization and high interest of the pain clinic experts in exploring innovative options, two additional therapeutic services are being researched in the KPNW Region: hypnosis and therapeutic touch. This expansion demonstrates evolution in both the collective exterior realm of the pain clinic and the individual interior of these subjective therapies.

Teams

Integrated health care teams are a crucial component of the KP health care system. A workgroup of the Interregional Care Experience Council recently conducted interviews of team members of the KP internal medicine teams that achieved high physician, practitioner, and staff satisfaction with work life and high patient satisfaction with care. Quotes from these team members bring alive the integration into collective exterior and interior: "Everyone shared, and everyone was listened to"; "Everyone has a voice"; "In a multidisciplinary team, if each segment of the team is working well, then the whole team works well"; "Everyone makes a contribution"; "Personal and professional relations improve when you work with people a lot; we see each other and know each other"; "We care about each other."

Patient and Physician

Patient-physician encounters in the conventional medicine office visit have been evolving from a traditional doctor-centered communication approach to a patient-centered communication and relationship approach and thus from objectivity to subjectivity. I would like to offer two examples.

Patient-Doctor Communication

Consider my poetic characterization of the evolution of the doctor-patient relationship, illustrated in Figure 3.[13]

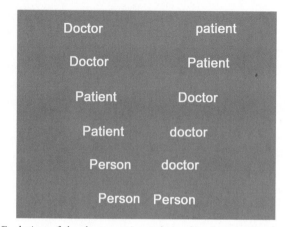

Figure 3 Evolution of the doctor-patient relationship. See text for description. (From Janisse T: Editors' comments. Primary care innovation, *Permanente Journal* 2(3):2-3, Summer 1998.)

Doctor-patient: Evolution begins with the traditional hierarchical physician-directed interaction, in which historically the patient–thinly gowned in a cold, lifeless room–has been diminished while waiting for the doctor. Required to state a chief "complaint," the patient is relegated at the outset of the encounter as a problem; then she is "examined." Few questions are permitted; there is neither time nor tolerance. "Yes, doctor. Thank you, doctor" is the appropriate refrain. Some may view this characterization as starkly accurate; some may view this as cynical. For some patients, this scenario may represent a comfortable and appropriate interactional dynamic.

Doctor-Patient: The patient assumes a certain stature, perhaps more recognized and regarded, or the doctor may have learned about customer service.

Patient-Doctor: A dramatic change occurs toward a patient-centered approach, in which both patient and doctor, however, are still possibly tense and rethinking the new model as well as their past and current communication behaviors. Partnership now begins to develop.

Patient-doctor: The doctor diminishes her(him)self in power and stature. Sitting down with hand off the doorknob, (s)he listens more, directs less, asks about the patient's preferences, and reformats "taking the history, making the diagnosis, and ordering the treatment" into a shared decision process. Partnership is more evident.

Person-doctor: The doctor recognizes the patient as a person from a holistic perspective: (S)he encourages expression of psychosocial-behavioral factors, family stories, and personal stories of vacations or hobbies or community involvement and includes these in a holistic diagnosis and treatment program.

Person-Person: The doctor reveals the person in her(him)self, the holistic nature of work as a doctor. Doctors may have lost a sense of the importance they play as a person in interactions with their patients. A purely intellectual exchange with only a physical outcome is often ineffectual in treating a patient's condition, which has both a physical component and a personal component (psychologic, emotional, social, and spiritual). In addition, evolution to this point prepares a person for a transpersonal encounter. Deep attention, presence, and compassion open to intuitive knowing and intentional caring.[14]

This model is dynamic. Patients and doctors may always find comfort and effective communication and relationship at one of these levels. Their communication may also evolve over time as their relationship builds. They may move from one level to the next during a single encounter.

In this evolution, the physician and patient each move from the exterior individual realm to the interior collective realm when they interact as people sharing a common moment of importance. Here in the realm of interpersonal interaction there is the potential to move to a transpersonal moment of either intuitive knowing or intentional caring. This place is that of intersubjectivity—a timeless moment of connection. Physicians, in that moment, may move from perceiving the visit as a diagnostic and treatment determination to perceiving the visit as a therapeutic moment. A caring act of intention may initiate the healing process before the first pill is swallowed, or this caring act may become the treatment itself (for example, validation of a self-care approach that could work instead of a prescribed pill).

Dimensions of the Interaction

Exploring dimensions of the patient-doctor interaction allows another perspective on this ancient encounter.

On the basis of Abraham Maslow's premise of a human's hierarchy of need—that lower-order needs must be satisfied before higher-order needs can possibly be satisfied—the model in Figure 4 shows a patient's hierarchy of need. The premise in shared decisions is that patients' needs, beliefs, and preferences (previously below the waterline of the doctor's awareness) must be recognized and met before medical evidence matters to them or before they are willing to follow the doctor's recommended treatment. This exploration in the interactive dialogue between patient and doctor exhibits movement from exterior dimensions of content, evidence, physical agents, and behavior to interior

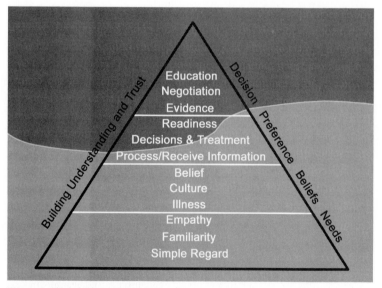

Figure 4 Shared dimensions of the physician-patient interaction show the hierarchy of patients' needs through the decision-making process. Historically, doctors were unaware of, or attended less to, those factors in the lighter region of the pyramid under the "waterline."

dimensions of needs, beliefs, and preferences. Not only is duality bridged, but integration also occurs.

The challenge for conventional medicine crosses a spectrum, from a physician becoming aware of the interior subjective and its importance in medical care to developing the skills to interact and engage in the subjective and intersubjective. The promise is that some physicians already practice that way: They practice integral medicine.

Physician

In Northern California, The Permanente Medical Group's physician health department created an educational videotape entitled "Mindfulness in Medicine," which focuses on mindfulness practice for busy doctors and health care professionals to reduce stress and increase work satisfaction.[15] The tape, made in conjunction with Jon Kabat-Zinn, Ph.D., founder of the stress reduction clinic at the University of Massachusetts Memorial Medical Center in Worcester, Massachusetts, highlights ways to work with patients and staff applying mindfulness practice in the clinic and hospital settings. Clinicians explain how focusing on breathing and body awareness, responding nonjudgmentally, and feeling less controlled by time improves their work and personal satisfaction.

Emil Dionysian, MD, an orthopedist in the Southern California Permanente Medical Group, learned how to meditate and, finding benefit, applied meditation in his daily practice with patients and colleagues. He now acts as a trainer at Deepak Chopra's Chopra Center for Wellness in La Jolla, California. Both these examples demonstrate the promise in conventional medicine to integrate the individual subjective into the primarily exterior objective practice of medicine for the benefit of patients and practitioners.

Patient

SELF-CARE David Moiel, MD, NW Permanente Chief of Surgery, developed a multidisciplinary team approach toward care of morbidly obese patients. Although his approach includes bariatric surgery, a writing course is now also included for these patients to express feelings about surgery, alteration of their diet and lifestyle, and transformation of their body image.[16] One patient quote is representative of the benefit patients have found: "In this group of like patients, writing about how I feel was more valuable for my health improvement than all of the years I spent in therapy." In San Diego, KP's Positive Choice Wellness Center similarly has used patient writing as therapy for various conditions.[17]

The challenge is that conventional medicine resorts to such physical means as gastric stapling to treat a medical condition. The promise is that the surgical team has chosen a multidisciplinary team approach, attention to psychosocial-behavioral issues, and a writing program to express feelings. This plumbs the subjective interior for improved health.

CHRONIC DISEASE SELF-MANAGEMENT In a multiyear, multi-region study,[18] David Sobel, MD, who practices primary care adult medicine with The Permanente Medical Group and is KP Northern California Director of Patient Education and Health Promotion, demonstrated that patients with chronic illness can be trained to give other patients structured educational support for behavioral change. These educational interventions can improve health behavior, quality of life, functional status, and health care utilization as well as costs in patients who have mixed chronic illness.[18] Although this self-management activity describes what is explicitly an exterior collective process, the beneficial outcomes from this activity represent a remarkable venture into the realm of patients teaching each other. This form of self-management may also include a component of intersubjectivity—an interpersonal activity between people with like issues in coping with chronic illness. The focus is on helping people lead as healthy a life as possible despite their illness.

Belief-Based Medicine

Essential to appreciating the value of subjective experience in medicine is to understand that people—patients and physicians—may behave on the basis of both their beliefs and their knowledge. These could be based on ancient wisdom or cultural practices, or they could be based on clinical experience and the conclusions of randomized controlled trials (science). Science does not always prevail in the minds of patients, in part because they do not understand the science and in part because their beliefs and preferences are not acknowledged, addressed, or met. Perhaps the high rate of patient "nonadherence" commonly reported in the medical literature is actually due to noncongruence of science and belief systems.

Physicians may not strongly consider patients' personal or cultural beliefs and experiences because they are not scientifically verified and may thus consider them ineffectual and unimportant. Some physicians may also avoid these beliefs because they find it personally threatening to leave the safety of their training experience and personally invoke their own life skills.

Furthermore, some physicians may not believe medical science, or incorporate it, because science does not fit their experience, practice, clinical judgment, or clinical belief system.[19] The troubling disconnection is that, because patients can't base their decisions on science, either because of unavailability of the information or lack of understanding, they must believe in and trust the physician. If the physician does not acknowledge and incorporate the patient's beliefs, then the patient's confidence in the physician may wane. There is a balance between personal and professional beliefs, experience, and scientific evidence for both doctor and patient that prevails in effective medical care.

The beliefs and subjective experiences of individuals and collectives are essential components of effective medical care and, when integrated with the exterior objectivity of conventional medicine, can result in effective integral medicine. The challenge is that physicians hold steadfast to the singular importance of scientific knowledge as seen in the public "evidence-based medicine" movement. The promise is that physicians and patients can admit the elements of belief and experience into their private decision processes. More substantively, with the increasing emphasis on culturally competent care to enhance medical outcomes, physicians and patients will find a common ground of understanding to improve their decisions together.

SUMMARY CONCLUSION

Although conventional medicine faces challenges in its evolution toward integral medicine, many signs promise progression. Using KP as a model that I know, my approach is intended to represent conventional medicine across the country, although KP's integrated system may differ in some ways. Noteworthy practices exist at the many levels of system, organization, group, team, physician and patient, physician, patient, and beliefs that indicate positive movement toward a future of integral medicine.

ACKNOWLEDGMENT

The Kaiser Permanente Medical Editing Department provided editorial assistance.

References for this essay are located on the DVD accompanying this book.

Transformation of the Healer: The Application of Ken Wilber's Integral Model to Family Practice Medicine

LAWRENCE E. GEORGE

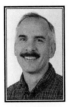

TRANSFORMATION OF HEALER AND PATIENT

A woman named Lynn (not her real name) came to see me about 10 years ago with the rather unusual complaint of excessive tearing—what in medicine is referred to as *epiphora*. The most common cause of this condition is obstruction of the tear ducts, which drain the tears down into the nose. A less common cause is excess production of tears from the lacrimal glands, which overwhelms the lacrimal ducts' ability to drain them away. Lynn was about 32 years of age and very attractive. She had been dealing with this condition for a number of years and was very annoyed with the constant tearing. I was not the first physician she had consulted for the problem, and, in fact, she had seen several ophthalmologists who had gone as far as probing her tear ducts several times, all to no avail. I listened carefully to her story and then replied that if the tear ducts were open and functioning, it would appear that the cause of the excess tearing was more likely from excess tear production. Furthermore, I suggested that I believed it was possible that if she was suffering with some type of subconscious issue, she might be, in effect, "crying" due to this buried emotional wound, causing the lacrimal glands to overproduce as in actual crying. She gave me a funny look and then rather abruptly announced she was leaving. At that point, it felt to me that I was in need of some emergency surgery to extract my size-11 foot from my mouth.

One year later Lynn returned to my clinic. She reported that during the visit of the previous year she left the office feeling that I was one crazy quack-of-a-doctor. Three months after that visit, however, she began having flashbacks about being sexually abused by her father. After 6 months of psychotherapy, the epiphora had resolved and she was coming to the office to thank me. My intervention that day provided an opening through which her healing could begin.

At that time, I was not really sure why I said what I did, but the experience taught me a couple of things. First, I was empowered to trust my intuition with my patients. As Alanis Morissette says in her song "You Learn,"[1] "I recommend sticking your foot in your mouth at any time." Second, I was motivated to expand the way I practice medicine to be more inclusive and holistic. I spent the next several years seeking in earnest for a model of health care that would make sense of what I was experiencing in the doctor-patient relationship.

KEN WILBER AND THE INTEGRAL MODEL

After years of searching and learning, I discovered the work of Ken Wilber, and immediately recognized that I had come across something worthy of extensive study. Here was a model of the evolution of human consciousness that included more truth, from more disciplines of discovery, than anything I had heretofore encountered. I began to apply the model and my new awareness to the practice of medicine, which is now referred to as *integral medicine*. Along the way, I often felt confused about how to prioritize and make sense of the complementary concepts that I was learning; Wilber's model did exactly that, and quite a bit more.

I think it is important to distinguish integral medicine from integrated or integrative medicine, which is the addition of alternative modalities of treatment (such as chiropractic, energy medicine, *Reiki*, herbology, homeopathy, etc.) to conventional or orthodox Western medicine. While these other treatment modalities certainly offer additional, often helpful approaches to patients, without a comprehensive model to make sense of how these diverse modalities fit in the overall approach to treating patients, it is a bit like adding more surgical instruments to the surgical tray without knowing how or when to use them during the operation, and whether or not they even apply to a particular operation.

It is difficult to summarize Wilber's model, which he has been refining for over 2 decades, in a short article, but a brief overview will help show its very useful application to medicine. The reader is encouraged to read Wilber's *A Brief History of Everything*[2] and *A Theory of Everything*[3] for a more complete description. After an extensive search of all the world's wisdom traditions, he delineated some twenty or so principles that guide evolution—what he refers to as *orienting generalizations*.

The first is that everything that exists is a holon. A holon is a whole/part—that is, everything that exists is a whole in and of itself and also a part of something else.

Another orienting generalization is that evolution proceeds in a transcending and including fashion. An example he commonly cites is that atoms are a part of molecules, which are a part of cells, which are a part of organisms, and so on, with each level transcending the former by including the component parts but adding something new and unique not present in the parts. In other words, each level becomes more significant as holons move up the evolutionary scale. A simplified version of the levels of evolution of a human being is the progression from body, to emotion, to mind, to soul, to spirit.

A third orienting generalization is that all holons exist in four aspects or quadrants simultaneously: (1) the individual external/physical aspect (upper right, UR), (2) the collective external/physical or social aspect (lower right, LR), (3) the individual internal/nonphysical aspect (upper left, UL) and (4) the collective internal/nonphysical or cultural aspect (lower left, LL)

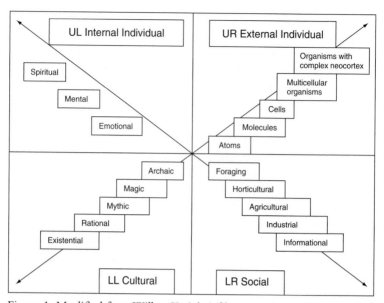

Figure 1 Modified from Wilber K: A brief history of everything, Boston, 1996, Shambhala Publications.

(see Figure 1; this is a greatly abbreviated version, with the lower left represented by cultural worldviews and the lower right by techno-economic base).

A simplified way of viewing the model, with regard to treating patients, is that each patient is to be viewed as a body, mind, and spirit (the levels) as he or she exists as a self in both cultural and social aspects (the quadrants). Now, the model is much more complicated and encompassing than this, as one will discover upon studying Wilber's work (e.g., lines of development, states and types of consciousness), but even these relatively straightforward principles can obviate some of the dissociation that is occurring in orthodox Western medicine today.

APPLICATION OF THE INTEGRAL MODEL TO MEDICINE

One can immediately see an application to medicine in the previously mentioned orienting generalizations. For example, since every thing that exists is a holon, all diseases can be considered to be holons. And since every holon exists in the four quadrants simultaneously, every disease has social, cultural, internal (the emotional, mental, and spiritual levels), and external/physical aspects. Furthermore, since each quadrant has multiple levels that increase in significance (also known as increased spiritual depth), each level (emotional, mental, and spiritual in the left upper quadrant) becomes more significant to both health and illness. What the model predicts for any individual is that each transcending level—for example, from physical to emotional to mental to spiritual—becomes increasingly significant to that individual's health and/or illness. As an example from the beginning of life, we know that you can feed an infant the highest quality breast milk (physical level, UR), but if the child is not loved and held (emotional level, UL), the child will not thrive and may even die.[4] At the other end of the spectrum, longevity studies have shown that one's attitude (emotional/mental/spiritual) is a better predictor of longevity than lifestyle or genetics (physical).[5-7] Based on my experience and study, as well as what the integral model predicts about the increasing significance of successive levels of development, I would estimate that genetics might be responsible for 10 percent to 20 percent of the illnesses we manifest (this obviously varies greatly from one disease entity to the next); environment (including smoking, excess drinking, pollution) approximately 30 percent; and emotional, mental, and spiritual issues the remaining 50 percent to 60 percent.

DIFFERENCES BETWEEN TRADITIONAL AND INTEGRAL MEDICAL APPROACHES

It is important to see that even though illness is usually viewed as emotional, psychological, or physical (i.e., not all of these at once), one will find internal (emotional, mental, and spiritual) and external (physical) representation, both individually and collectively, in every disease or illness. Western medicine typically treats medical, and often psychiatric illness, from a purely UR viewpoint and misses the really interesting aspects on the internal side.

A recent article from the American Academy of Family Practice reveals an approach to interstitial cystitis that is typical of the Western medical model.[8] The author states that there has never been an association with psychological issues in this condition, but goes on to say that there *is* an association with multiple other conditions and illnesses (e.g., fibromyalgia, migraine headaches, chronic fatigue syndrome, endometriosis), which, incidentally, *have* been shown to be associated with psychosocial issues.[9-12] It appears to be, in part, a case of not being aware of all of the diverse studies that are published, and certainly a lack of an integral awareness.

A psychiatrist once sent me a patient (whom he was treating for depression) for evaluation of chronic pelvic pain. Knowing that chronic pelvic pain has an association with a history of sexual abuse,[13,14] I questioned her as to whether this had occurred. She replied that, in fact, she had been sexually abused in childhood. I later called the psychiatrist to inquire whether any evaluation or treatment of her sexual abuse issues had been done, to which he replied, "We usually don't get into that." The problem tends to be that a thorough, dialogical, internal evaluation of the patient is usually not done, even by a psychiatrist who is traditionally trained for this type of intervention.

It becomes apparent, in an integral methodology, that treatments and therapeutic modalities should be specific to the respective level of the problem. Bill, a 47 year-old patient, came in for a physical exam and concerns regarding hypertension, chronic back pain, and migraine headaches. He had been engaged in regular meditation practice, 30 minutes a day, for more than 5 years; a yoga practice; fairly regular aerobic exercise; and a decent diet, and yet, his medical problems suggested to me that there were likely still unresolved emotional-level issues that were subconscious in nature. When I suggested this to him, he replied that he felt he had completed this work previously through reading, counseling, and workshops. I then offered that his spiritual practice would not heal old wounds (although the practice might loosen the lid, so to speak, on the subconscious and help bring these issues to the surface) and that the signs and symptoms of his physical body suggested that there might possibly be more emotional work to be done. He called a few days later to say that, after our discussion, he was beginning to experience some previously repressed emotion and would like to get back into psychotherapy. The typical Western medical approach would likely have limited the treatment to medication and perhaps physical therapy, missing the opportunity for a deeper and more comprehensive (i.e., integral/AQAL; "all quadrant, all level") approach. In effect, climbing two or three trees and completely missing the forest.

A precaution, of which the medical provider should be aware, is that certain interventions are not appropriate for all patients, depending on their level of development (this is true for interventions in physical, emotional, mental, and spiritual issues). For example, with regard to the spiritual line,[15] some Christians consider meditation to be evil, and therefore meditation would not be an appropriate therapeutic intervention for their particular spiritual level. The integral practitioner must be sensitive to each individual and avoid a one-size-fits-all type of intervention.

A young couple came to me with their 3-year-old daughter with the complaint that her behavior was so out of control that the father was on the verge of divorcing his wife to get away from all the stress associated with dealing with his daughter. He requested that I prescribe some type of medication for his daughter to make her more manageable. The child's mother was equally, if not more, stressed than her husband, and both were eager for a solution. The little girl was absolutely beautiful and, interestingly, very well-behaved during the visit. It became evident after a long interview that the problem began when the girl was approximately 18 to 24 months of age, during her toddler separation phase, and around the time that the father insisted that the child's pacifier be taken away. I pointed out that their daughter was going through a rather difficult psychological transition when they took away one of her coping skills, namely the pacifier. At this point, the father became angrier and insisted that under no circumstance would they ever give the pacifier back. He evidently preferred divorce to this rather simple intervention. In addition, the parents were using age-inappropriate discipline techniques, such as time-outs, which only further upset the girl. Since the father would not consider the pacifier, I suggested that, instead of alienating their daughter when she acted out, they try holding her, rocking her, and loving her. The mother seemed willing to try this intervention, but the father seemed rather disappointed that I had not simply prescribed a medication. I almost suggested that I might be willing to treat pharmacologically, that is for the parents, not the child (a little Xanax might go a long way for this particular father). I did see the mother about 6 months later and was pleased to hear that the intervention was very helpful.

Analysis of this problem from an integral perspective gives a more complete understanding of the factors involved and suggests a more comprehensive solution to the problem. Western medicine has increasingly moved toward a relatively exclusive UR pharmacologic approach. While this has certainly been very helpful in the treatment of numerous medical and psychological problems, there has been a dangerous and dissociated over-reliance on this UR quadrant approach. Certainly, knowledge of childhood psychological stage development (levels) is critical to helping the parents understand what their daughter might be experiencing and how to help them comfort her through this process. Equally important, however, is understanding the LL negative cultural attitude toward nursing beyond a certain age and widespread lack of acceptance of children's need to suckle to comfort themselves, which may continue to age 4 or 5. In addition, the parents would do well to begin to understand their own unmet emotional needs and family system cultural beliefs from their respective childhoods (UL and LL) to be more effective in their parenting.

PROBLEMS IN MEDICAL EDUCATION: GROSS AND SUBTLE REDUCTIONISM

A majority of medical schools today have included complementary and alternative classes in their curricula, but it is apparent to me, from working with medical students and family practice resident physicians in my office, that these courses are often optional and are treated as another tool one can consider using, but as with the previous analogy regarding the surgical instruments, there is no overriding model to help us see how all the instruments fit together or how and when they should be used.

Since the dawn of science, as Ken Wilber has pointed out, the entire internal aspect of the Kosmos (the left half of the model) has been reduced to its right hand correlates—what he refers to as subtle reductionism.[16] In my medical education, students would often discount courses in psychology or psychiatry, considering them to be much less important than the "hard" sciences we were learning. In addition (and this is particularly true in medicine), upper-level holons such as human beings are frequently reduced to their component parts. This is referred to as *gross reductionism.*[16] In other words, instead of treating a complex, highly evolved human individual who might be suffering with depression with an all-quadrant, all-level awareness, the patient is subtly reduced to a physical machine and grossly reduced to a chemical imbalance of neurotransmitters from a genetic defect. It is not that a reductionistic look at who humans are from the UR quadrant perspective is bad; it is simply that we must not ignore other aspects of human existence. Although science has uncovered the entire human genome (and this will lead to some wonderful new physical discoveries), it will never tell us much about love.

THE MIND-BODY SPLIT IN WESTERN MEDICINE

Family practice has attempted to be a more holistic approach in the Western medical model and has succeeded in at least acknowledging the importance of the internal aspect of individuals and the relevance of the collective sociocultural quadrants (LR and LL), such as the family. There is, however, a persistent tendency of mind-body splitting in Western medicine. For example, a patient has either a psychological problem or a physical organic problem but usually not a complex combination of both, which the AQAL model suggests. In addition, matters of spirit are nowhere discussed because the Western medical model, even in family practice, has no appreciation of how this might have relevance to an individual's health or illness. As Wilber would put it, everything transrational is discarded with everything prerational simply because both are nonrational.[16] What this amounts to is throwing out the spiritual baby with the mythologically and magically tainted bath water. It seems to me that much of the new age and some of the alternative therapies suffer from a similar failure to see where on the evolutionary spiral the various treatment modalities are located.

INTEGRAL MEDICINE DIAGNOSTICS: HOW TO PRACTICE INTEGRAL MEDICINE

For the last 10 years or so, I have routinely taken a psychospiritual history from my patients during extended visits, such as a complete history and physical, to get a sense of where they are from a developmental and cultural perspective. This history might include everything from what type of parenting they had in their youth; to current and past emotional stressors; to current and past mental stressors; to spiritual issues, such as their current beliefs, spiritual practices, and meaning and purpose in life; and issues concerning death and dying. This interview varies considerably depending on many factors, including the patient's age, beliefs, level of psychospiritual development,[16] receptiveness, illnesses, and so on. The point is, to be a more effective, integrally aware physician, one has to engage in dialogue to discover the internal quadrants of an individual patient. Although I use clinical examples that emphasize the UR, psychological aspects, this in no way is a reflection of my entire practice. I see patients with problems that range the full spectrum of family practice and only engage in psychotherapy on rare occasions. The whole point of this essay is that physicians (especially those in primary care) who want to be integral must at least be aware of the internal or UR quadrant issues and how they relate to the physical or UR quadrant manifestations, and vice versa. Not every physician will be comfortable in utilizing psychological therapies (patients can be referred to an appropriate therapist); the most important thing is the quality of the doctor-patient relationship (LL quadrant), and this is directly related to honoring everything that it is to be human—mind, body, and soul—in self, culture, and nature. The quality of the therapeutic relationship correlates with better outcomes regardless of the therapeutic modality.[17]

CLINICAL EXAMPLES IN INTEGRAL MEDICINE

A patient, whom I recently treated for hypertension, remarked that her blood pressure was only elevated when she was in a doctor's office—so-called "white coat hypertension." I commented that there are studies[18] that suggest that particularly labile hypertension, such as "white coat hypertension," can be correlated to subconscious emotional wounds, perhaps a bad experience as a child in a doctor's office (current recommendations for immunizations at some visits include up to 4 or 5 separate shots at each visit) or other childhood emotional traumas. She then said, "Doctor, I don't know if you believe in past lives or not, but I was a physician during the Civil War in a previous life and had to amputate limbs without anesthesia, and that is why I believe my blood pressure goes up in a doctor's office." Whether the doctor believes in past lives is not as important as the awareness that, for this particular woman, belief alone could be responsible for her "white coat hypertension." Past-life therapy might just cure her of hypertension and avoid an unnecessary medication—and thank God for anesthesia.

Another recent patient of mine was scheduled for a rotator cuff shoulder operation, but her orthopedic surgeon was reluctant to perform the operation until her blood pressure was under better control. During her pre-op physical, I asked her how she felt about having the operation, and she replied, "I feel fine about the operation, but I am just so damn mad at myself that I got up on that step ladder in the first place. If I hadn't done that, I wouldn't have fallen and injured my shoulder." I told her that it was very important that she forgive herself and go to the operation with self-love and not self-hatred. She smiled and seemed very relieved by this suggestion. I rechecked her blood pressure and it had immediately dropped 20 points. She said that she wished she could take me with her to the operating room to remind her of this. I then told her that she could, in fact, bring me with her by using imagery. She did this and sailed through the operation without a rise in blood pressure. Simply having an integral awareness when treating patients (and using this awareness to make some carefully considered remarks) can have a profound effect on medical outcomes.

THE SOCIOCULTURAL QUADRANTS IN MEDICINE

The collective or sociocultural aspects (LR and LL) of medicine today are more important than ever. The financing of health care (LR) is badly in need of an overhaul and is a huge factor in medical practice. Ten years ago, it was relatively easy to care for all patients, even those without insurance. Physicians were much more willing to give discounted or free care since financial margins were large. Since the advent of increased insurance "management" of health care, margins are thin and the willingness to give charitable care has significantly dropped. Approximately 40 million

Americans are without health insurance, and as many as 8 million more will lose their insurance in the coming year.[19] This will have an increasingly negative impact on access to health care, and, though there may be good treatments available for a particular disease, a patient may actually die from a lack of insurance (LR) in addition to the illness itself. A recent study has demonstrated that death rates for the uninsured are up to 25 percent higher than death rates for the insured.[19]

An example of how cultural beliefs (LL) can impact health and disease is exemplified by a young man who was dying of AIDS and was cared for by my wife, a hospice physician at the time. Although the newer AIDS drugs, which have made such a profound impact on survival of this disease, had become available, he had refused to follow through with treatment, which led to the terminal worsening of the disease. When he was admitted to hospice, as he became very near death, my wife learned that he had grown up gay in a Mormon community, where homosexuality is strictly proscribed. His culturally induced shame (LL) and self-judgment (UL) prevented him from accepting treatments for the disease and ultimately led to his death.

INTEGRAL AWARENESS

Providers of health care, whether in Western medicine, CAM, or some combination of both, need to become educated about the integral model so that they are at least integrally informed and can bring this awareness to each patient encounter. This might prevent some of the reductionistic approaches and single quadrant dissociations that currently affect the way that medicine is being practiced. It has been said that Western medicine treats the disease, and integrative medicine the patient. Integral Medicine incorporates both and also treats the doctor by offering a model that provides an integral awareness, which puts meaning, purpose, and love back into the practice of medicine.[20]

TRANSFORMATION OF THE HEALER

Most important, providers of health care must work on their own spiritual evolution to actually experience what the model represents.

As Wilber puts it, do not confuse the map with the territory; having a map of Hawaii is not like actually being there. As the saying goes, one cannot lead another where one has not gone him or herself. The ability to see the divine in everyone and treat each individual as though he or she were Christ or the Buddha himself can transform the suffering of illness into the grace of healing. In my early days in medicine, it was common to hear discussions of interesting patients in the hospital lounges and clinic hallways. Today, it is much more common to hear instead complaints of the deterioration of the medical profession, the interference from hospitals and insurance companies, and loss of income. To become integrally informed and take up an integral practice and then bring this new awareness to the practice of medicine can, I think, transform the practitioner in such a way as to bring back the enjoyment of the doctor-patient relationship. To see each patient as a luminous jewel, tarnished to be sure from the imperfect (from a relative perspective) unfolding process of human development, is to experience medicine as a spiritual path that transcends and diminishes the lower-level issues of the financing of health care. It also empowers us to begin to make changes in the sociocultural problems that we see in medicine today. This tarnish, which is manifested as disease ("dis-ease") in our patients, can be the grace through which both healer and patient can transform their respective lives.

References for this essay are located on the DVD accompanying this book.

Metaphysics of Virtual Caring Communities*

JEAN WATSON

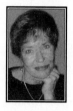

BACKGROUND OF THE ISSUES: "SPACE BETWEEN LIFE PASSAGES"

For the past 30 years or so, the University of Colorado has hosted the annual World Affairs Conference. During this time, invited distinguished scholars, thinkers, artists, musicians, scientists, writers, political journalists, and judicial leaders come to the Boulder campus from around the globe to grapple, free-associate, and brainstorm about a plethora of contemporary and future issues.

During this affair one year, I had an interesting experience. One of the invited speakers was my houseguest, a retired Supreme Court justice from California. During part of his stay, I had to travel to present a paper at a national conference. I explained that I was going to present a paper

*Adapted from Watson J: Metaphysics of Virtual Caring Communities, *The International Journal for Human Caring* 6(1):41–45, 2002.

on "Space Life or Life Space: The Rogerian Conference on Space Nursing," held at the University of Alabama, Huntsville (which, incidentally, hosted a tribute to Martha Rogers at the joint Rogerian Conference and American Holistic Nursing Association Conference during June 2001). When he heard the topic of the conference and the title of my paper, the justice's response was, "Is that the space between life passages?"

I share this little story because of the emerging relationships between and among space life, virtual realities, cyberspace, Rogerian science, caring science, and the wider notion, if not connection, between these concepts and the judge's innocent question, "Is that the space between life passages?" At this moment in history, these seemingly diverse concepts and theories are converging, for perhaps new reasons.

It struck me then, and continues to impress upon me now, that perhaps his question is the right one to ask. If so, then are people (a) moving from one level of being to another; (b) evolving from a humankind to a "spacekind" form of being, as the literature suggests; or (c) evolving from Homo sapiens to "Homospatials," as Rogers suggested? If so, what does it all mean? What is the metaphysics of such movement between life passages and evolutionary leaps in humanity? What does this have to do with caring science? With nursing? With creating communities of caring through global initiatives?

As a starting point, when one enters into the world of global space considerations and creating virtual communities of caring, one automatically enters the metaphysical realm in that one enters the nonphysical domain—the realm of connecting consciousness and information beyond time-space and physicality. When one introduces notions of caring and communities into the virtual realm, one is entering a reality that can and does constitute a new form of human experience—a space between life passages, to acknowledge the judge's innocent but astute question.

The potential impact of the shift from physical reality to virtual reality is so great that it is defining the culture that is resulting from its use—both positively and negatively. Virtual reality has already become a widely used metaphor for reality itself, and for its use and practice. Virtual world has led to a change in people's relationship with technology and knowledge and, ultimately, to a change in our view of others and ourselves.

It has been suggested by some that eighteenth-century German philosopher and mathematician Leibniz's vision of a community of minds actually anticipated the current data web, the Internet networks, and on-line relationships.[1] Thus this direction has been evolving in the human consciousness as part of the evolution of the species. Virtual reality itself has been traced back to hieroglyphics, to the petroglyphs, and to writing on papyrus and is evident in modern-day inventions such as the type-writer. As Heim points out in his book on the metaphysics of virtual reality, writing before the printing press was a form of worship.[1] But after Gutenberg, individuals and institutions owned the written word. Thus one revolution-evolution has led to another form of electronic, digital world and digital word, to word processing, to thought processing, and to postmodern deconstruction of text, words, and worlds.

The hypertext phenomenon breaks linear sequence, so disordered, nonlinear text replaces the straight logic of ordered thought. The reader interprets and interacts with the text, moving beyond what the author constructed, becoming part of the co-creation of the meaning of the text, beyond the original starting point of the author—this nonlinear, free-association format of hypertext, multimedia, multi-sensory juxtaposition of pictures and words creates a new form of expression: three-dimensional, colored, animated symbols for interaction versus an ordered, linear text that is passively read. This new order of human experiences and realities facing people in the twenty-first century is a quite different scenario from the mindset of the mid-to-late twentieth century.

The paradox of virtual reality is that, on the one hand, it becomes an intelligent technique that permits active use of the body in search of knowledge and a rejoining of mind and body for a possible evolution—a new breed of evolved consciousness or intellect. On the other hand, the mind-to-mind, consciousness-to-consciousness connection in the world of cyberspace creates a disembodied human-to-human connection and, often, an intense personal intimacy with strangers and friends alike, but is void of an embodied physical relationship.

The status of virtual experience raises many philosophical and meta-physical questions about an evolving ontology for humankind. Some of these rhetorical but nonetheless critical questions explore the following issues: (a) the nature of relationships and the meaning behind intimacy and connection; (b) the ambiguity between facts and fiction; (c) the blur-ring of intimacy and ethics; (d) the disembodied knowledge, connections, and relationships; (e) the authenticity versus artificiality of experience, relationship, and expression; (f) the inversion of reality whereby the simulated reality becomes a substitute for real experience and immediacy; (g) the extent to which humans can change and still remain human; and (h) whether a new form of humanoid is emerging through a symbiosis of machine and human, whereby the human is no longer outside the computer but is a looking glass to enter into.[1]

Thus, in this new territory one asks foundational, philosophical questions such as, "What is existence? How does one know? What is reality? Who am I? Who are you? What is space? Does space separate or connect?" These are no longer hypothetical questions, no longer remote or esoteric, but essential to consider in that it is part of the human evolution and destiny to redefine ourselves for the next leap in human experiences. As Myron Krueger says in his introduction to *Metaphysics of Virtual Reality*, "We have reached a point where 'what we have made, makes us'."[2] As humans enter into these new realities and new worlds of possibilities opening to us, it brings us to a crucial point in considering these life space passages and the relationship between space and life changes such as virtual reality and surrogate realities.

Part of what is unfolding might be thought of as a "metaphysics of being," an acknowledgement that any philosophical system expresses a truth and an apprehension of a real aspect of the reality of human life. These truths are mutually complementary. Conflict does not arise so much from the incompatibility of fundamental ideas as from the fact that different philosophical systems exaggerate one aspect of the world of human life, thus turning a partial truth into a whole or whole into a part. Exaggerations of a philosophy serve a useful purpose. They draw attention to basic truths; then once one digests the truth, then one can forget the exaggerations. Thus, one can use the truth as a source of knowledge and insight, forgetting the instrument by which it is attained. It is the metaphysical considerations of new ideas and their exaggeration to emphasize a truth that help one arrive at an insight or a new understanding.

Metaphysics pushes open the door that science and empiricism keep shut. The real role and function of metaphysics is to awaken one to an awareness of the enveloping being, in which all other finite existents are grounded. It is noted that the true and primary function of philosophy and metaphysics is to awaken one to an awareness of being that transcends being; it also reminds us that no metaphysical system can possess universal validity, due to the nature of metaphysics itself.[3]

DEFINITIONS

Metaphysics

Just what does metaphysics mean when considering virtual reality issues and global caring communities within a caring-science context? The best discussion of metaphysics I have discovered is that of Willis Harman and his work and writing through the Institute of Noetic Sciences. For example, he points out that the word *metaphysics* has two quite different meanings.[4] The first meaning of metaphysics is a branch of philosophy that encompasses both ontology (for example, "What is reality?") and epistemology (How do you know what you know?). An example might be, "I know that I am communicating with someone by sending them loving thoughts, in free space or cyberspace." The ontological question is: What and who is communicating? The epistemological questions are: Is the experience virtual or real? How do you know?

The second meaning of metaphysics is the study of the transcendent or supersensible, the contacting of reality that lies beyond the physical. This meaning is often associated with perennial wisdom traditions and the kind of knowledge that emerges from inward-looking, experiential, deep practice disciplines, such as meditation or yoga, or depth spiritual practices. Both meanings of metaphysics apply to virtual reality and creating virtual communities of caring at the global level. Indeed, human evolutionary leaps and cyberspace, hypertexts, and virtual surrogate realities lead to a union of technology and metaphysics, and new considerations of the importance of caring science in nursing and health.

Transpersonal

Transpersonal generally refers to a human-to-human connection that goes beyond the personal, physical ego self and connects with deeper, more spiritual, transcendent, even cosmic connections in the wider universe.

MODIFIED ONTOLOGICAL ASSUMPTIONS

The conventional assumption of separateness—of distinct separation between observer and observed, human and nature, mind and matter, and of separation of part of a system for organism to understand how it "really works"—no longer holds in the revised view of metaphysics and the notion of transpersonal. Such separatist thinking as a foundational, ontological assumption has to be overthrown in order to comprehend, grasp, and explain virtual reality, cyberspace, and other emerging phenomena, such as distant healing and prayer research. Indeed, such thinking of separation has kept earth and heaven, human and animal, environment and nature all separate, precluding any consideration of "action at a distance," either in time or space. The interface of technology and human technology changes the basic ontological position of separation and embraces—or is required to be open to—an ontological position of unity, connectedness, and a transpersonal consciousness and technology that transcend time, space, and physicality. The result is a transpersonal, metaphysical perspective for caring science and a new foundational, metaphysical principle for considering the creation of a virtual community of caring.

Willis Harman[4] outlined some of the aspects of self and consciousness that give new credence to the phenomenon of unity versus separation and that ultimately alter the separatist worldview or ontology and result in a new ontology and cosmology of unity. For example, he invited one to consider what I will call the concept of transpersonal caring consciousness. The emerging unitary views, which already are upon us from the human technology symbiosis, are at odds with the outdated, conventional metaphysical assumption of separation. The implications invite new horizons of human-technological evolution, which can embrace virtual and real, nonphysical and physical caring in a new order for new meanings. They include, among other areas, the following examples as directions. First, research on creativity and intuition reveals capabilities of the hidden, intuitive mind. Also, research on out-of-body experiences and near-death experiences seems to suggest that consciousness is something other than just physiochemical processes in the brain. Third, research on multiple-personality disorder, the shift from one self or consciousness to another, may be accompanied by measurable physiological changes, suggesting that personality is a holistic, nonreducible concept that can have real effects in the world, à la Martha Rogers's theory and science of the "unitary human being." Finally, lingering and growing bodies of evidence suggest that the personality, in some sense, survives after physical death and may subsequently communicate back to living persons in various ways.

CONSIDERATIONS OF TRANSCENDENCE, CONSCIOUSNESS, OR ACTION AT A DISTANCE

As Harman pointed out, there remain other puzzles about the metaphysics of separation that can no longer hold in a new world order of technology, cyberspace, and the virtual reality world. Elizabeth Targ's research at UCSF on healing at a distance and the collection of evidence Larry Dossey has compiled on prayer research are other examples of this revised ontology and metaphysical view of reality. This direction also encompasses native and ancient world traditions employing indigenous healing practices—for example, Brazilian healers' *Cueranderos* and other shamanistic practices around the world. In these ancient and contemporary practices, it was and is considered customary to send thoughts to others from a distance—to be in communication with a broader field of connectedness in the universe, beyond locality consciousness and even the physical, earthly plane.

Another category that upsets the separatist ontology of the metaphysics of reality is the phenomenon of "meaningful coincidences," according to one experiencing an unexpected event. Carl Jung referred to this phenomenon as "synchronicity." Other phenomena such as "telepathic communication," "remote" or "clairvoyant viewing," and connections and relationships between the act of prayer and the occurrence of the prayed-for, such as miracle healings, fall within a new relational metaphysics. Although there are no "scientific" explanations of these phenomena in the conventional metaphysical frameworks of separation, there are growing explanatory models related to field phenomenon, quantum physics, and mathematical devices that all are trying to link things in new ways. The result is an overturning, at some deep level, of the ontological assumption of separation and the epistemological assumption that all knowledge is based on physical-sense data. Thus one is confronted with new phenomena, so new models with a new and old metaphysical connection of unity are beginning to be contrived to account for nonconforming events. The emerging explanatory models generally are located within a new metaphysical foundation often referred to as a "transformative unitary framework." The emerging developments in technology, the Internet, virtual realities, and cyberspace all can be thought to reside in this new framework rather than the conventional separatist ontology of reality.

When this new view of reality, virtual or otherwise, begins to embrace the phenomena of consciousness and consciousness at a distance (for example, one can witness this emergence in the field of distance education), new rules and new metaphysical assumptions have to come into play. This shift leads one to consider virtual caring communities based upon new metaphysical, ontological assumptions of unity and transpersonal dimensions.

E=MC²: METAPHYSICS OF TRANSPERSONAL VIRTUAL CARING COMMUNITIES

"Someday, after we have mastered the winds, the waves, the tides, the gravity, we shall harness...the energies of love. Then for the second time in the history of the world, we will have discovered fire"

TEILHARD DE CHARDIN

David Bodanis's latest book, $E = mc^2$, can provide some new images and concepts for these ideas of love, energy, speed, and mass, even as metaphors. For example, as he makes clear, $E = mc^2$ is translated into E/energy = mass × celeritas/speed^2.[5] In using the metaphor and deeper understanding of $E = mc^2$, we can posit that the intellectual exchange of ideas (consciousness) that takes place underneath, in between, or beyond the verbal, cognitive word exchange is a more fundamental energetic exchange that can be communicated beyond time and space and physicality.

To play with these ideas within a transpersonal caring framework and new metaphysics, one could suggest another version of the equation that is E/energy = mass (caring consciousness) x caritas/love^2 (Figure 1).What results is a new formula, positing transcendent speed of nonlocal caring consciousness being sent at celeritas (speed faster than light) generated by energy of caritas/love, making new connections between words, such as cleritas x caritas. Thus, in this way one can imagine virtual caring communities as "vast energy sources" (caring-loving consciousness) hidden in solid matter itself (mass), waiting to be released into the universe. "All mass is really part of a connected whole, which is energy x celeritas/speed."[5]

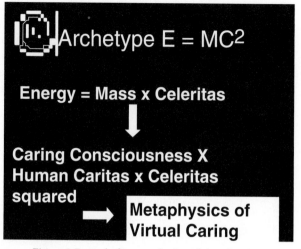

Figure 1 Formula for metaphysics of virtual caring.

VIRTUAL CARING AND TRANSFORMATIVE LEARNING

Continuing with the $E = mc^2$ thinking with respect to new learning approaches, Bache[6] noted that in transformative (virtual caring communities) learning, words not supported by the energy of personal experiences carry much less power to influence others than words that carry energy, consciousness, and intentionality (of love and caring). He indicated that this happens partly because when people communicate in person or at a distance, they unleash a tangible but invisible power into the space around them. This power comes from experience, consciousness, and ultimately, the energetic access that the experience has created in us. Higher energy thoughts such as love and caring carry higher frequency energy into the space, even if virtual. As Bache revealed this understanding, he suggested that words float on this power, like a canoe floating on a rushing stream.

However, in relation to caring community work, real, or virtual, the power of the teacher, or faculty, or leader alone is not the only power. The more important power is the power of the group, the community, and the learning circle. Thus, the intensity and authenticity of the community's individual and collective involvement in their own learning influence the strength of the energetic stream that underpins any of the content.

In this way of thinking, people begin to envision other dimensions of space, and words and communication offer extra dimensions with infinite facets. Instead of using linear, page-by-page, line-by-line, book-by-book approaches, we now learn to connect information. We seek the "text" in the intuitive; we find the associative manner, the intentionality and consciousness behind the words. We hear the stories and engage in the relationships of patients, nurses, students, and faculty. These stories and relationships can be turned over from different angles: different twists of the same text can be deconstructed and reconstructed for deeper dimensions of insight and understanding. We in turn begin to generate new archetypes for learning. We foster creativity, critique and literacy, intuition, and leaps of imagination, prompted by energetic jumps and "ahas" of insight and new associations. In this framework, virtual caring pedagogy can serve as a form of meditation, in the sense of the Latin word *meditar,* meaning "to be in the middle of, to hover in between."

The emerging metaphysics for both real and virtual caring learning and transformation is one of wholeness, of unitary awareness of a universe that is alive, unfolding, saturated with many more hidden orders of harmony than people can imagine, opening us again to the mysterious order that is organic and integrated and that has a beautiful design that we are just beginning to grasp. Thus, within the new metaphysics of transpersonal caring and virtual caring communities, one of the key criteria is whether individual and collective learning is being pursued n a way that supports powerful, positive, and enduring life transformations in individuals and in groups—not only in those present physically but also, perhaps especially so, in those persons not physically present but virtually there.

METAPHYSICS OF SPACE AND TOUCH IN VIRTUAL CARE

In this new transpersonal metaphysics of virtual caring, space is revisioned. Space can either separate or connect people, depending upon our worldview and the metaphysics position we select. In this same way, we can rethink caring touch. Touch can occur energetically at a distance or locally in person. Touch can be experienced virtually or actually and still be effective, depending upon the energy of the consciousness behind it—namely, caring and love or indifference.

Along these same lines of thinking, we consider "telecaring," "telepresencing," and "teletouch," making imagination and the virtual real by not being subject to the physical world alone and its limitations. This telecaring direction, however, calls forth our creative imagination, new explanatory models, and an evolving consciousness of our own human-field possibilities. Here we realize a deep understanding of field, which encompasses both outer and inner space. For example, virtual (caring) touch embraces all the senses—auditory, voice, visual, sensory, aesthetic, imaginary, olfactory, and meaning—not just the physical body. Touch in this framework includes feelings, emotions, and perceptions, be they physical or mindfelt or heartfelt.

However, within the model of virtual as well as physical touch, we must consider what we are intending: profane or sacred, good or harmful intentions. This heightened awareness of intentionalities becomes part of the metaphysics as well as the ethics of virtual caring communities. This framework still offers and needs to have an underlying logic, consistency, and coherence to it as part of a caring pedagogy and structure. It is here that the paradigm or framework shift is absolutely essential and must be made explicit. It, in turn, needs to be integrated, coherent, and made real in actual and virtual experiences. Because the cultural shift is rooted so deeply in our definition of reality (our metaphysics) and what is possible, a profound and comprehensive realignment of our mission and sense of self and other must be cultivated, sustained, and practiced. In doing so, we are still honoring the values and intentionalities of human preservation, human dignity, wholeness, alleviation of vulnerability, and so on. This conscious, intentional, values-based direction is intrinsic to nursing and the theory-guided practice of caring.

Finally, a new metaphysics for creating virtual communities of caring within a transformative learning paradigm is part of what is necessary for the future of nursing. What is required is to be consciously open to these potent energy sources of love and caring that are reaching into humanity from below and above. It is to consciously choose to participate, cooperate, and co-create with the creative process, making ourselves available to the rising energies of change and transformation that are fueled by a new consciousness of love and caring. It is to voluntarily step into the alchemical fire of our own energetic field resonance of *celeritas* and *caritas*.

References for this essay are located on the DVD accompanying this book.

The White House Commission on Complementary and Alternative Medicine Policy and the Future of Health Care*

JAMES S. GORDON

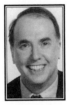

BACKGROUND AND PRECEDENT

Ninety years ago, at a time when medical education and the standards of physician practice were wildly variable, Abraham Flexner, a Carnegie Foundation consultant, issued a report titled "Medical Education in the United States and Canada." Aided by the American Medical Association, Flexner graded North American medical schools according to the scientific standards of Johns Hopkins, which in turn was basing its rigorous

---

* The Final Report of the White House Commission is available from the U.S. Government Printing Office (ISBN 0-16-15-1476-2).

curriculum on the German model. Flexner's report, with its emphasis on full-time faculty in the basic and clinical sciences and extensive laboratory and hospital facilities, set the standard for medical practice and licensing, as well as medical education, for the twentieth century.

In July of 2000, the newly appointed White House Commission on Complementary and Alternative Policy (WHCCAMP) began to undertake a study that I hoped would exercise as profound an effect on twenty-first century medicine.

The medicine that Flexner's report catalyzed, and the subsequent infusion of capital from John D. Rockefeller, helped to produce the extraordinary gains in scientific research, high-technology treatment of illness, and rigorous scientific education that became the hallmark and pride of American medicine. But the medicine of Flexner's heirs, though enormously powerful and precise, was, inevitably, incomplete.

In using a stringent set of criteria to judge medical education, Flexner, and those who followed his recommendations, eliminated some of the diversity that marked early twentieth-century medicine. Schools of homeopathy—and those emphasizing herbal and natural healing—disappeared, as did a number of those serving women and minorities. The scientific medicine of the ensuing 90 years made many advances, but in the process ignored or dismissed many other healing traditions and many practices as having only historical, anthropological, or sociological interest.

Beginning in the 1960s, increasing numbers of Americans—and others in developed and developing countries around the world—began to experience the limitations of the medical care they received and to look to these other traditions and practices to help them with their health care problems. In a very real sense, this search was stimulated by the success of the Flexnerian enterprise. It was, in fact, those who have had all the benefits of modern scientific medicine who have led the search.

These people were not turning their back on conventional medicine, but they were painfully aware of its limitations and side effects and therefore were exploring approaches that would complement this medicine—or be alternatives to it. They included men, women, and children with life-threatening illnesses like cancer and HIV, and many more with chronic pain, chronic fatigue, fibromyalgia, neurological disorders, chronic depression, and a host of other conditions. They were and are looking for therapies that are both more helpful and less toxic. As managed care becomes pervasive in the United States, many of these people are searching for something else as well. They want more time with the professionals who will provide care to them, a sustained healing partnership rather than a brief consultation, and an opportunity to participate in their own care as well as follow doctors' orders.

A survey published in the *Journal of the American Medical Association* in 1998 showed that 42 percent of all Americans were using therapies other than those their doctors prescribed, many along with and some without conventional care: chiropractic and massage for back pain; supplements and herbs for headaches, depression, diabetes, and weight loss; and a combination of dietary therapies, exercise, meditation, and group support as an option to cardiac surgery. In 1997 Americans made 649 million visits to alternative care practitioners, 243 million more than they made to their primary healthcare—MD—providers.

In recent years the movement to integrate complementary and alternative care and to create a more holistic and patient-centered approach has gained significant numbers of adherents among teachers of medicine and present and future health care professionals. Approximately three quarters of all U.S. medical schools have at least an elective offering in alternative medicine. Many thousands of practicing physicians are each year seeking advanced training in mind-body medicine, nutrition, herbal therapies, and Chinese and Ayurvedic medicine. And thousands of college graduates, many with excellent academic credentials, are now entering non-MD training programs in "complementary and alternative" approaches—among them chiropractic, acupuncture, naturopathy, herbalism, and massage therapy.

Congressional legislation, supported by an extraordinary bipartisan coalition, reflects the breadth and power of this movement. In 1991 Senator Tom Harkin (D-Iowa) created the Office of Alternative Medicine at the National Institutes of Health. In the years since then, the office's original budget of $2 million—a "homeopathic level of support," according to the office's first director—has risen to more than $100 million. The office has been upgraded to the National Center for Complementary and Alternative Medicine, and rigorous NIH-funded research on therapies that were ignored and disparaged 10 or even 5 years ago is proceeding apace at many of our leading academic medical institutions.

At the beginning of the twentieth century, Abraham Flexner worked with the American Medical Association to survey the medical landscape and to bring high scientific standards to the training of physicians as well as to the services they offered their patients. At the beginning of the twenty-first century, Congress and the president asked a commission of conventional physicians and researchers, complementary and alternative medicine pioneers, citizen advocates, and business people—men and women of many colors and ethnic backgrounds—to design a blueprint for a new medicine that is both scientific and inclusive.

THE WORK OF THE WHITE HOUSE COMMISSION

The job of the commission—our job—was to establish guidelines for scientifically exploring approaches that have come from other cultures and practices that have flourished outside of conventional care; to gather information about and describe models that can successfully integrate the most effective and safe of these practices into conventional care; to make this information—about what works safely and what doesn't—easily available to all Americans; and to recommend legislative initiatives that will make the best of these therapies, and training in them, an integral part of medical and other professional education.

The commission enhanced its mandate by assuming another responsibility: to address ways in which complementary and alternative therapies could enlarge and enrich a nationwide approach to health promotion and wellness.

Flexner's report established standards in medical education and practice and helped to give birth to generations of distinguished scientific physicians. The White House Commission's mandate was to help those scientifically trained physicians to turn their attention to other promising avenues for helping and healing; to formulate ways to bring together ancient wisdom and modern science, conventional practitioners with those whose primary training is in complementary and alternative approaches; and to educate the American public as well as professional caregivers. Flexner gave physicians an authority in which patients could trust. Even as it deepened that authority, the commission hoped to extend our national options for good care, enlarge the range of practitioners available to all Americans, and encourage patients and their caregivers to establish the kind of sustained healing partnerships we all want.

Many of the 20 presidentially appointed commissioners were conventionally trained health professionals. Others were trained purely as complementary and alternative medicine (CAM) practitioners. Several more were conventional health professionals who integrate complementary and alternative approaches into their work. The commission also included a number of academic physicians and health and mental health professionals who joined the commission interested in, but not experts in, CAM approaches. There were, as well, several business executives and patient advocates.

Though the commissioners came from diverse backgrounds, all swiftly agreed that our responsibility was to ensure the safety of products and practices that had been, or might be, labeled "CAM," as well as to maximize potential benefits of these approaches for the public. For 18 months we listened, in 14 meetings—10 in Washington and 4 "town halls" in San Francisco, Seattle, New York, and Minneapolis—to the testimony of over 700 individuals and organizations. We read over 1,000 written submissions. Commission members discussed what we had heard in subcommittees and in full commission meetings.

The range of those invited and the diversity of their testimony helped to ensure that the commission's recommendations would be broadly representative. At the commission meeting on Professional Education, Licensure and Credentialing (February 22-23, 2001), for example, well over 100 organizations—from the American Medical Association and the Association of American Medical Colleges to the American Massage Therapy Association, the National Breast Cancer Coalition, and the American College of Acupuncture and Oriental Medicine—submitted testimony. We had plenary session presentations and four working groups, which read through and discussed the positions we heard, the catalogues of institutional concerns, and the vast array of thoughtful proposals. We concluded with a full commission 4-hour discussion of all this material and a list of possible recommendations.

Directors of NIH institutes testified, as did CEOs and other executives of insurance and pharmaceutical companies. We heard representatives from broadcast networks and the world's leading medical journals, as well as ordinary patients and physicians who read the journals and watch the news.

The New York Town Hall, on January 23, 2001, was an open meeting in which testimony on all commission concerns—access, information and education, research, regulation and wellness—was welcome. One hundred and forty people—the regulators and the regulated, clinicians and patients, scholars and activists, healers from non-Western traditions, enthusiasts and skeptics—spoke to us.

Very few commissioners missed meetings, and all listened with remarkable attention to those who testified. Questioning was sometimes sharp but almost always respectful; self-proclaimed and sometimes combative "opponents" of alternative medicine were treated, I believe, with the same even-handed and thoughtful consideration as proponents.

The commission itself was a kind of community. Its members were generally respectful of one another and collaborative, but at times fractious as well. There were very real disagreements. Were we overreaching our mandate in dealing with the spiritual dimension of CAM, some wondered? Were we being too timid in our encouragement of parity among the different healing traditions, or were we ignoring scientific data on the efficacy of particular practices? Were we pushing for too much inclusion of CAM in conventional education or too little, too stringent regulation or not enough? From our first meeting we began to formulate principles that would guide our discussions and our recommendations. We continued to shape them over many months until we unanimously agreed on them, and they in turn came to shape and frame the final recommendations we would make. Here they are:

THE COMMISSION'S GUIDING PRINCIPLES

1. **A wholeness orientation in health care delivery**
   Health involves all aspects of life—mind, body, spirit, environment—and high-quality health care must support care of the whole person.
2. **Evidence of safety and efficacy**
   The commission is committed to promoting the use of science and appropriate scientific methods to help identify safe and effective CAM services and products and to generate the evidence that will protect and promote the public health.

3. **The healing capacity of the person**

The person has a remarkable capacity for recovery and self-healing, and a major focus of health care is to support and promote this capacity.

4. **Respect for individuality**

Every person is unique and has the right to health care that is appropriately responsive to him or her, respecting preferences and preserving dignity.

5. **The right to choose treatment**

Every person has the right to choose freely among safe and effective care or approaches, as well as among qualified practitioners who are accountable for their claims and actions and responsive to the person's needs.

6. **An emphasis on health promotion and self-care**

Good health care emphasizes self-care and early intervention for maintaining and promoting health.

7. **Partnerships are essential for integrated health care**

Good health care requires teamwork among patients, health care practitioners (conventional and CAM), and researchers committed to creating optimal healing environments and to respecting the diversity of all health care traditions.

8. **Education as a fundamental health care service**

Education about prevention, healthful lifestyles, and the power of self-healing should be made an integral part of the curricula of all health care professionals and should be made available to the public at all ages.

9. **Dissemination of comprehensive and timely information**

The quality of health care can be enhanced by promoting efforts that thoroughly and thoughtfully examine the evidence on which CAM systems, practices, and products are based and make this evidence widely, rapidly, and easily available.

10. **Integral public involvement**

The input of informed consumers and other members of the public must be incorporated in setting priorities for health care, health care research, and in reaching policy decisions, including those related to CAM, within the public and private sectors.

These guiding principles are consistent with the 10 rules for health care reform listed in the National Academy of Sciences' Institute of Medicine (IOM) report on ways to improve health care in the twenty-first century ("Quality Chasm: A New Health System for the 21st Century") and with the U.S. Department of Health and Human Service's most recent 10-year health objectives for the nation ("Healthy People 2110: Understanding and Improving Health").

These principles also point to a synthesis in health care that is both larger and more dynamic than that of "Quality Chasm" or "Healthy People" or any others that have been so far offered by an official U.S. government body.

Health care is generally regarded as a grim struggle of health professionals against disease and an uphill battle to educate the public about preventing illness and promoting health. The WHCCAMP's report suggests that illness is an ordinary part of life. It's as much a teacher as an opponent. It urges us to learn about the imbalances in our lives and in the natural and social world in which we live that may have created or contributed to our illness. It helps us to see how we can correct these imbalances. The healing traditions that we use are not only techniques to combat illness but systems to guide our physical, mental, and emotional transformation.

Patients are not simply recipients of others' professional expertise but also students of and active participants in their own care. Self-care is understood to be the true primary care and is central to all care. Physicians and other health professionals are engaged students of their own care and respectful teachers, not just authoritative "treaters."

The commission recognized that our Western medicine is an immensely useful and powerful system and that it is also one system among many. Its scientific methodology, which is as important as its specific achievements, may be put in the service of studying other systems of healing and care than the one that gave birth to it.

THE FINAL REPORT

The commission's work culminated in the 29 recommendations and over 100 action steps that are contained in its final report. These provide a blueprint for taking the next step toward a medicine that addresses the unique concerns of each person and embraces the benefits of all healing traditions. These recommendations and action steps are all clearly grounded in the commission's guiding principles.

There is, for example, a balance between scrupulous attention to scientific evidence and encouragement of courageous innovation. There are strong recommendations for reporting and disseminating information about dangerous side effects—"adverse events" related to CAM—and for penalizing false advertising and fraudulent practice. And there is an equally strong endorsement for providing public information about the demonstrated benefits of CAM approaches and for including those that are safe and effective in all service programs.

There is a faith in the ability of ordinary people, as well as health professionals, to understand and use good information to expand their therapeutic options. If people learn about the variety of approaches to healing that are available and have easy access to authoritative information about their efficacy and limitations, the commission believes, they are likely to make good decisions. If professionals are helped to understand the historical and social context of Western medicine and to see that it is but one tradition among many, they are likely to advise and treat their patients with more wisdom and modesty.

The role of government, which the final report discusses in some detail, is to ensure the provision of good information as well as to protect against fraud and help ensure public safety; to encourage collaboration among the different professions and between professionals and the public; and to stimulate the investigation of promising approaches regardless of the traditions in which they are based.

More specifically, there are recommendations that significant research spending should be shifted in the direction of approaches that cannot be patented and that may have wide applicability in the treatment of illness and the promotion of health—and away from the subsidy of studies on drugs and procedures that will yield huge profits to private enterprise. Research should no longer be restricted, as most of it now is, to the examination of single and partial treatments. It should be directed, increasingly, toward approaches that are truly comprehensive and individualized—toward the examination of the best possible and most integrated practices. The spirit of the report is respectful, democratic, adventurous, inclusive, collaborative, and participatory.

This last word is crucial. Flexner's report, some 100 years ago, reflected one man's perspective on medical education and his recommendations for shaping a profession in the image of the emerging science, its leaders, and their research methods. The White House Commission's report offers a blueprint for transformation based on collaboration between professionals and patients; an approach to health care that transcends any particular system; and an appreciation that medicine and healing are in the service of mental, emotional and spiritual fulfillment, as well as physical well-being, of personal wholeness and meaning.

Flexner's recommendations were implemented by a small group of powerful medical educators and philanthropists. For the White House Commission's recommendations to be implemented, the will and persistence of large numbers of the American people will be necessary. Collaboration will be required between open-minded professionals in all the healing traditions, philanthropists who are willing to help underwrite and implement the recommendations and study their consequences, and elected officials who are courageous enough to make sure the government fulfills its mandate to meet the health care and health needs of all people.

Sociopolitical Challenges of Integral Medicine

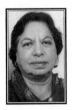

SUMEDHA KHANNA

INTRODUCTION

The driving force for writing this chapter comes from my evolving personal and professional life journey. Throughout this journey, a number of issues and questions about the medical field have arisen in my mind. While I have not been able to find answers to many of my questions, I have been visualizing the possibilities and feeling sometimes excited, at other times discouraged. Yet I have continued my personal professional enquiry because I truly believe that a new vision of health, healing, and medicine is not only needed but absolutely imperative. The rising cost of providing high-quality health care and the growing burden of disease and disability on individuals and society present a critical challenge to our collective consciousness to seek new ways to create and sustain health and prevent disease and disability.

A PERSONAL QUEST

I graduated in clinical medicine in India. Even though India is a land with a rich tradition of indigenous medicine, throughout my medical education not a word was spoken about other systems of healing. My medical education was based completely on the Western dualistic model. The curriculum was imported from England. The teachers were educated in England, and the exam papers were created in England. I spent 6 years in England completing my postgraduate specialization in obstetrics and gynecology. My deep concern for prevention and early care motivated me toward the social side of obstetrics, and I came to the United States to study public health, with a major in maternal and child health and population dynamics. This launched me into the international health arena, and I joined the World Health Organization. Over a period of 25 years, I had the opportunity to serve in 60 countries of the world, providing technical and managerial expertise in diverse areas of health such as safe motherhood, reproductive health, the training of rural health workers, the design of national health plans and strategies to provide basic health care to all, the reorientation of medical and other health professional education programs, the evaluation of national and international health policies, and the development of leadership for health.

THE GAPS IN HEALTH CARE

My extensive international health experience made me even more aware of the fact that, despite all the resources, technology and managerial potential, no country in the world has been able to provide a continuum of health care to all its citizens from birth to death. The situation no doubt is far worse in the developing and poor countries of the world, but health care gaps are also notable in the richest countries. Modern medicine has made significant progress in the treatment of certain conditions. Its contribution to increased life expectancy is invaluable. But the general health of the population has not improved to the degree that might be expected considering the enormous cost and efforts that sustain modern health care systems. The prevalence of chronic diseases continues to increase, especially after midlife. Technological advances have certainly contributed to earlier and more precise diagnoses of conditions and early interventions, especially if surgical measures are required. Yet a majority of these conditions are attributed to the choices we make in our lifestyles or are forced to make because the opportunity of choice is not there.

NEED FOR INTEGRAL THINKING

Over the past decade I have been learning about other systems of health care and healing. I didn't want to become a practitioner in any particular field. My main objective was to explore how we could enhance our health through integrating body, mind, and spirit practices in our daily life. What do the various systems of health care and healing have in common? How can we associate integral thinking in relation to health?

Integral thinking is based on the principle of unity of all things. It views the universe as a whole and human being as an integral part of Being, the dynamic unity of all opposites. Integral thinking represents a dynamic integration of the scientific, phenomenological, dialectical methods of the West and the self-analytical, psychointegrative, and nondual value disciplines of the East. Practically all other systems of health care except the conventional, or the Western, model emphasize healing rather than curing. They give a higher significance to the role of mind in health and healing and treat the person as a whole, as well as consider the environmental and other social influences on the person's health and healing. They consider human beings as an integral part of the cosmic energy, the Universal Life Force.

CHALLENGES

Conceptual

The most important challenge for us is to redefine or clarify the concept of health in the twenty-first century. The World Health Organization's definition of health—"Health is a state of complete physical, psychological, spiritual and social well-being, and not merely an absence of disease or infirmity"—is a generally accepted definition. In the public health sector, much thought and action are influenced by this definition, but in the practice of medicine it seems to remain a theoretical concept. The daily work of doctors is dominated by finding a diagnosis for the presenting symptoms and taking measures to treat the condition.

There is no doubt that over the past 2 decades our concept of health has evolved. Health is increasingly recognized as a multidimensional phenomenon, involving interdependent physical, psychological, social, and spiritual aspects. Nevertheless, it is hard to convey this understanding to the public at large.

In recent years there has also been an evolution in our understanding and acceptance of the value of different systems of health care practice other than the ones associated with conventional medicine. Our definition of these systems has evolved from traditional (as they have originated and are practiced by various traditional peoples around the world), to alternative (as they have often been used as alternatives to conventional medicine), and more recently to complementary (as some of the practices are advocated to complement conventional medicine) and holistic (as they consider the person as a whole and as an integral part of the cosmos). A new set of values is taking hold in the field of medicine, values that incorporate the wisdom of ancient traditions and the scientific knowledge of modern medicine.

Scientific research in recent years has also provided valuable insights into the influence of the mind on health. There is growing evidence that mind-body techniques not only improve the quality of life, particularly for someone dealing with a serious illness, but also affect the course of disease itself. Recent studies have also opened the way toward identifying the links between the immune system and the central nervous system. In fact, mind-body medicine has emerged as one of the most powerful fields of science in recent years. The use of mind-body approaches such as relaxation, hypnosis, and biofeedback is becoming more widespread and is gaining more respect and interest from researchers in major medical institutions. Other healing practices, such as Hands on Healing, Reiki, and distant healing through intention and prayer, incorporate the role of spirit in healing and are also receiving the attention of the scientific community.

Putting Concepts into Practice

Therefore we are in a much better position today to launch the concept of integral medicine. However, a major challenge is to clearly define the concept, and this concept has to be understood and accepted at all levels of society—by individuals, by health care practitioners, by health care organizations, and by society as a whole.

Individuals and Society

Integral medicine is characterized by an integrated approach to the individual. It focuses on the treatment of the whole person rather than treatment of the individual parts. It places emphasis on the individual's personal responsibility in creating and maintaining health. But how do we clearly explain this concept to individuals? How do we shift the current way of thinking about illness and healing?

Our conventional medical system defines disease as mainly caused by external organisms and conditions and not by an imbalance between individuals and other factors in their lives and the world. That is not an easy concept to explain to someone suffering from symptoms that are causing discomfort. Most people seek quick alleviation of their symptoms and, once these are relieved, forget about them until they reappear in one form or another. Very rarely do individuals take time to examine the underlying reasons for their "dis-ease." They expect their medical care provider to cure their illness and do not take adequate responsibility for their health. Even when it is clear that the underlying reason for their illness is embedded in their lifestyle choices, it is difficult for them to sustain a healthy lifestyle.

This understanding of health and disease as being a product of imbalances in the general harmony between the individual and the world has to be taught to children at a very young age. Our children need to grow up with respect for maintaining their health being one of the most important goals of life. They need to learn about their personal role in creating and maintaining their health and to understand that it is a lifelong responsibility. They need to learn and integrate health-creating practices such as a healthy diet, exercise, and relaxation techniques in their daily lives. Yet how many schools have integrated health in their curriculum? And how many educators are prepared to teach integral health?

Integral health begins at home. Parents have a major responsibility in this respect. They must be the role models for their children and pay attention to diet, nutrition, environment, and daily health-creating practices for themselves and their family. The role of the media is crucial in sensitizing society to the concept of integral medicine. This represents one of the most difficult challenges for society.

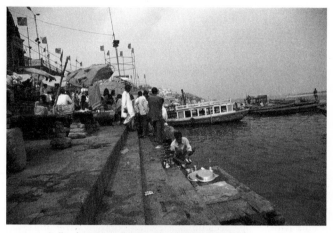

A, "Indian Steps." (Courtesy David "Dudi" Shmueli.)

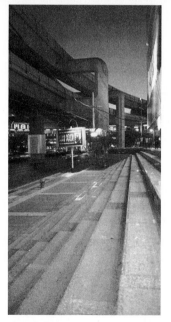

B, "Paris Steps." (Courtesy David "Dudi" Shmueli.)

Health Care Practitioners

The development of modern medicine has made the partnership between practitioners and people increasingly difficult to achieve. Over the past 4 decades medicine has become centered on high technology. Physicians have become more specialized in narrow fields, and economic considerations have forced doctors to spend less time with each patient. Most health care practitioners are educated in their unique system of medicine. While some medical schools are beginning to include some aspects of body-mind medicine, this is still far from adequate.

Integral medicine promotes a model of equal partnership between doctors and complementary health care practitioners who are skilled and experienced in their own field of specialization. While it is not feasible that all health care providers are trained in all systems of medical care, it is important that they have some understanding of the complementarities of different systems. Respecting one another's contributions to health care is also crucial. This requires openness, trust, nondefensiveness, and respect on all sides. Health care practitioners from all fields have to recognize and honor the part each plays in ensuring the overall well-being of the patient.

Health Care Organizations

Our current system of medical care is not conducive to the application of the integral medicine approach. The majority of primary care physicians are organized and equipped to provide only conventional medicine. A fairly well-established system of referrals to medical care specialists and hospitals is in place. Government-supported public health systems take care of preventive and environmental-related services. Providers of complementary care also are specialized in their particular fields and operate independently. The respective professional associations regulate the standards and codes of ethics and conduct. More recently, some hospitals and comprehensive health clinics have begun to offer some complementary therapies such as acupuncture, chiropractic, biofeedback, and relaxation techniques upon referral from the primary care physician or the medical care specialist. There are very few operational models of integral medicine in place. We would need to define what a true integral medicine model looks like and examine the feasibility of reorienting our current systems of providing medical care.

Who Pays for What?

One of the biggest challenges to integral medicine will come from those who determine and manage the financing of medical care, most importantly, the health insurance companies. Health is one of the biggest businesses and involves influential stakeholders such as pharmaceutical companies, health insurance agencies, health maintenance organizations, and the government. Patients have very little power in this business. The health insurance companies determine what payments will be made for what services, as well as individual benefits and liabilities. It is relatively easier to get coverage for advanced technological diagnostic and intervention procedures than it is to obtain preventive services and simple, inexpensive health maintenance modalities.

It is estimated that nearly half of all U.S. adults now go outside the health system for some of their care. They make more visits to nonconventional healers than to medical doctors and spend more of their own money for the privilege—about $30 billion a year, by recent estimates. Each year more money is spent on supplements and herbal remedies that are considered to be beneficial in the prevention of certain health problems and that can complement conventional medications. Yet, medical insurance companies are willing to pay for the more expensive medications but not for inexpensive supplements and herbs. Some medical insurance companies may partially pay for some of the complementary therapies if they were prescribed by a referring physician and if they were administered in a primary care clinic or a hospital.

Part of the problem is the dearth of sound research to determine the value and effectiveness of complementary therapies. Several reputable scientific and medical establishments are pursuing such research. But it is not enough. Medical insurance and pharmaceutical companies should contribute to this research, since in the long run it will influence the cost of health care.

We need to look at the cost of complementary practices. Relaxation and meditation can cost next to nothing. Self-help groups are available in many communities, and individuals make a small or no financial contribution for joining them. Thanks to the baby-boomer generation, the awareness and availability of such health-enhancing and complementary practices have expanded rapidly over the past decade. How much of the cost of mind-body practices will be covered by medical insurance? There is no clear answer to this question.

CREATING A NEW VISION
Clearing the Way

As stated earlier, one of the most important tasks facing those who advocate integral medicine is to clarify the concept. What does it mean to the individual, society, health care practitioners, health care organizations, health care policy-makers, and health insurance agencies? Fortunately, many renowned physicians, scientists, and healers representing reputable institutions have initiated the dialogue on many complementary modalities that contribute to health. The rich contributions from several of these pioneers to this anthology serve as a testimonial to their commitment to advance this concept.

It is an opportune moment for the Institute of Noetic Sciences to take a lead in sponsoring a Noetic Conference dedicated to integral medicine. It would serve to open a dialogue among the many stakeholders in the business of health, including representatives of the clients. It would clarify the conceptual basis and advocate practical ways of shifting from the fragmented to the integral medicine model. It will bring to light some creative examples of practical models and experiences of what works and what doesn't.

Clearly, the concept of integral medicine has to be understood and accepted by society as a whole. I believe that people are already embracing the idea and are willing to take primary responsibility for their health. Advocacy by such well-known experts as Carolyn Mays, Larry Dossey, Deepak Chopra, Andrew Weil, Kenneth Pelletier, Rachel Naomi Remen, and Joan Borychenko, to name a few of the pioneers in this field, will go a long way toward legitimizing the concept of integral medicine.

Education and Training of Health Care Practitioners

Integral medicine has important implications for the education and train-ing of health care practitioners, whether they practice conventional med-icine or one of the complementary therapies. Though many medical schools now offer elective courses in integral medicine, few of today's doctors have learned to look beyond laboratory tests to grapple with the patient's experience of illness and quest for health. The future looks hope-ful: Several leading medical schools have formed a consortium to push for fundamental changes in the way future physicians are to be trained.

It will not be enough to offer an elective course or a lecture here and there in complementary systems. It is also not practical to expect that doctors have to learn all complementary therapies to which they want their patients to have access. It is especially important that the primary care physician or family doctor have a good understanding of the value and effectiveness of major complementary therapies so that he or she can offer patients a choice or a more comprehensive approach to prevention and treatment of disease. One can visualize several approaches for such training.

According to one scenario, an entire year of medical education might be spent studying about health—what creates it, what destroys it, and what protects it. These medical students would learn about the human body as an integral part of the cosmos. They would learn about the body's energy and immune system and its innate capacity for healing. They would learn about mind-body medicine. They would become more aware of the individual's personal responsibility for health and learn how to communicate with their patients about this. They would also develop some basic understanding of other major complementary therapies— what they have to offer and their relative effectiveness.

Another approach would be that the doctors who choose to pursue a primary care or family practice would spend 1 year as an intern with some complementary care practitioners. Yet another possibility is to offer fellowships to those interested in more in-depth learning about some of the complementary therapies, especially the mind-body practices, that they can integrate in their practice. Another useful approach would be to have joint seminars and workshops for conventional and complementary care practitioners to enhance their understanding and respect for one another's approaches and values. In fact, these should become an important aspect of their continuing education program.

These approaches are not mutually exclusive, nor are they entirely new. It is possible that some of them are already in practice. We need to learn more about them and advocate a fundamental change in the preparation of our future health care practitioners.

Organizational Changes

The vision of integral medicine asserts that all parties will benefit from a respectful co-operation and integration of health care models. Our current structures of health care will require modification to allow access and movement across the boundaries of conventional and complementary medicine. This has to become the norm within the modern health care system. The role of the primary care physician or family doctor will be crucial. A well-prepared primary care physician who is familiar with all the different aspects of the patient's life is an important gatekeeper and care-coordinator of an integral health care system.

We need to learn about the well-functioning integral medicine models and how they can be replicated. One example is the Health and Healing Center of the Institute of Health and Healing, at the California Pacific Medical Center, in San Francisco, California. The center integrates self-care with expert care and the best of conventional medicine with proven healing practices from around the world. The center's physicians and practitioners are experts in many of the world's great healing traditions, including Western medicine, all backed by research. The center offers a personalized approach to health care that combines conventional and complementary approaches. The Institute of Health and Healing also offers classes to teach individuals and practitioners fundamental tools for wellness.

There are ethical and legal considerations in the practical application of integral medicine. These would have to be clarified by the health care policy-makers. The involvement of respected professional bodies such as the American Medical Association, the American Public Health

Association, and other professional health practitioners associations is crucial. The leaders of these professional bodies would need to be asked to include this topic in their meetings, to encourage active discussions among the various professional organizations, and to sponsor operational research in creating models of integral education and practice.

International Response

The concept of integral medicine has to be universally applicable. In some of the European and Asian countries, many of the complementary medicine modalities are already well-accepted along with those of conventional medicine. There is scanty information available on any integral medicine models in practice. Here the role of the international organizations, especially the World Health Organization, is crucial. The latter has the global responsibility for defining health and validating, as well as launching, innovative concepts and initiatives to health care. So far, its initiative in complementary medicine has been limited principally to some research and evaluation of indigenous herbs and medicines. There has been no concerted effort in evaluating the effectiveness of complementary medicine therapies in the prevention and treatment of diseases.

In 1978 the World Health Organization launched the "Goal of Health for All by the Year 2000." It defined the basic components of this goal and the strategy of primary health care for achieving it. Today, 25 years later, progress toward this goal has been very uneven, and inequalities in health persist and in some cases have even worsened. Deteriorating health conditions (especially in the poor countries of the world), gaping inequalities in access to health care, rising cost of health care, and emerging new diseases present major challenges to the World Health Organization in advancing its goal of universal health care. It is an opportune moment for the organization to take a leadership role in promoting and defining new and creative ways of providing integral health care using all available resources and expertise in the countries, including traditional and complementary approaches. The leadership of the organization should be approached about the prospect of convening an expert consultation on integral medicine in the near future.

CONCLUDING COMMENT

In the complex world of twenty-first-century health care, no single therapeutic practice should have the monopoly on the effective diagnosis and treatment for all conditions. Scientific, psychological, nutritional, environmental, and spiritual insights must surely be fully employed to restore and maintain health. The two paradigms (conventional medicine and complementary medicine) should be looked at side by side and their benefits continuously evaluated. The choice does not have to be "either/or" but instead can be "both/and."

References for this essay are located on the DVD accompanying this book.

The Ecozoic Era [*]

BRIAN SWIMME
THOMAS BERRY

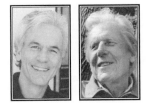

INTRODUCTION

Presently we seek to remedy the devastation of the planet by entry into a new period of creativity participated in by the entire Earth community. This new period we identify as the Ecozoic era: a fourth biological era to succeed the Paleozoic, the Mesozoic, and the Cenozoic eras. These last three terms are conceptual expressions invented in the nineteenth century that enable us to think about the larger patterns of functioning of the biosystems of the planet. The terms are subjective, "mythic," organizational expressions with a basis in the observable world, although they are themselves not found in the observable world. Since we are terminating the last of these periods, there is a need for a fourth term along the same

---

[*]Adapted from Swimme B, Berry T: *The universe story: from the primordial flaring forth to the ecozoic era, a celebration of the unfolding of the cosmos*, New York, 1992, HarperCollins, pp 240-261.

lines of expression. This fourth term we designate as the emerging Ecozoic era.

THE EMERGING ECOZOIC ERA

That the universe is a communion of subjects rather than a collection of objects is the central commitment of the Ecozoic. Existence itself is derived from and sustained by this intimacy of each being with every other being of the universe. We might even suggest that the Earth functions as an organism, provided that we understand we are using the term *organism* here as an analogous expression, since the Earth is not simply an enlarged organism at the same level as a tree or a bird. Yet there are similarities between the unity of Earth's functioning and the unity of functioning of any other living being that justifies the use of the term *organic* to describe the inner coherence and integral functioning of the planet Earth. Indeed, the Earth is so integral in the unity of its functioning that every aspect of the Earth is affected by what happens to any component member of the community.

Because of this organic quality, Earth cannot survive in fragments. This is one of the most significant aspects of the emerging Ecozoic era. The integral functioning of the planet must be preserved. The well-being of the planet is a condition for the well-being of any of the component members of the planetary community. To preserve the economic viability of the planet must be the first law of economics. To preserve the health of the planet must be the first commitment of the medical profession. To preserve the natural world as the primary revelation of the Divine must be the basic concern of religion. To think that humankind can benefit from a deleterious exploitation of any phase of the structure or functioning of the Earth is an absurdity. The well-being of the Earth is primary. Human well-being is derivative.

While it is true that the various members of the natural community nourish one another and that the death of one often means the life of the other, this relationship is not ultimately one of enmity but one of intimacy. The total balance in this process is preserved. If there is a taking, there is a giving. Without reciprocity the Earth could not survive. Failure to understand this is one of the reasons for the devastation of the late Cenozoic era by its human component. We thought that we could be nourished by the soil without in turn nourishing the soil in accordance with its own organic processes and its own rhythms of renewal. We thought that we could exploit the petroleum in the oil fields of the world through our petrochemical industry when we had no way to replace the carbon in a contained area so that the chemistry of the air could be adjusted for the proper functioning of the climate and for the benefit of the life systems of the planet.

This lack of reciprocity is due to treatment of the nonhuman world as an object of exploitation rather than as a subject to be communed with. Especially with the soil: there must be a human communion with the life principles in the soil if there is to be any ultimate benefit for either the soil or the human. The soil is a magical place where the alchemy takes place that enables living forms to survive. So, too, there is the intimate rapport that humans have with the animal world as this comes down to us from the tribal peoples with their totemic traditions of animals as our venerated ancestors.

This intimacy of relatedness extended beyond the living world to the various natural phenomena whereby the universe functions, especially to the sequence of the seasons, to the rain and the wind, to the thunder and lightning and surging of the sea, to the stars and all the other heavenly beings. Everything existed within the single embrace of this immense world, where the primordial mysteries of existence were shared in common. In the early civilizations the cosmological order was consistently experienced in terms of human society, and human social order was conceived in terms of the cosmological order. These were different aspects of a single universal order of things.

When we propose that the future might be designated as the Ecozoic era, we have in mind the restoration, in a new context, of this primordial mode of human awareness.

One important aspect of this new view of the universe is our new realization that the Earth is a one-time endowment. It is indeed an ever-renewing planet, but within limits. Just what these limits are we do not know. But whatever the limits of this planet, it is infinitely precious. No other such planet exists in the solar system. We know of no other such planet in the universe.

The pathos is that we, even now, are deliberately terminating the most awesome splendor that the planet has yet attained. We are extinguishing the rainforests, the most luxuriant life system of the entire planet, at the rate of an acre each second of each day. Each year we are destroying a rainforest area the size of Oklahoma. Not only here but throughout the planet, we are not only extinguishing present forms of life, we are eliminating the very conditions for the renewal of life in some of its more elaborate forms.

We have moved from such evils as suicide, homicide, and genocide to biocide and geocide, the killing of the life systems of the planet and the severe degradation, if not the killing, of the planet itself. We have moved from simple physical assault of the planet to disturbance of its chemical balance through our petrochemical industries, to questionable manipulation of the genetic constitution of the living beings of the planet through genetic engineering, to the radioactive wasting of the planet through our nuclear industries.

In the terms of the biologist E.O. Wilson,[1] we seem to be bringing about "the greatest impasse to the abundance and diversity of life on Earth" since the earliest beginnings of life some 4 billion years ago. In the estimation of Paul Ehrlich,[2] another eminent biologist, we are probably extinguishing some ten thousand species each year. Yet another distinguished biologist, Peter Raven,[3] indicates that we may be killing our world.

It has been difficult for humans to appreciate that the planet is given to us as a one-time endowment. Although the Earth is resilient and has extensive powers of renewal, it also has a finite and a nonrenewable aspect. Even the seasonal renewal aspects of the planet can be extinguished—species of plants and animals, for instance. Once a species is extinguished, we know of no power in heaven or on Earth that can bring about a revival. The law of entropy is a formidable law.

HUMAN INFLUENCE IN THE ECOZOIC ERA

It is already clear that in the future the Earth will function differently than it has functioned in the past. In the future the entire complex of life systems of the planet will be influenced by the human in a comprehensive manner. If the emergence of the Cenozoic in all its brilliance was independent of any human influence, almost every phase of the Ecozoic will involve the human. Although humans cannot make a blade of grass, there is likely not to be a blade of grass unless it is accepted, protected, and fostered by the human. These are the three controlling terms in human-earth relations for the foreseeable future: acceptance, protection, and fostering.

Acceptance of the given order of things is a more complex affair for humans than it is for other components of the life community since the human has, apparently, a greater capacity for critical reflection on the universe, the Earth and its proper mode of functioning, and our own human role in this larger context of things. Yet for the human, as for every other being, existence is not something acquired or merited by any positive act on the part of either the species or the individual. It is a pure receiving that brings with it conditions determined by the larger course of earthly events, not by the subject brought into existence. This involves the acceptance of existence by the species, by the society, and by individuals within the larger context into which they are born.

For the human, existence brings with it immense possibilities of delight and yet a series of never-ceasing anxieties concerning survival, both physical and psychic. Despite the satisfaction experienced in breathing air, drinking water, gazing at the stars in the darkness of the night, awakening to the dawn, or communing with the sunset in the evening; despite the joy we have in natural phenomena, such as the song of the mockingbird or the taste of a peach; despite the mutual fulfillment in the embrace of child and parent and humans with one another; despite the folk songs we sing and the music of the great composers, the visual and performing arts, our dances and religious rituals; despite the inner spiritual experiences available to us, we find in the Western psyche what might be designated as a deep hidden rage against our human condition. There are, of course, the more ordinary pains to be endured, the heat of summer and the chill of winter, periods of abundance and scarcity, the disappointments in human relationships. There are indeed the distortions, the pains we endure personally and the pains of others. Eventually, we discover, death is the price we pay for life.

For all these reasons there tends to develop a pervasive sense of the pathos of existence. Yet if the delights of existence came with pure, unalloyed joy, with no price to be paid, if death were not the condition of life, then the whole of existence might tend toward the trivial. Danger and death are conditions for adventure, and life without adventure can be a dull experience. The very structure and functioning of the universe do not permit such a mediocre existence.

Yet such a mediocre mode of being is precisely what has been invented in the terminal phases of the Cenozoic. With newly acquired power for mechanistic control over the natural world, we have discovered the power to protect ourselves from the elements, to produce food in enormous quantities and transport it anywhere in the world, to communicate instantly throughout the planet, and even to delay death by artificial contrivances. With all this knowledge and our corresponding skills, we have created a less threatening, human-controlled world, a world deprived of the great natural challenges of the past. It also goes with a devastated natural world, for, in the process of protecting ourselves from the natural conditions of things, we have done away with many of the most delightful and creative aspects of our existence. What we have gained by controlling the world as a collection of objects we have lost in our capacity for intimacy in the communion of subjects. We no longer hear the voices of all those natural companions of ours throughout the Earth. Nor is it clear that we have really gained the satisfactions we sought.

This new world of automobiles, highways, parking lots, shopping malls, power stations, nuclear-weapons plants, factory farms, and chemical plants; this new world of hundred-story buildings, endless traffic, turbulent populations, mega-cities, and decaying apartments has become an affliction perhaps greater than the more natural human condition it seeks to replace. We live in a chemical-saturated world. It is not a life-giving situation. If not deadly, it is degraded. Humans now live amid limitless junk beyond any known capacity for creative use. Our vision is impaired by the pollution in the atmosphere. We no longer see the stars with the clarity that once existed.

Yet there has developed a mystique of this sort of existence, especially by those most protected against the full force of the destitution consequent on the total process. There is a feeling of accomplishment, an irrevocable commitment that this is the way into a more creative mode of being for the entire planet, since, after all, we are ultimately in control and the planet is here to serve human needs and purposes. Our sciences and our technologies seem fully capable of providing a remedy for any ill consequences of what we are doing. We have extraordinary powers, such as those associated with genetic engineering.

FROM THE CENOZOIC TO THE TECHNOZOIC OR ECOZOIC?

A newly developed mystique of our plundering industrial society is committed to moving out of the Cenozoic—not by entry into the Ecozoic but by shaping an even more controlled order of things that might be designated as the Technozoic era. The greater part of contemporary industrial society, it seems, is oriented toward the Technozoic rather than to the Ecozoic. Certainly the corporation establishment, with its enormous economic control over the whole of modern existence, is dedicated to the Technozoic.

From this it is clear that a mystique counter to the commercial-industrial mystique must be evoked if the Ecozoic era is to come into being. The future can be described in terms of the tension between these two forces. If the dominant political-social issue of the twentieth century has been between the capitalist and the communist worlds, between democratic freedoms and socialist responsibility, the dominant issue of the immediate future will clearly be the tension between the entrepreneur and the ecologist, between those who would continue their plundering and those who would truly preserve the natural world, between the mechanistic and the organic, between the world as a collection of objects and the world as a communion of subjects, between the anthropocentric and the biocentric norms of reality and value.

Only a comprehensive commitment to the Ecozoic can effectively counter the mystical commitment of our present commercial-industrial establishments to the Technozoic. There is a special need in this transitional phase out of the Cenozoic to awaken a consciousness of the sacred dimension of the Earth. What is at stake is not simply an economic resource but the meaning of existence itself. Ultimately, it is the survival of the world of the sacred. Once this is gone, the world of meaning truly dissolves into ashes. We will be living in a lunar situation, for on the desolate expanse of the moon our only conception of the divine would reflect the lunar landscape, our imagination would be as bleak as the moon, our sensitivities as dull, our intelligence as blank. We cannot change the outer world without also changing our inner world. A desolate Earth will be reflected in the depths of the human.

HUMAN CONSCIOUSNESS, RESPONSIBILITY, AND APPRECIATION

The comprehensive objective of the Ecozoic is to assist in establishing a mutually enhancing human presence on the Earth. This cannot, obviously, be achieved immediately. But if this is not achieved in some manner or within some acceptable limits, humans will continue to exist in a progressively degraded mode of being. The degradation both to ourselves and to the planet is the immediate evil that we are dealing with. The enhancement or the degradation will be a shared experience. We have a common destiny—not simply a common human destiny but a common destiny for all the components of the planetary community.

The immediate goal of the Ecozoic is not simply to diminish the devastation of the planet that is taking place at present. It is rather to alter the mode of consciousness that is responsible for such deadly activities. When we fail to recognize the primary basis for survival in uncontaminated air, water, and soil, and the integral community of life systems of the planet; when we insist on altering the chemical constitution of the atmosphere; when we begin to affect the beneficent climate and the life-giving sequence of the seasons that has brought about the luxuriance of the Cenozoic period into which we were born, then we must consider that we are into a deep cultural pathology. It is particularly pathetic when we bargain over these issues of life and survival for monetary gain or some commercial advantage for a few individuals or a corporative enterprise.

The basic obligation during any historical moment is to continue the integrity of that creative process whence the universe derives, sustains itself, and continues its sequence of transformations. To alter this in some significant manner or to seek to control this process under the assumption that we know how the planet functions in its comprehensive context is the ultimate folly. This sequence of transformations is too mysterious for comprehensive understanding by ourselves or by any form of consciousness that we are acquainted with.

The human mode of understanding, however, does bring with it a unique responsibility for entering into this creative process. While we do not have a comprehensive knowledge of the origin or destiny of the universe or even of any particular phase of the universe, we do have a capacity for understanding and responding to the story that the universe tells of itself, how it emerged in the beginning, the sequence of transformations leading to the wondrous world spread out before us in the heavens, and the vast spectacle presented to us by the Earth in its geological, biological, and human manifestations.

As with all other earthly beings, we are expected to enter into this process within those distinctive capacities for human understanding and appreciation that provide our human identity. We are expected to enter into the process, to honor the process, to accept the process as a sacred context for existence and meaning, not to violently seize upon the process or attempt to control it to the detriment of the process itself in its major modes of expression.

It is critical that we develop and act from a pervasive human responsibility at every level of the human, from the individual person through all manner of social and political communities throughout every profession and human association, since our responsibility is to life itself, to the planet Earth, and to the role assigned our existence as a species. Our responsibility now, at the end of the twentieth century and the beginning of the twenty-first century, can be fulfilled only by assisting in the emergence of the Ecozoic era, which is coming into existence out of the ruins of the Cenozoic.

By entering into the control of the planet through our sciences and our technologies in these past 2 centuries, we have assumed responsibilities beyond anything that we are capable of carrying out with any assured success. But now that we have inserted ourselves so extensively into the functioning of the ecosystems of the Earth, we cannot simply withdraw and leave the planet and all its life systems to themselves in coping with the poisoning and the other devastation that we have wrought.

The primary need is to withdraw from our efforts to impose a mechanistic overlay on the biosystems of the planet, to step back from what we have been doing. Then we might listen to the natural world with an attunement that goes beyond our scientific perceptions. However helpful these may be, they cannot deal with those spontaneities that ultimately determine the course of things in the biosystems of the planet. In understanding this process something more than science is needed, or a new mode of science, such as that suggested by the title *A Feeling for the Organism,* a biography of the biologist Barbara McClintoch.[4]

Our proposal, then, is not that we walk away from the natural world but that we follow our own instinctive sensitivities in relating to the natural world. That humans have not, in fact, abandoned the Earth is increasingly evident in the multitude of movements throughout the various regions of the Earth. The orientation we have outlined here is in general the commitment of all serious ecology movements throughout the human community. A multitude of such movements in our social institutions are already functioning.

FROM DENIAL TO REVELATION

That our Western civilization should be the principal cause of such extensive damage to the planet is so difficult a truth for us to absorb that our society in general is presently in a state of shock and denial, of disbelief that this can possibly be the real situation. We are unable to move from the conviction that as humans we are the glory and the crown of the Earth community to the realization that we are the most destructive and the most dangerous component of that community. Such denial is the first attitude of persons grasped by any form of addiction. Our Western addiction to commercial-industrial progress as the basic referent for reality and value is becoming an all-pervasive attitude throughout the various peoples and cultures of the Earth.

Efforts to present the full reality of the situation generally are being met with intense opposition, an opposition due in large measure to the subservience of our religious, educational, and professional establishments to our industrial culture. These major determinants of our cultural forms are manifesting minimal concern for the catastrophic situation that is before us.

The remedy would seem to emerge, as in most denial situations, after a crash so severe that we are suddenly confronted with a choice between death and abdication of our addictive mode of functioning. In this case, the impending crash is of immensely greater dimensions and more definitive consequences. The crash that faces us is not the crash simply of the human; it's a crash of the biosystems of the Earth and, indeed, it is in some manner the crash of the Earth itself.

We do not imply here that the more elementary life systems of the planet are in danger of extinction. These, the microforms of life—along with the insects, rodents, plants, and many of the trees and animals—will surely continue, probably in ever-greater abundance. What is indicated here is that the conditions of the planet in any foreseeable future, or in that phase of historical or biological time available to human understanding, would suffer severe deterioration in terms of their present mode of expression. The water and air and soil pollution could remain for a significant period, along with the decline of the rainforests and the diminishment of life species.

Yet the tendency to minimize the difficulties before us is the obstruction to any radical change in human consciousness, a change at the order of magnitude required for entry into the creative phase of the Ecozoic. This change requires something of a different order but equivalent to a new religious tradition. Our new sense of the universe is itself a type of revelatory experience. Presently we are moving beyond any religious expression so far known to humankind into a metareligious age, one that seems to be a new comprehensive context for all religions.

THE WELL-BEING OF THE EARTH IS PRIMARY

The Ecozoic era requires a comprehensive human consensus. It needs such support for its planet-wide programs. The entire planet would then be considered as a commons. Already the atmosphere, the seas, and the space above the Earth are being recognized as areas of universal relevance. There are also biological areas of global concern.

The human professions all need to recognize their prototype and their primary resource in the integral functioning of the Earth community. The natural world itself is the primary economic reality, the primary educator, the primary governance, the primary technologist, the primary healer, the primary presence of the sacred, the primary moral value.

In economics it is clear that our human economy derives from the Earth's economy. To glory in a rising gross domestic product with an irreversibly declining gross earth product is an economic absurdity. As long as our patterns of consumption overwhelm the upper reaches of Earth's sustainable productivity, we will only drive the Earth community further into ruin. The only viable human economy is one that is integral with the Earth economy.

Education is already late in its revision, but we can expect that it will be extensively altered in the future. Education might well be defined as knowing the story of the universe, of the planet Earth, of life systems, and of consciousness, all as a single story, and recognizing the human role in the story. The primary purpose of education should be to enable individual humans to fulfill their proper role in this larger pattern of meaning. We can understand this role in the Great Story only if we know the story in its full dimensions.

In our governance we are moving from a limited democracy to a more comprehensive biocracy. Already we can envisage a constitution not simply for humans on this continent but for the entire North American community, including both the geographical structures and functioning of the Earth and the various life systems dispersed over the Earth. A beginning has been made in the legislation requiring environmental impact statements before any major project affecting the environment can be undertaken. Among the challenges that face governance in the human order is the relationship of national governments with each other, with particular reference at the present time to the more industrialized northern nations of the planet that are exploiting the less industrialized southern nations. Currently this is not only negating human advancement but is bringing about a pervasive devastation of human societies.

The engineering profession begins to learn that human activity is most effective and most enduring when it is in accordance with the natural functioning of the ecosystem into which it is inserted. Human engineering needs to be guided by the masterful technologies of Earth. In the transport systems of vascular plants, in the energy conversions of photosynthesis, in the efficiencies of the hydrological and mineral cycles, in the communication systems of the genetic codes are technological models of great power and elegance. Needed now are biocentric human technologies that are coherent with Earth technologies and that would enable our agricultural, energy, and architectural projects to be carried out in an integral relationship with Earth's functioning.

The medical profession begins to see that the well-being of the ecosystems of the planet is a prior condition for the well-being of the human. We cannot have well humans on a sick planet, not even with all our medical science. As long as we continue to generate more toxins than the planet can absorb and transform, the members of the Earth community become ill. Human health is derivative. Planetary health is primary.

Religion begins to appreciate that the primary sacred community is the universe itself. In a more immediate perspective, the sacred community is the Earth community. The human community becomes sacred through its participation in the larger planetary community.

In morality we are expanding our moral sensitivity beyond suicide, homicide, and genocide to include biocide and geocide, evils that were not recognized in our civilization's traditions until recently.

Beyond all this, and in a sense more encompassing than any of these, is the role of women in the future. The present need is recognition of women in their capacity to interpret the human venture at its most basic level in the context of the universe and the planet Earth. The family—child-bearing and child-rearing—will always be a central focus of human concern. Yet for women especially a new range of activities is needed, both for themselves and for the larger destinies of the human-Earth venture. We cannot do without the special insights that women offer in every phase of human existence.

The need to limit population growth and even to consider a possible decrease in population has altered in a definitive manner one of the most basic aspects of the entire human situation. This leads immediately to new possibilities for women's participation in the course of human affairs, which has been consistently thwarted in most traditional civilizations. The rise of movements such as feminism and ecofeminism has already altered all the basic professions and social institutions throughout the industrialized countries of the world. As this participation increases throughout the world, as women are liberated from the oppressions they have long endured, as women reach new levels of personal fulfillment, a new energy will undoubtedly be felt throughout the Earth. While we cannot know just what the consequences will be, there is reason to hope that this will be a vast creative and healing energy.

DEVELOPING AN ECOZOIC LANGUAGE

So far we have had a human-centered language. We need an Earth-centered language. A new Ecozoic dictionary is gradually taking shape as we begin to articulate our new vision more clearly. All the more substantive words in the language are undergoing a transformation, words such as *society*, *good* and *evil*, *freedom*, *justice*, *literacy*, *progress*. All these words need to be extended to include the various beings of the natural world—their freedoms, their rights, their share in the functioning of the Earth.

Our Cenozoic dictionary cannot deal adequately with the realities of existence in this new period. We need an Ecozoic dictionary.

Beyond any formal spoken or written human language are the languages of the multitude of beings, each of which has its own language given to it generally, in the world of the living, by genetic coding. Yet each individual being has extensive creativity in the use of the language. Humans are becoming much more sensitive to the nonhuman languages of the surrounding world. We are learning the mountain language, river language, tree language, the languages of the birds and all the animals and insects, as well as the languages of the stars in the heavens. This capacity for understanding and communicating through these languages, until now enjoyed only by our poets and mystics, is of immense significance since so much of life is lived in association with the other beings in the universe.

Among the greatest linguistic changes is the change from our present efforts in an exclusively univocal, literal, scientific, objective language to a multivalent language much richer in its symbolic and poetic qualities. This is required because of the multivalent aspects of each reality. Scientific language, however useful in scientific investigation, can be harmful to the total human process once it is accepted as the only way to speak about the true reality of things. A more symbolic language is needed to enter the subjective depths of things, to understand both the qualitative differences and the multivalent aspects of every reality.

Indeed, all our basic words are multivalent terms that are used analogously. This simply means that there are qualitative differences in their various meanings. Precisely because of its organic mode of being, the Earth is not a global sameness; Earth is a highly differentiated unity as is every organic reality, so that each component bioregion has its own unique mode of integration and its own special role to fulfill that needs to be recognized and responded to if any well-being is to be achieved by the planet in its integrity.

The sciences and the humanities, business and religion, the arts and sciences—all these divisions of learning are beginning to overcome their isolation from one another. Even though the distinctive roles of each need always to be recognized, they will ideally become much more integrated with one another in the future. All our professions and institutions need to be appreciated in the light of the single story that governs the basic functioning of the Earth as well as the entire human process.

HUMAN—A SPECIES AMONG SPECIES

We begin to rethink the structure and functioning of our cities. No longer must we endure without protest the oppression of the automobile as the primary factor in our city architecture. Already cities are being redesigned to bring the streams above ground rather than condemning them to flow through our sewers. Our cities begin to be places for habitation not merely by humans but also by other life forms. We begin to make provision for the birds and the various animals that are proper to the region.

There is no reason why the various life forms—the fish in the streams, the flowering plants, the animals proper to the region—should not share in our common habitat. We diminish the grandeur of the human habitat once we exclude other living forms from sharing in the single life community. The need of things to be distant from one another at times need not indicate that the variety of living forms can be diminished without harming the inherent vigor of the community itself and all its component members.

Earlier we were concerned simply with our own limited area. We withdrew from the major forces of life into the realm of our own limited controls. We developed our individual self with a neglect of our community self, our relationship with the planet Earth, and with the entire natural order that constitutes the larger self of our own being.

What we seldom think about is the human as species. We will never come to appreciate the full significance of human adjustment in this new biological era until we begin to think of the human as a species among species. We have thought about the human as nations, as cultures, as ethnic groups, as international organizations, even as the global human community, but none of these articulates the present human-Earth issue so precisely as thinking about the human as a species among species.

We need an interspecies economy, an interspecies well-being, an interspecies education, an interspecies governance, an interspecies religious mode, interspecies ethical norms. Until we begin to think of our human story as integral with the larger life story and the larger Earth story, we will not be fully into the Ecozoic period. We will not have an Ecozoic governance.

THE CELEBRATORY EXPERIENCE OF EXISTENCE

A final integration of the Ecozoic era with the larger pattern of the Universe Story, such as we are narrating it here, has to do with the curvature of the space-time continuum. The nature of this curvature is bound up with the energy of the universe's primordial Flaring Forth. Had the curvature been a fraction larger, the universe would have immediately collapsed into a massive black hole; had it been a fraction smaller, the universe would have exploded into a scattering of lifeless particles. The universe is shaped in its larger dimensions from its earliest instant of emergence. The expansive original energy keeps the universe from collapsing, while the gravitational attraction holds the component parts together and enables the universe to blossom. Thus the curvature of the universe is sufficiently closed to maintain a coherence of its various components and sufficiently open to allow for a continued creativity.

This balance of forces is again what gives to the Earth its special qualities. Its own gravitational attraction holds the Earth together. The resultant inner pressures, combined with the Earth's inner nuclear energy, keep the Earth in a state of balanced turbulence whence its continued transformation takes place. Because this balanced turbulence was not achieved in the other planets, they were unable to bring forth such living forms as emerged on Earth.

We might say that the industrial age, from its human influences, has so upset this balance that the planet has gone into a burnout phase of its existence. The industrial plundering of the planet has increased the toxic condition of the Earth to a point beyond that which the Earth can manage creatively. The Earth cannot dispose adequately of the chemical residues spewed into the atmosphere by the burning-off of the fossil fuels that the Earth had kept stored for millions of years in order to achieve the chemical balance needed for the expansion of the life systems of the planet.

What the Ecozoic era ultimately seeks is to bring the human activities on Earth into alignment with the other forces functioning throughout the planet so that a creative balance will be achieved. When the curvature of the universe, the curvature of the Earth, and the curvature of the human are once more in their proper relation, then Earth will have arrived at the celebratory experience that is the fulfillment of earthly existence.

References for this essay are located on the DVD accompanying this book.

Living in the Earth: Ecopsychology, Health, and Psychotherapy*

SARAH A. CONN

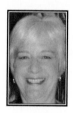

THIS ESSAY WAS DEVELOPED from an insight expressed so well by Joanna Macy[1]:

> We are living cells in the living body of Earth. Our collective body is in trauma and we are experiencing that. Even though we try to suppress it or drown it out or cut a nerve so we don't feel it, the collective plight exists at some level of our consciousness.... We need to listen to ourselves as if we were listening to a message from the universe...There is no private salvation.

"I feel terrible again, and I can't figure out why. Is it my medication or my upcoming evaluation at work or the anniversary of my mother's death? I feel so inadequate. I should by now be able to figure it out myself. I should be able to pull myself together."

---

*Adapted from Conn SA: Living in the Earth: Ecopsychology, Health, and Psychotherapy, *The Humanistic Psychologist* 26(1-3):179-198, Spring/Summer/Autumn 1998.

How many times have we heard ourselves or others individualize and pathologize our experience in the way demonstrated by this client? Our notions of health in this culture are based on being able to "figure out" what is causing our distress, singling out one cause close to home so that we can "fix it," "pull ourselves together," "get over" it by ourselves once and for all. True to our mechanistic indoctrination and our Cartesian baptism, we tend to look for "private salvation" by focusing on separate parts, emphasizing the importance of the mind and striving for control. Our linear notion of time leads us to expect to be able to "fix" our distress once and for all; if it returns, we must have failed in some way. The field of possible explanations and methods does not include our participation in the larger context of the living earth, our "collective body," as Joanna Macy names it.[1]

Ecopsychology, which focuses on the ways human beings experience themselves within the larger context, invites us to consider that collective body. The principles and practices of ecopsychology invite us to hear the earth speaking through our pain and distress, "to listen to ourselves as if we were listening to a message from the universe."

WHAT IS ECOPSYCHOLOGY?

Ecology is the study of connection, of the interrelationships among all forms of life and the physical environment. Psychology is the study of the human psyche, of the human mind and soul as it perceives, feels, thinks, and acts. Ecopsychology brings psychology and ecology together to study the human psyche within the larger systems of which it is a part.

The theoretical base of ecopsychology sees the earth as a living system. Human beings, their psyches as well as their products and cultures, are integral and crucial parts of that system. The practice of ecopsychology is based on the recognition that the needs of the earth and the needs of the human individual are interdependent and interconnected and that human health and sanity must include sustainable and mutually enhancing relations with the natural world.

One aim of ecopsychology is to develop new models of health that articulate and promote sustainable and mutually enhancing relationships, not just at the intrapersonal level (within humans) or the interpersonal level (among humans) but also at the level of "interbeing" (between humans and the nonhuman world). The goal of ecopsychological practice is to develop methods and forms that enable individuals to sense, think, feel, and act as interdependent beings, interconnected within the whole community of life at all levels, from the individual psyche to a particular place on earth to the earth as a whole to the universe. Many psychotherapeutic approaches agree that the experience of connectedness is crucial to health. Broadening the field within which this connectedness is investigated and encouraged is one major contribution of ecopsychology.

Ecopsychology is a developing perspective with diverse approaches within it. Common to each of these approaches is attention to the modern human psyche's disconnection from the nonhuman world and to the ways this separation has truncated and deadened human experience, both individually and collectively.

In our Western Euro-American culture, the dominant psychology of the self is still based on the Cartesian worldview. Humans are seen as separate from and hierarchically superior to the nonhuman world. Individual humans are seen as separated from each other, and some humans are thought to be superior to other humans. Most of us describe ourselves by our occupational, family, gender, racial, or ethnic roles. Most of our descriptions of ourselves are nouns preceded with an "a." "I am a woman, a psychologist, a mother, a wife, a WASP." This way of describing ourselves emphasizes separateness, boundedness, fixedness, reification, nonfluidity. We think we can locate ourselves as a "thing" in space and time, separate from other "things" in other spaces and times. This is the dominant version of reality: The world is a collection of separate entities that are related mechanically, if at all. We have narrowed the experience of connectedness to dominance, manipulation, and control.

This narrowing has had consequences both ecologically and psychologically. As Brian Swimme and Thomas Berry point out, "What humans do to the outer world, they do to their own interior world. As the natural world recedes in its diversity and abundance, so the human finds itself impoverished in its economic resources, in its imaginative powers, in its human sensitivities, and in significant aspects of its intellectual intuitions."[2] Or as ecologist Donald Worster states, "Besides losing so many of the larger animals, we have lost a considerable range of human

feelings—the delight and the joy, the humility that may come from standing in the presence of what we have called the wilderness. In most parts
of the country such feelings are gone forever."[3]

The psychological consequences of our disconnection from the natural
world are showing up in our psychotherapy practices as symptoms in our
clients. As we begin to see these symptoms not as enemies to be conquered
or eliminated, as modern Western medicine so often does, they appear as signals, as feedback within a larger system that includes the more-than-human
world. We can then begin to hear the "earth speaking through" the client's
problems. As therapists, we can become "naturalists of the psyche,"[4] appreciating each experience with the client for its part in the whole, exploring the
landscape—in both "inner" and "outer" dimensions—thoroughly. This
involves learning to hear, see, and feel the "earth speaking through" the
symptom and developing ways it might be pointing toward the symptom-
holder's fuller, more mindful participation in the larger community. We can
as therapists learn to let "the earth speak" through our practices as well as our
understandings, to broaden the field in which we work. Ecopsychology is
beginning to articulate the concepts and methods for this endeavor.

ECOPSYCHOLOGY AND HEALTH

What lenses can we use that will focus our efforts to find an ecopsychological view of health? One possibility emerges from a native-American
way of viewing insanity. In one indigenous tribe of North America, the
word for madness or insanity has four syllables. This Okanagan language is
not written but spoken, and each syllable of the word for insanity carries
a depth of meaning that is ecopsychologically profound.[5,6] Each of these
syllables points to an arena of difficulty related to some kind of disconnection from the web of life. Each of these four arenas of disconnection
points to a constellation of elements we believe are essential for health in
an ecopsychological context. Within and among each of these interrelated
constellations, specific practices for healing must be developed.

The first syllable of the Okanagan word for insanity points to the tendency to "talk, talk inside your head." We have been described as a "disso-
ciative culture," showing cultural signs of the trauma of profound
disconnection from our bodies and from the larger body of the earth.[7]

Often what our clients present to us can be seen as psychic monocultures, ways of thinking and feeling that are rigid, inflexible, and truncated. We need to look at ways of knowing that augment the cognitive, intellectual, abstract methods we have used to "figure things out." Ecopsychological health requires us to make lively, unmediated, direct contact with the world, listening and looking and sniffing and touching and feeling our connections not only with ourselves and each other but also with the earth, the sun, and the moon and the stars, as we learn to take our place in the interdependent web of life. We need to attend to the ecology of experience, to look at how our feelings and sensations fit together with the talk inside our heads.

The second syllable of the Okanagan word for insanity refers to being "scattered and having no community." In many ways, this is a description of modern industrial life, with its support of bounded, separate, so-called self-contained individuals who experience themselves as "empty," needing to be filled up by continually consuming goods and services and "virtual" experiences. Ecopsychological health invites us to bring relationality to the foreground of our lives. This will involve recognizing the communities of which we are a part, developing rituals that enliven and maintain those communities, and practicing citizenship in new, more direct ways.

The third syllable of the Okanagan word for insanity refers to "having no relationship to the land." When we in modern industrial society do look at community, we tend to leave out the nonhuman world. We do not see the land as part of the community. Ecopsychological health will include recognition of our embeddedness in the land. We will become familiar with the place in which we live. Our "ground" will include the flora and fauna native to our particular place, as well as a knowledge of the stresses and strains from non-native imports and the human-made world. Human health must include active participation in a community of living beings. There is no such thing as "individual" health separate from the systems within which the individual exists. As Elizabeth Roberts,[8] an "eco-immunologist," puts it, "Every act of healing has one obligation: it must create a pattern of health around itself.... Our health is created by helping other systems to become healthy."

The fourth syllable of the Okanagan word for insanity refers to being "disconnected from the whole-earth part." The root of the word *health* points to being whole or making whole. In an ecopsychological context, an individual is psychologically healthy when he or she is able to experience a deep inner coherence and at the same time an alive, ongoing connection with the larger systems of which he or she is a part. Health is thus remaining whole in the face of constant flows of the larger systems through us. As parts of the larger air, water, soil, meaning, and feeling systems around us, both biosphere and culture, nature and nurture, this means to know ourselves as wholes in our constant "partness." Maybe this means to know ourselves in our unique "particularity" and to be able to tack back and forth between our wholeness and partness. The challenge is honoring our uniqueness as we learn how "to listen to ourselves as if we were listening to a message from the universe."

To be healthy is to become who one really is, an authentic, unique and connected being, exercising both assertive and integrative abilities. The balance between these two tendencies is crucial to health. To be healthy means opening to and claiming one's unique part in the whole, letting the whole express itself in oneself in unique ways. It means dwelling in the boundaries between our wholeness and our partness, knowing ourselves as both and each.

In sum, direct contact with the world around us, embeddedness in community and in the land, and living out of "the whole-earth part" of ourselves constitute essential aspects of ecopsychological health.

ECOPSYCHOLOGY AND PSYCHOTHERAPY

Many schools of psychotherapy teach us what to look for as we sit with our clients and learn about their pain and their problems. How we hear their stories and with what questions we direct their story-telling can vary considerably depending on our training. One way that ecopsychology invites us to expand the psychotherapeutic context is by attending to the interplay between the inner and the outer landscapes, to include the community, the land, and the "whole-earth part" in the stories we hear and request from our clients.

In this endeavor the contributions of ecology can be very helpful. Writing in the 1950s, Eugene Odum, considered a father of ecology, introduced the idea of an "ecosystem," defining it as "any unit that includes all of the organisms (i.e., the 'community') in a given area interacting with the physical environment."[9] Besides inclusivity and interconnectedness, which includes the physical environment, the conditions for a healthy ecosystem include diversity and adequate nourishment patterns.

How might this particular ecological frame, combined with the four arenas described above, contribute to the direction of a particular therapy? The following client story demonstrates how we can use this frame when exploring both the inner and outer landscapes in which the client is embedded and looking for the connections between these realms, which have been artificially disconnected within our culture.

My client, Adrienne, found that her connection to the land enabled her to redefine the meaning of "trust" in her life. Adrienne had completed therapy and had moved to the country a year before. Then she called for a consultation because she was having an anxiety attack. In the midst of several major transitions in her life, she was suddenly faced with two major crises at the same time. Her mother, who lived 2,000 miles away, had fallen and broken her hip. She had done major work around her childhood experience of being rejected by her mother, but this occurrence stirred up the family dynamics, and she was pulled by her siblings into the fray. At the same time, the negotiations she was in with her former husband about her children's college bills had turned ugly; communications had broken down. Adrienne was frightened and was not sure of what. She felt the return of old feelings—that she was not good enough, that she was doing something wrong, that she might be crazy.

True to the American way, Adrienne was individualizing and pathologizing her experience. When I asked her what she noticed about the larger context of both these crisis situations, she was able to see that they both had to do with money in some way. Her trust fund from her family of origin was getting low, and the battle with her ex-husband for more support of her children's education felt crucial to her. And her mother's situation reminded her that she had no more inheritance, either financial or emotional, to fall back on. She indicated that the "ground" felt pulled out from under her. I reminded her that she had moved to the country for more contact with the "ground." She had developed psychological resources in her contact with the land—special places where she walked, animals she had gotten to know—that she could connect with now, while she worked with the question of what all of this was calling for from her. Because of our previous work in therapy, I knew I could ask her to consider the following question: What movement in her life was being called for by these current circumstances? As she contemplated this question, a strong feeling passed through her. She felt enormous grief: the necessity to let go of her past, of her family as it had been, of a previous ground of being that no longer worked for her. I wondered if she now needed to develop a trust in the universe, a new ground that did not depend so much on money, especially family money. She needed to look at the ways she could support herself now. She immediately related this task to letting go of dependence on the family "trust" fund, to learning to trust herself in her new landscapes, both inner and outer.

Our consumer culture encourages this narrowing of emotional experiences to money and the things it can buy. "Trust" for Adrienne had become so attached to family finances that other sources of confidence in herself and in her relationships, both human and more-than-human, had fallen far into the background. She needed to pull them forward again.

Connecting with the land became an important part of the psychotherapeutic process for Adrienne, as it has for many clients, enabling each of them to become more grounded, both actually and metaphorically. Health in an ecopsychological framework involves finding our ground in our home landscape as a way of finding ourselves within the larger context of the earth as a living system within an evolving ecological universe. Connecting with the community of living beings and with the land can support us in honoring our part in the whole while we move and change with the changes in that larger context.

"THE WHOLE-EARTH PART"

Ecopsychology, in its focus on the human psyche within the larger systems of which it is a part, can be said to look at what James Hillman has called "the soul's need to place itself within the great scheme of things." Who are we in the larger picture of the earth as a living system? In our consumer culture, learning to know and to honor our "whole-earth part" can be extremely difficult.

Many of my clients' experiences point to what I have referred to as a "materialistic disorder," the tendency to define oneself in terms of material possessions. This disorder is encouraged by the consumer culture supported by massive corporate advertising, which encourages what Kanner and Gomes have called the "consumer false self."[10]

The modern American version of the bounded, masterful self-contained individual is the "empty self." Since the 1940s, there has been a steady deterioration of tradition and community in American culture. People no longer define themselves in terms of their role in their communities or center themselves in the rituals of their traditions. They are bombarded constantly with images from the consumer culture, which now define success and "the good life" in homogenous ways, with little difference across communities and traditions. The result is a sense of self that is empty of meaning and purpose, needing to be filled up with goods, substances, services, and celebrities. Philip Cushman,[11] in a seminal article on this subject, contends that the two institutions that have grown up since World War II to minister to the "empty self are advertising and psychotherapy."

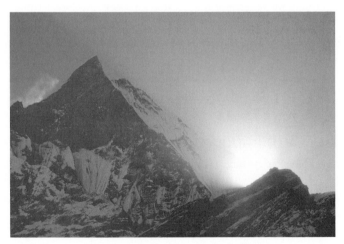

"First Light." (Courtesy Michael Eller.)

The challenge for ecopsychology is to find ways for psychotherapy to respond to the empty self—not by providing another way to soothe or to fill it up but by discovering and supporting the person's unique contribution to the larger context of the earth as a living system. Brian Swimme, in his *Canticle to the Cosmos* video series, describes the "yearning within each human to participate with the powers of the universe."[12]

What might be the routes to the "whole-earth part" in psychotherapy? How might psychotherapists enable their clients to explore the following questions: What is my heart's desire? How can I honor it? How does it connect me to the world? Access to these questions can emerge through ecological exploration of the inner landscape. Sometimes this access can emerge through exploring connections to the land. And with clients suffering from materialistic disorders, it can emerge through focusing on the sources and flows of nourishment in their lives, as in the following story.

Linda had been working for some time on the connections between her compulsive consuming and her traumatic, abusive childhood. As she worked through the trauma of her personal history, she began to notice her tendency to overwork and to then feel that she deserved a treat. She was dedicated to her work with poor elderly people, a calling she had discovered during a period in her life when money was not a concern. She wanted to continue doing it, but she realized that she had to learn to attend to what would truly nourish her rather than stuffing herself with candy when she was tired. By exploring her "hunger" at those times, she realized that she wanted and needed more interactions with people around her. As she began to honor this desire or need, she discovered that she had a real ability to establish and maintain community. She first began to arrange gatherings of all the people in her apartment building. She then became a prime mover in establishing groups that met regularly to address issues important in her life. One of these groups attended specifically to members' relationship to the consumption of food and other products.

In learning with the support of others to open to and live with the question of what her heart desired, Linda discovered that another source of nourishment was solitude. In a crowded apartment in a crowded city building, this is not always easy to achieve. But she began to carve out time alone almost every day, by walking to a nearby park, or hiking along the river, or sitting in the back yard of a friend's apartment building. This solitude enabled her to connect with the nonhuman world. As Linda has begun to notice and develop sources of true nourishment, she is able to explore more deeply her cravings for things, for food. Recently, for example, she attended to a craving for ice cream when it arose (instead of immediately getting the ice cream and eating it). She was able to sit with the craving, paying attention to where in her body she felt it and staying with it long enough to notice that what she really needed was to put on a piece of music, close her eyes, and be still for 10 minutes. Linda is now beginning more consistently to explore her cravings, to befriend them, to ask them questions, and to learn that they are connected to several specific needs that can be satisfied without overspending or overeating.

A key to sustainability in one's life is to establish balance in the physical, psychological, and spiritual nourishment cycles, within individual and community life. Linda knows something about her "whole-earth part" through doing what she is "called" to do in the world—working with poor, elderly people. Her challenge has been to honor her individual needs for nourishment in order to sustain her work for the world. Thus, with regular contact in community and with the land around her, she is beginning to restore a balance to her psychic ecology, to be able to honor the work for the world that expresses her "whole-earth part." Through this contact with land and community, she begins to be able to hear the larger context speaking through her own and others' experiences.

CONCLUSION: NO PRIVATE SALVATION

Ecopsychological perspectives on health and psychotherapy invite us to rediscover ourselves as dwellers within the earth as a living system. When we consider the human psyche from this perspective, we can begin to view personal pain as both unique to the person and as a signal from the larger context, as "the earth speaking through us." Exploring the inner and the outer landscapes within which we live and the connections between them, we look for diversity, interconnectedness, and flows of nourishment in the system of which the pain is a part. How does the pain represent a signal, an opportunity for movement, a call for participation in the larger system?

The failing health of the earth as a living system affects us all. The challenge of attending to our larger selves is a formidable one, impossible to accomplish without the support of and nourishment from diverse communities of living beings connecting to the land around them. Ecopsychology invites psychotherapy practice to expand its focus beyond the inner landscape, to explore and foster connections within community and with the land, to view the development of ecological identity and an active participation in the world as essential aspects of health.

The evolving ecological story about the world tells of continual change. The healthy individual does not develop a fixed identity in a world of continual change. Instead, in the process of opening to the inner and outer landscapes, one can become more harmonious with the larger wholes within which one exists. In so doing, a healthy individual's identity changes continually, expanding and contracting according to the context of the moment. And the possibilities extend beyond the family, the neighborhood, the country, or even the planet to include the sense of being a part of the evolving ecological universe at the same time that one's sense of coherence, uniqueness, and connectedness is sustained.

References for this essay are located on the DVD accompanying this book.

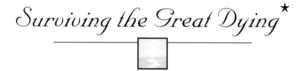

Surviving the Great Dying[*]

MICHAEL LERNER

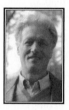

"In the future, the Legend of the Great Dying will be recited to the children of the Third Planet:

It happened thusly. First, there was the Great Explosion in human numbers and in technological prowess. In 200 Earth years, all the wild places were degraded or destroyed. Next, the chemicals and gases released by agriculture and industry impaired the health of the surviving species and changed the climate. The Great Heat then occurred, as did the Second Great Flood. Simultaneously, thousands of species of plants and animals were transported across natural barriers and became invasive species in their new surroundings; this was known as the Great Mixing. Near the end of that era, there were many new plagues—the Great Sickness—that ravaged the weakened, unprepared human beings and other species.

---

*From Lerner M: Medicine and Environment/Surviving the Great Dying, Spring 2003. Reprinted from YES! PO Box 10818, Bainbridge Island, WA 98110. Subscriptions: 800/937-4451. Web: yesmagazine.org

Our ancestors learned too late the simple, karmic law of ecology:
all is interdependent and all is interconnected. As bad philosophers
continued to debate whether human beings were part of nature or its
butcher, a spiral of dreadful causation erased this illusory dualism,
and it became evident that the destiny of humanity on Earth was to be
both victim and executioner of creation. At the end, all earthly beings
became joined in an intimate, slow dance of death."

FROM MICHAEL SOULE'S INTRODUCTION TO *CONSERVATION*
MEDICINE: ECOLOGICAL HEALTH IN PRACTICE.[1]

AGE OF EXTINCTIONS

Scientists know with clarity this, our deepest truth: We live in an Age of Extinctions. This is the sixth great spasm of extinctions in the history of our planet. We are driving biodiversity back 65 million years, to its lowest level of vitality since the end of the Age of Dinosaurs. Climate change, ozone depletion, toxic chemicals, habitat destruction, and invasive or infectious species are five of the principal drivers of this Age of Extinctions.

None of this is controversial in conservation biology, the parent discipline of conservation medicine. Less well-known are the future possible drivers of extinction. Bill Joy, chief scientist for Sun Microsystems, proposed in his historic *Wired* magazine article, "The Future Does Not Need Us," that biotechnology, nanotechnology, and robotics hold the tragic promise of creating unnatural entities that can self-replicate out of control. Nature is already being flooded with genetically modified organisms from agricultural biotechnology. The comparable modification of humanity's germline draws ever closer. It is conceptually possible that nanotechnology and robotics will lead to the creation of unnatural entities capable of self-replication as well. How can we save as much life as possible in this Age of Extinctions? Some so-called conservative commentators scoff at the question. They believe that there is no real threat to life from any technologies other than nuclear, chemical, or biological warfare. The enthusiasts of a posthuman future, by contrast, quite happily accept the possibility that the future has little need for carbon-based life forms and actively look forward to the convergence of the computer, the robot, and genetically modified posthumans.

The question of how much of life we can save in this Age of Extinctions has real meaning only for those of us who neither celebrate nor embrace the end of nature. We are, we should recognize, the true conservatives of our time. We are conservative in the root sense that we are dedicated to the conservation of the tried and true ecosystems and life forms of the Earth. We are conservative in that we want our children and their children to be genetically unmodified, to live surrounded by nature in all its glory, and to live lightly and justly on Earth. We, believers in natural law in the deepest sense, regard the question of who and what can be saved in this Age of Extinctions as the greatest religious, philosophical, and practical question of our time.

I believe that the path to saving all that we can of life on Earth—the path to what David Orr calls the Ecological Renaissance—lies with the emerging environmental health movement. I believe, for example, that the right of women to gestate and breast-feed their babies toxic free will be one of the great human rights issues of the new millennium. I believe that as the science linking human health to environmental health grows stronger, our experience that our personal health is being affected by the environment will drive the scientific lessons deep into our consciousness. This potent combination of scientific evidence and direct personal experience of wounds inflicted upon us and those we love by a degraded environment will, I believe, energize the emerging environmental health movement, making it into a global force.

Take chemicals and health as an example. There is growing evidence that there are over 100 diseases and conditions of our time in which chemical exposures either do or may well play a contributing role. The list includes asthma, allergies, autism, many cancers, learning disabilities, endometriosis, infertility, Parkinson's disease, and much more. Scientists are beginning to understand that all human beings on Earth carry hundreds of persistent bioaccumulative toxins in their bodies (chemicals that stay in our bodies over time), some at levels that are associated in animal studies with diseases similar to those that are endemic in the human population. Similarly, scientists have begun to establish that low levels of these chemicals in our bodies, once thought to be safe, can have significant health effects.

Let me speak of my own family's experience. In my family, learning disabilities are common, both of my parents have had cancer, one of my half-sisters died in her 20s of cancer, there are four family members on the autistic spectrum, and none of the children born to me and my brothers would be alive today without intensive medical intervention at conception or birth. While we cannot know the causation of any of these conditions with certainty, all of them may plausibly be linked to exposure to environmental chemicals. One thing I know for certain is that my mother was given DES when she was pregnant with me to prevent miscarriage. If I had been a girl, I would have had a high risk of reproductive tract cancer. DES is a potent endocrine-disrupting chemical.

Likewise, climate change is ever more powerfully and rapidly entering collective consciousness, not as an abstraction but as a direct threat to our health, our welfare, and the economies that sustain us. Changing vectors of infectious disease like West Nile virus, droughts that are killing crops, glacial melts that are destroying drinking water sources—these are no longer distant abstractions but increasingly direct realities.

The impact of poverty on health is an overwhelming reality, especially in developing countries. But even in the United States the power of this issue is rapidly increasing. Again, scientific data on "disparities in health outcomes" increasingly demonstrate that income disparities are one of the most powerful of all predictors of public health, with countries that promote greater equity enjoying better health and countries with a growing divide between rich and poor—such as the United States—suffering from worse public health. As a practical matter, greater equity promotes better health everywhere in the world, and the consciousness that promotes equity also tends to preserve the environment. It is the consciousness of the interdependence of all life.

The environmental health movement both differs from and shares much with the environmental movement. Many analysts of the environmental movement now recognize that this great shift in global consciousness, for all its accomplishments, has largely failed to connect its passionate advocacy for nature with the immediate concern of most people living in an increasingly urban world: the preservation of their own health. Yet the truth is that human health, animal health, and ecosystem health are inextricably connected.

Millions of people around the world intuitively share this apprehension of the essential unity of life. The great Buddhist poet Thich Nhat

Hanh calls this the consciousness of InterBeing. It is a venerable consciousness shared by many indigenous peoples, an ancient knowing that has been driven to the periphery of modern consciousness by industrial interests, the specialization and fragmentation of the scientific enterprise, corporate control of the global media, and other forces. But InterBeing is a way of knowing the world that is ineluctably returning to the center of post-post-modern discourse. The Law of InterBeing is, as Michael Soule says so beautifully, "the simple, karmic law of ecology: all is interdependent and all is interconnected."[1]

The emerging environmental health movement is the prose that is putting the poetry of InterBeing into practice. When breast cancer patients, women with endometriosis, mothers of children with asthma and birth defects, and representatives of dozens of other disease tribes begin to recognize their shared interest in reducing chemical contaminants in the environment, they form a potent new social force. When they are joined by the physicians, nurses, and other health professionals who care about them, their power is further amplified.

Like the civil rights movement, the emerging environmental health movement is a complex social phenomenon. It brings together, in often uneasy alliance, many groups with different primary concerns. Patient groups, for example, are first concerned with service delivery and the search for a cure. But as they begin to recognize that environmental factors are either a known or highly suspected contributor to the disease they share, their concern with prevention begins to rise.

Since patient groups are at the heart of the emerging environmental health movement, women are destined to play a central role in its leadership. Public opinion research confirms that women are much more likely to care about threats to the health of their families than men.

Environmental justice advocates have long understood that the incinerators, toxic waste dumps, and chemical plants across the street are making them sick. So do occupational health scientists who work with trade unions. Environmental groups, by contrast, may have as a primary concern what is happening to wildlife and ecosystems. But they are beginning to recognize the power of joining forces with patient groups, health professionals, scientists, environmental justice groups, occupational health advocates, religious groups, and others with a shared concern for environmental health. This is not the place to discuss at length the organizing principles of the emerging environmental health movement. It would take too long to describe how grassroots-based, market-focused campaigns with the real power to change corporate behavior in the marketplace have become the new tool of many groups working for environmental health goals. People have discovered their power in the marketplace, even when legislatures, the courts, and the executive branch have become dominated by special interests. Corporate brands contain much of the value of global corporations; hence they remain fundamentally vulnerable to grassroots-based, market-focused protest campaigns. These market campaigns cannot resolve the fundamental question of how an ecological society should be organized. But they do represent one of the instruments for peaceful change in our time.

Human health is the common language of those who would disagree on everything else. We may or may not care about spotted owls, or about the struggles of low-income Americans, or about famines in Africa. But we all—progressives, Libertarians, and conservatives—care about whether we and those we love are healthy or sick.

A TEACHABLE MOMENT

For those who think the dream of a just and sustainable future is a utopian fantasy, it is worth remembering the history of the last 250 years in its positive as well as its many negative aspects. In this extraordinarily brief period of time, countries around the world established democracies as their dominant form of government, brought to an end slavery as a norm that had been accepted for millennia, recognized the rights of women and organized labor, and extended legal rights to prisoners, to the mentally ill, and to children. Many of us have seen in our own lifetimes the power of the civil rights movement, the environmental movement, the gay rights movement, and many other movements of consciousness. What all these movements have in common is the gradual extension of respectful awareness of what we share with other people and with other life forms.

How do we summon the collective will to make this great transition in consciousness and technology when the forces opposed to it dominate every sector of the global system? Twenty years of work with people with cancer has taught me that when we face our mortality, we enter one of the great teachable moments of our lives. It is in the contemplation of our mortality that we often begin truly to live from our deepest consciousness.

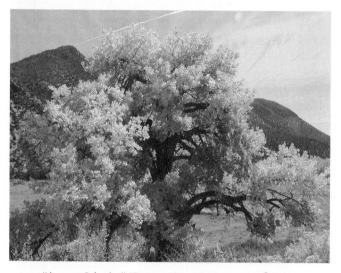

"Autumn Splendor." (Courtesy Convivial Design, Inc. © 2004.)

I believe that as recognition of the reality of this Age of Extinctions enters human consciousness, we may collectively enter into a teachable moment in the evolution of human consciousness. As our collective consciousness deepens, we may begin to discover the collective will to bring the global system back to the principles of living in harmony with nature.

We know the hour is late. Much of our inheritance of life has already been destroyed. Far more will be heedlessly squandered before we have any hope of consolidating an ecological renaissance. We also know that we may not succeed. The forces of destruction may overwhelm our bravest efforts. But the question of whether we will succeed is not the deepest question for us. The question we must ask ourselves concerns how we choose to live during this Age of Extinctions. What do we tell our children? What do we tell ourselves?

My friend Rachel Remen once asked the great philosopher Gregory Bateson who he was. "I am," Bateson said, "a friend of evolution." Bateson was a friend not only of genetic evolution but equally of the evolution of consciousness. I believe that the way to live in this Age of Extinctions is to find for ourselves that core of meaning that has always been essential for people living in dark and difficult times. For some, that core of meaning is religious or spiritual; for others, it centers on family and friends, whereas for others, it is found in nature or music or art or service to others.

My most fundamental hope is that, as we come to recognize the reality that we are living in an Age of Extinctions, we as a species will find the core of meaning that helps each of us move through this dark collective night of the soul. My hope is that the individual and collective searches for meaning will begin to form a larger pattern. I believe that the emerging environmental health movement symbolizes this movement toward shared meaning. A line in a James Taylor song says

> "Let us recognize that we are bound together/All men and women/Living on this Earth/By our desire to see the world become a place where our children can grow free and strong."

I believe it is the recognition of the truth of those words that may bring us through.

The reference for this essay is located on the DVD accompanying this book.

Healing Through Collective Consciousness: The Therapeutic Nature of the Human/Animal Bond

WILLIAM BENDA
RONDI LIGHTMARK

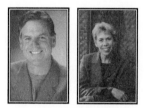

> *"What is man without the beasts? If all the beasts were gone, man would die from a great loneliness of the spirit. All things are connected."*
>
> CHIEF SEATTLE, 1854

INTRODUCTION

In this paper we address the challenge of creating a comprehensive conceptual model for healing from the point of view of our interwoven relationship with nature. Our focus is the field of interspecies therapeutics, an extraordinarily effective and little recognized contribution to the recovery and maintenance of human well-being.

The descriptive trinity of *body, mind, and spirit,* although rather overutilized in the integrative medicine literature, still affords both academic and lay audiences a comprehensible representation of what the field is attempting to address. Examination of healing in a historical context, however, reveals these concepts to be simply a resurgence of past cultural philosophies. For example, it is common to point to indigenous cultures like the Native American as examples of a philosophy and lifestyle that seem to achieve greater dimensions of holism than does our Western model. From such a cross-cultural point of view, *body* is not only our physical vessel, representative of how our physicality is reflected in nature, but also a reminder of how the "body" of the natural world sustains our very existence. *Mind* is both the result of the neurological processes transpiring within our cranium and the interplay of the consciousness of all living things, ultimately personified through reciprocal, balanced, harmonious interplay among and between species (and perhaps phylogenetic kingdoms). *Spirit,* while made physically and philosophically manifest through various religious incarnations, must also remain, by definition, indefinable and includes all of the ways we are inspired and nourished by our experience of the natural world.

Unfortunately, the evolution of institutional settings has resulted in a disruption of the familiar textures of life and sense of place, separating us from the meaningful landmarks we use to orient ourselves. The natural world has always given us a sense of context, weaving together the themes of seasons, patterns, places, and cycles into a connected structure, a larger perspective, the "view from 50,000 feet" that Ken Wilber uses to describe his integral approach in the introduction to this book.

When it comes, therefore, to creating a model of healing that fully addresses the question of what it is to be whole, we suggest that the world of nature may well be the most inclusive example. By including our relationship with nature, we find not only the I, we, they, internal, and external perspectives, as in Wilber's design, but also acknowledgment of our integration into a universal dynamic pattern that persists to support and nurture human existence—no matter how much we interfere with its processes. Indeed, the shaman might consider any model that did not integrate the human into "the web of life," as evoked by Chief Seattle in 1854, to be but a sophisticated evolution of the Cartesian viewpoint.

Let us, for a moment, revisit the four kingdoms of nature—mineral, plant, animal, and human—that we studied in elementary school. At the present time, the field of complementary and alternative medicine (CAM) is deeply engaged in investigating the first two kingdoms, mineral (supplements) and plant (botanicals), to the tune of multimillion-dollar NIH grants and controversial congressional legislation. It is fascinating that this same field has generally ignored the benefits of the third kingdom, the one most closely associated with us in a teleological as well as social context. The human/animal bond, more dramatically than any other relationship, demonstrates the healing power of living in harmony with nature. It is the very exercise of engaging with life in *all* of its manifestations on this planet that truly moves us in the direction of wholeness.

A glance at the chapter headings in this book reveals topics representing great gains in the understanding of esoteric, intuitive, and non-physical dimensions of healing. We read about the power of positive support and the therapeutic relationship; the gifts that come from being in service to life; the benefits of inner stillness and being in the moment; how sharing and lending energy to another can support and sustain; the lessons of death and dying; the question of psychic awareness and healing; perspectives on healing in different traditions; and the loss of connection with nature.

The curious thing to note is that the concept of the human/animal relationship comfortably resides in most of these categories. The animal can be, for example, a preeminent model of unconditional devotion and service, as well as an energy balancer, a tutor in opening the heart, an inspiration for being in the moment, a teacher about death, and a psychic who knows when you are sad, who can find the way home in the dark, tell you if you have skin cancer, or warn you if you are about to have a seizure.

From an ecological point of view, relationships between humans and animals have been ongoing as long as there have been records inscribed on the cave wall, and undoubtedly far earlier. The human/animal connection may in fact be the oldest and most time-proven therapeutic modality in existence—while also the least recognized, both by those in the mainstream and also by a majority in the CAM profession. It is not as if the concept of, for example, seeing-eye dogs for the blind or companion animals for the elderly is utterly unknown. The problem, however, is that a comprehensive understanding of the numerous ways that animals benefit human health issues does not exist in the medical field in such a way that the knowledge can be applied to an existing model. The use of animals in scientific medicine is predominantly considered to involve (depending on one's bias) either torture in the name of research or sacrifice for the common good.

Despite such oversight, we intend to use this chapter to demonstrate how multiple diverse approaches to healing with animals are being used with great success by a significant number of well-organized and credentialed organizations and institutions across the globe. What is most notable, and often least appreciated, is that this kind of therapy often works when other methods fail. Animal companions and trained "animal therapists" provide outcomes that not only rival many modern medical advances but also bestow help and comfort for chronic conditions that have yet to be satisfactorily addressed by our current technology-based paradigm. And to complete the integral picture, this therapy is noninvasive, devoid of adverse side effects, and surprisingly cost-efficient. Yet, when we visit our doctor with stories of physical and emotional duress, this simple approach is rarely recommended as an option, most likely because the doctor never heard of it in medical school, residency, or in the countless journal articles that cross his or her desk each year. When compared with more conventional and even alternative modalities, the amount of academic research on these protocols is extraordinarily limited.

Of course, the pleasures of bonding with another species may at first appear self-evident to those who enjoy close association with the nonhuman world. This includes not only those beings with fur, fins, or feathers but also reptiles and even insects—from spiders to honeybees. Our common view of the relationship of the animal kingdom to human evolution, however, has been quite limited, and our actions often exploitative rather than synergistic.

Fortunately, there have been changes in scientific perspectives. Over the past 2 decades, research studies have demonstrated that the benefits animals provide to *Homo sapiens* are far greater than simply pleasure or assistance with daily labor. In the last 10 years, we were introduced to the concept of the "horse whisperer," a person who by training and intuition can communicate nonverbally with his or her equine counterpart and thus experience harmonious connection from the "equine viewpoint." What our culture is just beginning to realize now (but mainstream science has not yet grasped) is that animals themselves are by nature "people whisperers," and they have, whether innately or intentionally, the capacity both to restore and to sustain us in ways that we have either forgotten or never imagined.

HISTORICAL BENEFITS OF THE HUMAN/ ANIMAL BOND

Cultural records in the form of cave paintings of animals first appeared about 30,000 years ago, and the conventional view is that domestication of wolves, the first "pets," began between 10,000 and 20,000 years ago. However, more recent evidence from the study of ancient DNA samples suggests that the evolution of wolves to dogs may have taken place up to 100,000 years in the past, assigning the animal an indispensable role in the evolution of Homo sapiens. Some have hypothesized that people did not domesticate wolves so much as wolves domesticated people, hanging around human settlements replete with attendant supplies of food and activity and eventually proving themselves mutually beneficial in hunting and protection. Those with canine pets today would not argue the likelihood of this scenario.

Cats were probably domesticated (if that is actually possible) around 5,000 years ago in ancient Egypt and held sacred in agricultural societies for their abilities as mousers. Horses were also domesticated at about the same period, probably in the geographical area of Turkestan. Recognition of the psychological and physical benefits of pet ownership is reflected in the fact that in ancient Tibet and China large breeds of dogs were used for hunting and protection, while small dogs were kept inside homes and monasteries as companion animals. Although many animals were domesticated to ease human burdens, the likelihood that the relationship was not merely exploitative is suggested by the sacred place various species hold in some contemporary cultures.

Animals as healers is a concept as old as the written word. Asklepios, the Greek god of healing, wielded divine power through sacred dogs and serpents. Pliny the Elder in the first century extolled the psychological benefits of the companionship of lap dogs. The earliest written documentation of the potential health benefits of animals may have been inspired by the horse, perhaps beginning in the fifth or sixth century with Hippocrates' chapter on "Natural Exercise," which describes the benefits of horseback riding.

In the 1790s the Society of Friends founded York Retreat in Yorkshire, England, incorporating interaction with rabbits and poultry in the treatment of mental patients. Florence Nightingale recommended small pets for the chronically ill in 1859. In America, shell-shocked veterans of World War I were given dogs for companionship and comfort, and in the 1940s a cooperative effort between the Red Cross and the Army Air Corps convalescent hospital in Pawling, New York, included snakes, frogs, turtles, and farm animals in treating soldiers recovering from injuries or operational fatigue.

In 1966 in Beitostolen, Norway, physiotherapy and sports utilizing dogs and horses were incorporated in the treatment plan for the disabled, including riding and skiing for the blind. Also in the '60s, psychologists began to note changes in human behavior patterns in people who had acquired animal companions, which inspired the serious study of the human/animal bond and stimulated research in the fields of social work, sociology, and veterinary medicine.

In sum, animals benefit the body, soothe the soul, and evoke a sense of sacred connection to the mystery of life. Although we are given this gift whole, it is instructive to take a moment and examine specific areas where the human/animal bond is especially beneficial.

HUMAN/ANIMAL INTERACTION AND PHYSICAL HEALTH

Perhaps the most measurable effects of any therapeutic modality lie in the physical realm, and perhaps the best-studied effects of relationships with animals are demonstrated by improvements in human cardiovascular health. Friedmann et al.[1] looked at survival rates of patients hospitalized with myocardial infarctions, or unstable angina, and found that only 5.7 percent of pet owners died within 1 year of discharge compared with 28.2% of non-pet owners, all other medical and demographic factors being equal (p < .05). This study was later expanded to 369 patients, where it was found that dog owners in particular were 8.6 times more likely to be alive in 1 year as compared with those who did not own dogs.[2]

In Melbourne, Australia, cardiac risk factors such as high cholesterol (p < .01), triglycerides (p < .01), and systolic blood pressure (p < .01) were determined by researchers to be higher among nonowners than pet owners.[3] After the investigators employed the Australian Department of Human Services and Health 1995 Statistical Overview to estimate cost savings that could arise from owning pets, they hypothesized economic savings of $26.244 million from decreased medical visits, $18.856 million from pharmaceutical savings, and $99.792 million from hospitalizations, which amounted to a total health care savings of $144.892 million annually.[4,5]

The effect of pet ownership on blood pressure, a major risk factor for several of the leading causes of death in this country, is of particular interest. One of the most telling studies, by Allen et al. at the State University of New York, investigated 48 New York City stockbrokers with hypertension. They found that acquiring a dog or cat resulted in half the increase of blood pressure under artificial stressful situations than in those without pets. These effects were noted even when the subject was not in the same locale as his or her animal.[6] Interestingly enough, it has been noted that *dogs themselves* undergo a 50 percent reduction in blood pressure when petted by humans, suggesting that the physical benefits of the human/animal bond are not unilateral.

Recent research by this author on the benefits of hippotherapy (physical therapy on horseback) utilized remote surface electromyography (EMG) to measure muscle activity in truncal musculature of children with spastic cerebral palsy.[7] Fifteen children were randomized to either hippotherapy or sitting on a stationary barrel, and EMG readings were taken during sitting, standing, and walking before and after the intervention. Reduction in spasticity after only 8 minutes resulted in an average of over 60 percent shift toward right/left symmetry in children on the horse but not on the barrel, suggesting a most desirable alternative to invasive neurosurgery and injection of botulinum toxin for this condition.

The physiological basis for such effects in these examples are myriad and, as of yet, not clearly delineated. It most likely falls into two categories, the first being purely physical. For example, the three-dimensional movement of the horse is so similar to normal human gait that the disabled child imprints this on his or her nervous and musculoskeletal system, while at the same time truncal muscles are strengthened and contracted joints loosen and move more freely. With regard to the cardiovascular effects of dog ownership, the daily walks required by the canine companion result in patterns of daily physical exercise beneficial to heart health.

The second physiological effect is stress reduction; the very act of communing with an animal companion results in decreased release of stress hormones from the adrenal medulla and therefore mitigated blood pressure escalations.

Although published data of the physical benefits of animal-assisted therapy are minuscule compared with more traditional approaches, anecdotal evidence abounds. We should indeed remember that anecdotal observations are more than fleeting descriptions of random experience but are in fact the ubiquitous origin of randomized controlled trials.

HUMAN/ANIMAL INTERACTION AND PSYCHOLOGICAL HEALTH

Although we may attribute many of the physical benefits of animal-assisted therapy to sound physiological theory and reasoning, improvements in emotional and psychosocial function have been more difficult to measure and document. This is interesting given the fact that the majority of outcomes research has focused on this area, perhaps because of the large numbers of therapy and service animals used specifically to provide companionship in hospitals, nursing homes, prisons, mental health institutions, and in home health care. Such studies consistently note positive improvements in emotional stability, self-esteem, and identity and worth in patient populations of all ages and with a wide variety of psychological dysfunctions.

A NEW STORY FOR HEALTH AND HEALING

Why should this be? If we look beyond the rigid constraints of the scientific method and tap into our own emotional experience, we will see how a deep connection can be achieved with a different species. Although

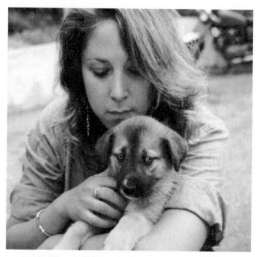

A, "Dawn." (Courtesy David Scott May.)

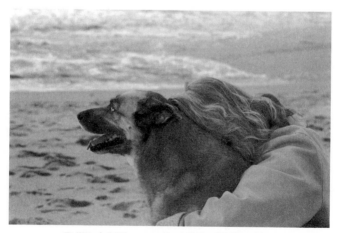

B, "Dusk." (Courtesy David "Dudi" Shmueli.)

we may normally prefer our own kind, under duress the quality of connection becomes more important than the origin of such support. When we are ill—and especially when we are chronically ill—we feel lonely, isolated, and out of contact with the normal routines of everyday life. Longstanding chronic illness or disability, with its attendant specter of social and cultural rejection, serves to intensify our fears and sense of separation and isolation. Our emotional state is often contagious, reflected as fear, concern, and, at times, feelings of guilt in our loved ones, further disrupting our social fabric and magnifying overall stress.

By contrast, when we are sick, disabled, depressed, cranky, grieving, or afraid, our animal companions not only continue to accept us just as we are but are delighted to have unlimited "alone time" with us, letting us know that we are still loved and needed no matter how we look or feel. An emotional lift during bouts of the flu for most of us, yes. An absolute soul-saving presence for those afflicted with disabilities lasting months, years, or lifetimes, as well as for those who are trapped within dysfunctional families, an aging body, or the prisons of stone or of the mind.

The gift is not unilateral—life is as much about caring as it is about being cared for; if a sick or disabled person can make an animal happy, alive, and thriving, the individual experiences a sense of empowerment that can only enhance health and healing. This occurs not only with companion animals but also through connections with wild animals, birds (we have all seen, for example, the image of the elderly woman in the tattered coat feeding pigeons in the park), and fish.

In the end, the song says, the love you take is equal to the love you make. When one feels useful and needed, one strives to become and remain healthy in order to continue caring for those that need us. It is not uncommon for the health care system to find pet owners insisting upon early discharge so that they can get back to their species-specific responsibilities.

HUMAN/ANIMAL INTERACTION AND SPIRITUAL HEALTH

Animals have been used as symbols for different spiritual qualities by shamans, medicine men, and religious scribes since the first recorded word. Animals have also historically been associated with fertility, power, the cycle of life, and numerous other mythical and archetypal images. We all have experienced how a magnificent landscape or dramatic sunset can evoke deep emotion and a sense of the sacred; if the sunset had its own heartbeat and palpable life force, if the landscape demanded presence and engagement from the viewer as an essential part of the experience, the effect would likely be far more moving. Looking deep into the eyes of an animal, whether tame or wild, can evoke a nameless thrill, a sense of recognition of one's own sacred, ultra-dimensional, natural self.

Jung identified the *collective unconscious* as a transpersonal realm, outside our egocentric perspective of everyday reality and inhabited by commonly shared archetypal images and patterns of behavior. In his writings, animals are ascribed a significant place in the process of soul development, appearing in our dreams as guides and leading us through the dark valleys of life's journey. Jung believed such creatures to be symbols of true devotion and suggested that how we relate in the physical realm to such emissaries reveals how we relate to our higher Self, which in turn is a direct measure of wholeness and health.

If animals do indeed hold therapeutic power, what is the source of such power? The answer may come from more recent psychological theory and discourse. One can argue that it is particularly in the human/animal bond (and most frequently in the human/canine relationship) that we encounter that elusive force we call *unconditional love.* Let us put aside for a moment the connotations found in song, poetry, and Hollywood and examine this rather esoteric ideal a bit more objectively.

Considering love in its purely energetic form, we can dispense with the adjective *unconditional* as redundant. Fundamentally, to love is to be open, to surrender, to drop all personal boundaries that cause distance and separation. To love is active; it does not exist in the past or future but manifests only in the present moment. Unfortunately, such love generally eludes those of us at the pinnacle of the food chain; we tend not to live in the present but in the intellectual, time-bound fantasies of past and future. Animals, however, not only live in the moment but can live nowhere else (unless made susceptible to human neuroses through overbreeding or abuse). Of course, more is involved here than being capable of love; the creature must have the desire to participate in the relationship, and many will, despite the neglect of their human companions. It is often said that a dog, for example, is the only thing on earth that loves you more than he loves himself, reflected by its number-one ranking in animal companions.

Exactly how does the presence of an unconditionally loving, living-in-the-moment fellow creature like the dog contribute to emotional and spiritual healing? The field of psychology has come to the conclusion that this kind of healing can rarely take place in isolation, because viewing ourselves and our life dramas through our eyes only provides far too distorted a reflection, due to our inherent limitations of perspective. Our culture supports the livelihood of so many therapists because we find we need the context of relationship in order to transform. We need an open-hearted, in-the-moment witness. An exceptional therapist will have the capacity to be present, remain objective, and demonstrate total acceptance while simultaneously opening a space of unconditional love for his or her client.

Human practitioners with these attributes are not easy to find. There are, however (to continue for a moment our paean to the dog), thousands of four-legged therapists all around us, and their services are given freely and without any expectation, except one. Dogs are incapable of lying and will never fully accept a human who is attempting to gain through deception. Dogs expect the truth.

Freud wrote, "Dogs love their friends and bite their enemies, quite unlike people who are incapable of pure love and always have to mix love and hate." Indeed, your dog will follow you to the ends of the earth no matter what your behavior, but he or she will *fully* engage with you only when you can manage to enter that same domain of unconditional presence. Many devotees of other species of animals would very likely hold this to be true of the object of their affection as well.

If it is true that unconditional love and acceptance of our self is the road to psychological and emotional healing, then being in the presence of one who lives always in that space can show the way. On these terms, the look in the eyes of our animal companion takes on a whole new meaning. We are looking into the soul of nature, where we all live, regardless of shape, hide, or number of legs.

THE STATE OF THE ART OF ANIMALS AS HEALERS

We have already referred to the countless nonhuman therapists working incognito as household pets. From 1980 to 2001, the number of dogs and cats in the U.S. grew from 98 million to 130 million, and Americans are found to spend nearly three times as much money caring for their pets as the federal government spends on welfare. It is far from uncommon for people to forego their own medical treatment out of cost considerations but to write any check necessary to preserve the life and health of their pets. Sixty-three percent of pet owners say, "I love you" to their pets daily, and 83 percent refer to themselves as their pet's "mom" or "dad."[8] Research shows that we use exactly the same facial expressions and vocal characteristics in speaking to a puppy as we do to a human infant.

Although this may be the first time the healing potential of animals has been explored in this kind of academic text, we have already acknowledged that the field of animal-assisted therapy is far from new. Institutions from schools to prisons to nursing homes have long employed dogs, rabbits, birds, and a variety of other species to help people of all ages and disability. There are currently over 2,000 canine programs and 650 equine therapy centers in the United States alone, and countless others abroad, because the movement did not originate in this country but in central Europe. Not only are a large percentage of such centers and their human therapists trained and certified under national guidelines, but numerous not-for-profit organizations exist to ensure the continued quality, credibility, and viability of the field.

The best and most concrete evidence of interspecies therapeutics having a significant impact upon public health occurs in two demographics at particular risk. Animals can and do transform the lives of children and the elderly, the latter being a major source of social and economic challenge in American life, and with the graying of our baby boom generation only increasing this burden in the not-too-distant future. The most common theme in health-based literature concerning this demographic revolves around loss, whether loss of spouses to death, children to adulthood, employment to retirement, or sense of worth to a culture that does little to counter this perspective. Fortunately, however, humans appear old, ugly, and sick only to themselves and other humans, and never to their animal companions.

Outcomes research is quite definitive with regard to the physical, emotional, and psychological benefits of pet ownership. From studies of independent-living older adults, dog owners report less depression after the loss of a spouse.[9] Pet ownership is a significant predictor of improved health and morale,[10] and dog owners in mobile home parks are twice as likely to go for walks, talk about activities occurring in the present, and report less dissatisfaction with their social, physical, and emotional states than non-dog owners.[11] Seniors currently institutionalized suffer from the same cultural stress as do their more independent peers, with the additional loss of personal freedom. It has been shown that dogs increase interactive behaviors among nursing home residents[12-14] and that birds can decrease depression among elderly in rehabilitation settings and adult day care centers.[15,16]

Although medical science has yet to come up with a satisfactory treatment for the increasing incidence of Alzheimer's disease, those patients with pets at home exhibit fewer episodes of verbal aggression, anxiety, and mood disorders, and among institutionalized patients, socialization is increased and behavioral distress is decreased in the presence of companion animals.[17-19] Economic indicators reveal significant potential monetary savings as well, as dog owners report fewer health problems, and a study of 938 Medicare enrollees in a HMO revealed fewer doctor contacts among those who owned pets.[20,21] If a pharmaceutical company could come up with a pill that would achieve even one of these outcomes, it would without a doubt become an immediate best-seller.

As significant to society as the health and well-being of our elderly are, the true measure of our future lies in how our children fare as they travel the road to adulthood. We need not enter into a lengthy discussion of the increasing social and environmental stresses that will permanently imprint upon young minds and souls, but we can examine how interspecies relationships may mitigate such effects.

Animals have always been, and will always be, a constant presence and consistent influence in a child's life. It is said that children who throw stones at birds and children who feed birds are both responding to an inherent tendency to focus attention on living beings. Which choice they make is a learned behavior, and the animal itself can be the source of learning and therefore affect present and future choices.

Pets always have time for play, conversation, and listening, even when parents and siblings do not. A majority (79 percent) of fourth-grade students in one German study reported confiding in their pets when they were sad, and almost half preferred the company of their pets to other children.[22] Forty-two percent of 5-year-olds spontaneously elected their pets when asked to whom they would turn when feeling sad, angry or afraid or needing to tell a secret.[23] From a societal point of view, the presence of a companion animal has been shown to increase social contact between children, especially when the animal owner is disabled. Several studies suggest that the more dysfunctional or disruptive a child's social context, the more positive the benefits of pet ownership.

Although children and the elderly appear to reap significant benefits from the human/animal interaction, research also supports improved quality of life in groups with other physical and psychological challenges, such as patients with cancer or AIDS and the homeless. Probably best known, because they have been the most socially visible, are demographic populations like the blind and neurologically impaired, who depend upon trained service animals for independent living on a daily basis.

THIS IS PROGRESS, BUT WHY ISN'T THERE MORE?

Given these kinds of preliminary research findings, combined with the existence of thousands of companion and service animals attending to tens of thousands of impaired people in this country alone, plus the potential savings to a cash-strapped health care system, why isn't animal-assisted therapy part of every hospital's formulary? Unfortunately, it is likely that science turns a blind eye because, were it to accept the concept of emotional give and take in animals, it would be forced to acknowledge that animals can feel. And the problem here? If the scientific establishment were to confirm the existence of an emotional life in animals subjected to pain, suffering, and imprisonment in the name of research, if it were to acknowledge that each day we humans create terror, rage, and despair in creatures who share a part of our psyche, the entire academic system would be faced with a unfathomable ethical predicament.

Thus the mainstream argument hinges on discussions of anthropomorphism, the misguided transference of human characteristics to another species, and the field of healing via the human/animal bond remains unexplored territory in the highest echelons of medical science. It is ironic, however, to think that the most insistent critic of interspecies therapeutics very likely reaps the benefit of the energy field of an animal companion at the end of a long and tiring day.

A NEW VISION AND MODEL FOR HEALING

Despite the contradictions, companionship with animals is abiding. Without them, said Chief Seattle, we would suffer "a great loneliness of spirit." Beginning with the 1960s research of Jane Goodall and her work with chimpanzees in Africa, the old anthropomorphic argument becomes weaker by the day. Animal activism continues to improve conditions for animals in the lab, on the farm, and in the shelter, and books about the human/animal bond are on the best-seller lists.

As medical professionals with a goal of facilitating wholeness in the highest and best sense of the word, to push for a medicine that is integrative and healthcare that is integral, our perspective needs to embrace not only the human up close and personal but also the human in context with the natural world, specifically in relation to other sentient beings.

This can come to pass only with continual inquiry into the meaning of nature, life, and our existence on this planet. We must foster respect not only for the patient we meet in the clinic or the reflection we greet in the mirror but also for every other form of life, even including those beings that nourish our bodies *and* our spirits. This is not impossible— indigenous cultures who once lived on the very land we walk upon embraced such a model for living.

Our call for a new paradigm of health care has paraphrased Chief Seattle in evoking that all things are connected. The time has come to live what we speak; otherwise, the evolution we are seeking can never fully materialize. And those who will help us reach such a goal may well be waiting for us patiently at home. . . .

References for this essay are located on the DVD accompanying this book.

Social Healing: Herald of a Shift in Human Consciousness

JAMES O'DEA

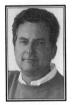

TRANSFORMING OUR RELATIONSHIP TO THE PAST

"Love sees what is invisible,"[1] writes Simone Weil. But what if you could not make the fullness of your humanness visible to others? What if you cared for your children with the passion of a loving parent but others took your children from you because they failed to recognize this profoundly humanizing quality in you?

This is precisely what happened to the Aboriginal people of Australia: They were made invisible by their colonizers. Maybe the colonizers were unable to classify the continent's indigenous people because they lacked the tools of cross-cultural analysis. Even today we are by no means free of major blind spots with regard to understanding diverse cultures.

Umberto Eco[2] notes that the early colonizers of Australia somehow squeezed the platypus, an undeniably confusing animal, into the category of mole despite its strange beak and other unusual characteristics. It just didn't fit any known category for them; thus, in a certain sense, they could not see it for what it was. Before we dismiss this as a trivial insight, we might want to consider the pervasive problem of inadequate or nonexistent cognitive categories for many domains of human experience. Our evolution into more expansive conscious often requires us to embrace or "discover" new categories that in turn help us to enter new worlds of meaning.

Whether based on false perception, lack of understanding, greed, or all of the above, the native peoples of Australia were dispossessed and oppressed because they were not visible to the colonizers. The indigenous worldview was simply incomprehensible to those who saw themselves as the vanguard of progress and civilization. The notion of belonging to the land rather than owning it and exploiting its resources for one's own gain somehow fell, for those arriving from the "civilized world," into the category of less intelligent or less evolved. It took a few hundred years for this worldview to begin to appreciate the wounds it had, in its ignorance, inflicted on a peaceful society.

As recently as 1997, a compelling report to the Australian parliament, entitled *Bringing Them Home,*[3] described the magnitude of the suffering of Aboriginal families whose children had been forcibly removed by the State up until the 1960s. Half a decade earlier, in 1992, the High Court of Australia delivered a judgment, known as *Mabo*, which gave Aborigines native title to ancestral lands taken from them during the colonization of the continent. Both the report and the court's decision marked the need for social healing in Australia. They created the context to deal with the wounds carried from the past.

The basis for the acquisition of the Aborigine lands had been a legal justification on the basis of *terra nullius*—a doctrine that the land was empty, uninhabited by humans. At the close of the twentieth century the justices in their wisdom made the Aboriginal people fully visible before the law. In a boldly stated judgment they also recognized the full humanity of these ancient peoples and the depth and integrity of a culture that the dominant culture had hitherto been unable or unwilling to recognize.

The justices declared the treatment and dispossession of the Aborigines "the darkest aspect of the history of this nation. The nation as a whole must remain diminished unless and until there is an acknowledgment of and retreat from these past injustices."[3]

By addressing the past in this manner, the justices were paving the way for a more integrated, and thus healthier, future for all the people who live in Australia today. While the past cannot be altered, there are ways that we can transform our relationship to it so as to prevent the repetition of its most egregious ills and the repetition of cycles of suffering and abuse. The past need not forever be the trigger of patterns that wound us in the present and inhibit our future potential. We can heal.

WHAT IS SOCIAL HEALING?

Social healing is an emerging field that seeks to deal with wounds created by conflict, collective trauma, and large-scale oppression. It seeks to identify areas of collective experience, which remain unresolved, neglected, and repressed within the psyche of groups and even nations. Its domain is centrally within consciousness rather than politics per se; it is psychospiritual in nature and activist only in its consequences.

Its primary modalities are truth, reconciliation, forgiveness, and restorative justice. It requires individuals to assume the responsibility to become healing agents themselves, and as such it is experiential rather than ideological.

Social healing is an affirmation of our power to create meaning, relationship, and health from seeking truth and reconciliation with our fellow human beings. It invites us to see ourselves as empowered to dialogue with history—and history in the making—and not simply experience it as a series of externalized events or enactments that are beyond our reach. It is a form of self-actualizing democracy; it requires the participation of our inner lives. It places high value on the quality of being that we manifest together. It begins in our awareness and is an expression of our longing for greater wholeness.

Social healing aligns itself with the emerging consciousness movement that strongly validates subjective lived experience. We have discovered that the world configures itself to our best interpretations of it. And this understanding has brought us into a much more intimate relationship with the universe. We know more clearly now that whatever we describe in the activity of atoms and molecules is threaded with meaning and woven with interpretation from our experience.

We are only beginning to imagine what it might mean for us to really wake up inside evolution and consciously pulse it with new meaning. As yet, it seems, we do not know the extent or the limits of our power either for good or ill. Duane Elgin[4] and others have suggested that this is akin to being in the adolescent phase of our species' development. Maturity brings an understanding of the injury we can cause others through an inappropriate exercise of power. It also brings greater clarity about ways to harness our creative engagement with others as well as the power to heal, transform, and generate well-being for ourselves and others.

Much of our lives is spent in exploring the relationship between self and others, and yet there are such significant variances both within and between cultures as to make this a truly complex issue. In many ways we cannot avoid giving offense and even hurting each other, but we can learn not to oppress and exploit each other.

The development of a global curriculum around exploitation and oppression is under way, but it would be an understatement to say that it is near completion. Race, ethnicity, gender, sexual orientation, and disability continue to be arenas of oppression, which result in violent death, extreme poverty, avoidable disease, and dehumanizing social rejection.

People are often unsure about how to change systems, cultural patterns, or religious beliefs without getting entangled in rancorous dispute, divisiveness, and, for some, the justification for violent retaliation.

This is a central challenge for social healing as an emergent field: It must get inside the roots of oppression, feel its emotional texture, its psychological structure and the humanness of victims and perpetrators alike in their numerous guises and settings. It deconstructs systems in order to access the experiential reality that they create. To do so, it attempts to be perceptive, understanding, and compassionate rather than taking a stance of blame and accusation. Social healing requires us to go more deeply into what it means to be human.

Jacob Needleman points out that "Western civilization has operated under the assumption that we can understand the universe without understanding ourselves."[5] He suggests that "both within and outside the sciences a new sense of the unknown has appeared. The unknown is ourselves." What is increasingly known is that we are more interconnected than we had ever imagined. When we shift our awareness toward an appreciation of our deep relatedness, we begin at the very least to transform structures that feed off of separation and division. Both the inner and outer discovery and confirmation of the nature and degree of our relatedness may be the path whereby we can transform dysfunctional and oppressive systems from the inside out.

As the world continues to shrink, we are beginning to understand that we are relational beings who generate meaning together. The new frontier of social transformation is one in which both scientific and spiritual worldviews meet in confirming the charged, creative, and generative nature of great masses of individuals communing together and creating webs of meaning and networks of influence. The World Wide Web is both a vehicle and a symbol for this sea change in human consciousness. Even though there are major forces that seek to make the Internet the new commercial frontier, viewing it as a kind of prime real estate to capture, it is demonstrating a resilient capacity to be a global commons where a great multiplicity and diversity of voices can be heard. People are participating in a global conversation as never before.

The shift in awareness from being spectators of a collective human drama that is primarily influenced by superstars in the political, intellectual, and religious spheres to one in which each of us begins to recognize ourselves as participants and even as "players" is indeed a very significant one.

As many have noted, this shift in consciousness is one where our interior life may still be beautifully private, but it is also an arena in which we can source the collective in ways that we had never previously imagined. We can experience a shift from passive spectators to imaginatively and compassionately engaged participants in designing healthier and more sustainable lifestyles. This shift entails a de-conditioning of worldviews that are sustained by artificial constructs that maintain a strict separation between the inner life of individuals and the external or "objective" life of society.

The process of moving from spectator to conscious participant is particularly evident in the field of health with the dramatic rise in complementary and alternative approaches. Take the classic medical model, for example. In the past, crudely speaking, you got ill and something was done to you by a trained professional to make you better. Now, there is widespread understanding that you must take responsibility for promoting your own health and well-being. In the words of mind-body medicine pioneer Kenneth Pelletier:

> Essential to all complementary and alternative medicine is the point that the intervention or cure does not exist 'outside' the individuals, independent of 'inside' changes in attitude, lifestyle, and orientation toward self and environment. Such an approach demands internal, psychological transformation and the active ongoing involvement of the individual.[6]

It is easier to see that the outside/inside analogy holds true for the social body when we are referring to people directly caught up in violent trauma such as brutal conflict, flagrant denial of human rights, and various kinds of political oppression. In these contexts they are clearly not spectators watching events in history unfold—as though they were happening on the "outside." They are caught up inside events, which, if they survive, permanently change their basic orientation "toward self and the environment."

It is more difficult to see how internal transformation can come about in relation to events that one always perceived as happening on the "outside," or out of a past with which one experiences little connection. Events abstracted from direct experience seem to occur beyond "the fragile geometry" of the self, and as such they are the stuff of theories and conjectures, fiction, movies, or the evening news.

Social healing has much to say to those who survive the fires of violent trauma and those who inherit or who even inhabit the nightmares of history. But it also addresses itself to those who live at various degrees of separation in time and space from historical trauma, to those who live the illusion that they have no relationship to the suffering of others, and to all who have dreams and a longing for better days.

HEALING FROM THE FIRES OF GENOCIDE

Here is a story of social healing from "inside" from a survivor of the fires of genocide. Arn Chorn Pond was a young child when he was picked up by the Khmer Rouge as they began their genocidal rampage through Cambodia. He survived because the murderous men who smashed the heads of other children a few feet away from him were moved by the beauty of his flute playing. He was forced to witness the killing of hundreds of people on a daily basis for a very prolonged period. Arn eventually fled the killing fields and was fortunate enough to be brought to the United States by his adoptive father, Peter Pond.

For Arn, his journey inside the cauldron of these events left him with deep psychological scars and emotional wounds. The world had violently invaded his inner space, and he knew that he would self-destruct unless he found healing. Initially he did so by telling the truth of what happened in his country to audiences across the United States. Eventually, he was able to say,

> I'm not just alive today because bullets failed to reach my brain or because I wasn't butchered by the awful Khmer Rouge genocide. I'm alive, finally, after all these years because I love again. I can feel the pain of others, not just my own, who are suffering the pain of human madness.[7]

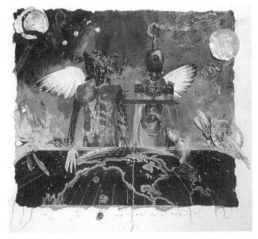

"With Only One Wing." (Courtesy Eileen Hyman.)

Arn would not say that his healing is complete; his own healing has become inextricably linked to healing others, including those who experienced the genocide and those who were born into its aftermath. His capacity for love has translated itself into work with gang kids in some of America's cities; he has co-founded one of the largest youth volunteer organizations in Cambodia and has spearheaded remarkable work to save the work of masters of traditional Cambodian music. His story is told in a contemporary documentary entitled *The Flute Player*.[8]

A SOCIAL HEALING MOVEMENT EMERGES

The movement toward a healing paradigm in the social domain during the last century was stimulated by charismatic leaders such as Mahatma Gandhi and Martin Luther King. Their emphasis on nonviolent approaches to conflict, their efforts to diffuse hatred, their refusal to demonize opponents, and their ability to affirm unifying principles undergirded their lifelong efforts to promote social harmony and reconciliation. Their passionate quest for justice was held within a ground of being suffused with creativity and compassion. They were not so much concerned with blame and retribution as with more healing forms of restoring fairness and justice. They stand in marked contrast to the divisive tactics of mere ideologues and demagogues.

Nelson Mandela and Desmond Tutu have taken on their mantle in our time to demonstrate the power of forgiveness and reconciliation in the social domain. They recognized that forgiveness and reconciliation require truth telling. And for the truth to really be told it has to be so much more than the official story. People must be able to speak the truth of events as they experienced them. Their work gave potent affirmation to the significance of individual human experience. The Truth and Reconciliation Commission set a new benchmark in human affairs by placing such great value to the expression of raw experience. Through its work, South Africa stands a far greater chance of healing the wounds of the past than if it had simply adopted the model of triumphalism still so dominant in global politics.

Through the commission's work, South Africans were able to explore and describe the nature of their wounds and, by so doing, begin to address them. Social healing concerns itself particularly with the intergenerational transfer of wounds. If unaddressed, these wounds are fed rather than healed and can become an unhealthy aspect of an individual's or a group's self-definition. They can also be submerged in the collective psyche only to be triggered by historical events. Tito, for example, was able to repress the wounds and divisions between ethnic and religious rivals in the former Yugoslavia, which had stretched back hundreds of years. But once the repressive lid was removed, the old unhealed wounds surfaced with a vengeance.

People have different narratives of the past. Social healing accepts the complexity created by the impact of lived experience and is subsequently influenced by the screens of collective perception and potentially selective memory. Nonetheless, narratives are often sacred and core to individual and group identity; as such, they are not susceptible to casual revision. If anything, an exploration of our narratives leads more to an understanding of mass psychology, deeper motivations, and the power and influence of myths and worldviews.

It appears, however, that if we feel heard, we are more likely to listen to others. Initiatives such as One by One, which brings together Holocaust survivors and former Nazis, and the Compassionate Listening Project, which facilitates the sharing of experience by Israelis and Palestinians, demonstrate that profound understanding can flow from hearing one another's stories. In these examples truth is not made relative in a moral sense but in an experiential sense. Social healing does not seek to arbitrate moral questions and make determinations about who is right and who is wrong. It concerns itself with revealing our capacities to restore community and create the basis for future peace and harmony.

There may be hope for an evolutionary shift in consciousness that will both heal and transform our relationship to the past. It is a shift that requires humility and an exploration of the science of being itself. Needleman speaks to this shift when he writes:

> Now fitfully, and with great uncertainty, it seems we are being called back from the impulse to believe we can stride into nature with our mind pointed like an unsheathed sword. And the discoveries of science about the organic interconnection of all things, from the atomic nucleus to the unfathomed psyche of man [sic] to the inconceivable entities of cosmic space, in a like manner invite us to something greater than the search for additional facts and information.[5]

"ADDITIONAL FACTS AND INFORMATION" WILL NOT SUFFICE TO HELP US HEAL

In order to heal we will also need heart and soul and the love that sees beyond the visible surfaces of our existence into the deep space of our individual and collective being. Even the idea that social healing is beginning in various parts of our planet allows us to imagine that a future without brutality and oppression is a real possibility. Even more dizzying for me is the notion that I, as an individual, can make a contribution to that future and that we all can: a healing by the whole system, for the whole system.

References for this essay are located on the DVD accompanying this book.

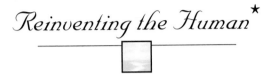

Reinventing the Human [*]

THOMAS BERRY

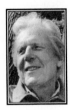

W̲E MIGHT DESCRIBE THE challenges before us by the following sentence: The historical mission of our times is to reinvent the human—at the species level, with critical reflection, within the community of life systems, in a time-developmental context, by means of story and shared dream experience.

I say *reinvent the human* because humans, more than any other living form, invent themselves. Other species receive their basic life instructions at the time of their birth. With this endowment they know how to obtain their food, how to defend themselves, how to obtain shelter, how to carry on their mating rituals, how to care for their young. Some species, especially the mammalian species, do need some teaching and guidance from an older generation. Young bears need to be taught how to fish. Many

[*] Adapted from Berry T: *The great work: our way into the future,* New York, 1999, Bell Tower, pp 159–165.

animal species need to be taught how to hunt. Yet this is minimal when compared with the extent of teaching and acculturation that humans need to arrive at maturity. That acculturation process is the purpose of the long childhood distinctive of humans. With their genetic endowment the other life forms are, from an earlier age, much more fully equipped than humans to carry out their basic patterns of survival and propagation.

We need to reinvent the human *at the species level* because the issues we are concerned with seem to be beyond the competence of our present cultural traditions, either individually or collectively. What is needed is something beyond existing traditions to bring us back to the most fundamental aspect of the human: giving shape to ourselves. The human is at a cultural impasse. In our efforts to reduce the other-than-human components of the planet to subservience to our Western cultural expression, we have brought the entire set of life systems of the planet, including the human, to an extremely dangerous situation. Radical new cultural forms are needed. These new cultural forms would place the human within the dynamics of the planet rather than place the planet within the dynamics of the human.

We must find our primary source of guidance in the inherent tendencies of our genetic coding. These tendencies are derived from the larger community of the Earth and eventually from the universe itself. In Jungian terms, these tendencies identify with those psychic energy constellations that take shape as the primary archetypal forms deep in the unconscious realms of the human. Such forms find expression in the symbols of the Heroic Journey, Death-Rebirth, the Sacred Center, the Great Mother, the Tree of Life. Although these symbolic forms are broadly the same in their general meaning, they each take on various modes of expression in the different religious and cultural traditions, modes that are analogously the same in their essential meaning.

The necessity of rethinking our situation at the species level is clear in every aspect of the human. With regard to economics, we need not simply a national or a global economy but local subsistence economies wherein the variety of human groups become acquainted with the other species in the local bioregion.

Our schools of business administration at the present time teach the skills whereby the greatest possible amount of natural resources is processed as quickly as possible, put through the consumer economy, and then passed on to the junk heap, where the remains are at best useless and at worst toxic to every living being. Now there is a need for humans to develop reciprocal economic relationships with other life forms, providing a sustaining pattern of mutual support, as is the case with natural life systems generally. Especially as regards law, we need a jurisprudence that would provide for the legal rights of geological and biological as well as human components of the Earth community. A legal system exclusively for humans is not realistic. Habitat of all species, for instance, must be given legal status as sacred and inviolable.

Thirdly, I say *with critical reflection,* because this reinventing of the human needs to be done with critical competence. Originally, there was a certain instinctive, spontaneous process whereby the early cultural formations were established. Now we need all our scientific insight and technological skills. We must, however, see that our sciences and technologies are coherent with the technologies of the natural world. Our knowledge needs to be in harmony with the natural world rather than a domination of the natural world. We need the art of intimate communion with, as well as technical knowledge of, the various components of the natural world.

We insist on the need for critical reflection as we enter the ecological age in order to avoid a romantic attraction to the natural world that would not meet the urgencies of what we are about. The natural world is violent and dangerous as well as serene and benign. Our intimacies with the natural world must not conceal the fact that we are engaged in a constant struggle with natural forces. Life has its bitter and burdensome aspects at all levels. Yet its total effect is to strengthen the inner substance of the living world and provide the never-ending excitement of a grand adventure.

Fourth, we need to reinvent the human *within the community of life systems.* This is the central phrase, the primary condition for reinventing the human. Because the Earth is not adequately understood either by our spiritual or by our scientific traditions, the human has become an addendum or an intrusion. We have found this situation to our liking since it enables us to avoid the problem of integral presence to the Earth. This attitude prevents us from considering the Earth as a single community with ethical relations determined primarily by the well-being of the total Earth community.

While the Earth is a single community, it is not a global sameness. Earth is highly differentiated into arctic as well as tropical regions, into mountains, valleys, plains, and coastlands. These geographical regions are also bioregions. Such areas can be described as identifiable geographical regions of interacting life systems that are relatively self-sustaining in the ever-renewing processes of nature. As the functional units of the planet, these bioregions can be described as self-propagating, self-nourishing, self-educating, self-governing, self-healing, and self-fulfilling communities. Human population levels, our economic activities, our educational processes, our governance, our healing, and our fulfillment must be envisaged as integral with this community process.

There are great difficulties in identifying just how to establish a viable context for a flourishing and sustainable human mode of being. Of one thing we can be sure, however: Our own future is inseparable from the future of the larger community that brought us into being and sustains us in every expression of our human quality of life, in our aesthetic and emotional sensitivities, our intellectual perceptions, our sense of the divine, as well as in our physical nourishment and our bodily healing.

Fifth, reinventing the human must take place *in a time-developmental context.* This constitutes what might be called the cosmological-historical dimension of the program I am outlining here. Our sense of who we are and what our role is must begin where the universe begins. Not only do our physical shaping and our spiritual perception begin with the origin of the universe, so too does the formation of every being in the universe. This human formation is governed by three basic principles: *differentiation, subjectivity, and communion.*

Our present course is a violation of each of these three principles in their most primordial expression. Whereas the basic direction of the evolutionary process is toward constant differentiation within a functional order of things, our modern world is directed toward monocultures. This is the inherent direction of the entire industrial age. Industry requires a standardization, an invariant process of multiplication with no enrichment of meaning. In an acceptable cultural context, we would recognize that the unique properties of each reality determine its value both for the individual and for the community. These are fulfilled in each other. Violation of the individual is an assault on the community.

As a second imperative derived from the cosmological process, we find that each individual is not only different from every other being in the universe but also has its own inner articulation, its unique spontaneities. Each being in its subjective depths carries that numinous mystery whence the universe emerges into being. This we might identify as the sacred depth of the individual.

The third cosmological imperative indicates that the entire universe is bonded together in such a way that the presence of each individual is felt throughout its entire spatial and temporal range. This capacity for bonding the components of the universe with one another enables the vast variety of beings to come into existence in that gorgeous profusion and yet comprehensive unity we observe about us.

From this we can appreciate the directing and energizing role played by the *story* of the universe. This story that we know through empirical observation of the world is our most valuable resource in establishing a viable mode of being for the human species as well as for all those stupendous life systems whereby the Earth achieves its grandeur, its fertility, and its capacity for endless self-renewal.

This story, as told in its galactic expansion, its Earth formation, its life emergence, and its self-reflexive consciousness, fulfills in our times the role of the mythic accounts of the universe that existed in earlier times, when human awareness was dominated by a spatial mode of consciousness. We have moved from cosmos to *cosmogenesis,* from the mandala journey toward the center of an abiding world to the irreversible journey of the universe itself as the primary sacred journey. This journey of the universe is the journey of each individual being in the universe. So this story of the great journey is an exciting one that gives us our *macrophase identity,* with the larger dimensions of meaning that we need. To identify the microphase of our being with the macrophase mode of our being is the quintessence of human fulfillment.

The present imperative of the human is that this journey continue on into the future in the integrity of the unfolding life systems of the Earth, which presently are threatened in their survival. Our great failure is the termination of the journey for so many of the most brilliant species of the life community. The horrendous fact is that we are, as the Cambridge University biologist Norman Myers has indicated, in an extinction spasm that is likely to produce "the greatest single setback to life's abundance and diversity since the first flickerings of life almost four billion years ago."[1] The labor and care expended over some billions of years and untold billions of experiments to bring forth such a gorgeous Earth are being negated within less than a century for what we consider "progress" toward a better life in a better world.

The final aspect of our statement concerning the ethical imperative of our times is *by means of the shared dream experience.* The creative process, whether in the human or the cosmological order, is too mysterious for easy explanation. Yet we all have experience of creative activity. Since human processes involve much trial and error, with only occasional success at any high level of distinction, we may well believe that the cosmological process has also passed through a vast period of experimentation in order to achieve the ordered processes of our present universe. In both instances something is perceived in a dim and uncertain manner, something radiant with meaning that draws us on to a further clarification of our understanding and our activity. This process can be described in many ways: as a groping or as a feeling or imaginative process. The most appropriate way of describing this process seems to be that of dream realization. The universe seems to be the fulfillment of something so highly imaginative and so overwhelming that it must have been dreamed into existence.

But if the dream is creative, we must also recognize that few things are so destructive as a dream or entrancement that has lost the integrity of its meaning and entered an exaggerated and destructive manifestation. This has happened often enough with political ideologies and religious visionaries. Yet there is no dream or entrancement in the history of the Earth that has wrought the destruction that is taking place in the entrancement with industrial civilization. Such entrancement must be considered as a profound cultural disorientation. It can be dealt with only by a corresponding *deep cultural therapy.*

Such is our present situation. We are involved not simply with an ethical issue but with a disturbance sanctioned by the very structures of the culture itself in its present phase. The governing dream of the twentieth century appears as a kind of ultimate manifestation of that deep inner rage of Western society against its earthly condition as a vital member of the life community. As with the goose that laid the golden egg, so the Earth is assaulted in a vain effort to possess not simply the magnificent fruits of the Earth but the power itself whereby these splendors have emerged.

At such a moment a new revelatory experience is needed, an experience wherein human consciousness awakens to the grandeur and sacred quality of the Earth process. This awakening is our human participation in the *dream of the Earth,* the dream that is carried in its integrity not in any of Earth's cultural expressions but in the depths of our genetic coding. Therein the Earth functions at a depth beyond our capacity for active thought. We can only be sensitized to what is being revealed to us. We probably have not had such participation in the dream of the Earth since earlier shamanistic times, but therein lies our hope for the future of ourselves and of the entire Earth community.

The reference for this essay is located on the DVD accompanying this book.

PHOTO AND ART CREDITS